East African Doctors

A History of the Modern Profession

John Iliffe's latest book is the first history of an African medical profession in Uganda, Kenya and Tanzania from the earliest training of modern medical staff in the 1870s to the present day. Based on extensive research, and dealing exclusively with African doctors, it offers a new understanding of professionalisation in the Third World. It describes the recruitment and education of doctors, their understanding and practice of modern medicine, their struggle for international recognition of their qualifications, their efforts to develop East African medical systems after independence, and their experiences during a period of political and economic difficulty. The book ends with an account of the significant work of East African doctors in the study and control of AIDS. This is a major contribution to the social history of Africa and to the social history of medicine more broadly.

JOHN ILIFFE is Professor of African History at the University of Cambridge and formerly Reader in History at the University of Dar es Salaam. His publications include *A Modern History of Tanganyika* (1979), *The African Poor* (1987), which was awarded the Herskovits Prize of the African Studies Association of the United States, and *Africans: The History of a Continent* (1995).

East African Doctors

A History of the Modern Profession

John Iliffe

CAMBRIDGE
UNIVERSITY PRESS

PUBLISHED BY THE PRESS SYNDICATE OF THE UNIVERSITY OF CAMBRIDGE
The Pitt Building, Trumpington Street, Cambridge CB2 1RP, United Kingdom

CAMBRIDGE UNIVERSITY PRESS
The Edinburgh Building, Cambridge, CB2 2RU, United Kingdom
http://www.cup.cam.ac.uk
40 West 20th Street, New York, NY 10011–4211, USA http://www.cup.org
10 Stamford Road, Oakleigh, Melbourne 3166, Australia

First published 1998

Printed in the United Kingdom at the University Press, Cambridge

Typeset in 10/12 Times New Roman [SE]

A catalogue record for this book is available from the British Library

Library of Congress Cataloguing in Publication data

Iliffe, John.
East African doctors: a history of the modern profession / John Iliffe.
p. cm. – (African studies series)
Includes bibliographical references and index.
ISBN 0 521 63272 2 (hb)
1. Physicians – Africa, East – History. 2. Physicians – Africa, East – Biography. 3. Medicine – Africa, East – History. I. Title. II. Series.
R653.A35314 1998
610′.9676–dc21 97–51551 CIP

ISBN 0 521 63272 2 hardback

For
TERENCE RANGER
on his retirement

Contents

Acknowledgments

One of the successful aims of this research project has been to renew my links with Kenya, Tanzania, and Uganda. In Kenya I received kindness from Godfrey Muriuki, Henry Mutoro, Shirin Walji, John Karanja, John Sutton, and Justin Willis. In Tanzania I was grateful to Frederick Kaijage, Nestor Luanda, Issa and Beatrice Omari, and Nicholas Westcott. In Uganda I enjoyed the support of the Makerere Institute of Social Research and its Research Secretary, Patrick Madaya, while Juliet Kiguli of the Institute made the translations from Luganda, which I have altered occasionally in wording but not in sense. Musila Musembe and Richard Ambani in Nairobi, J.M. Karugila in Dar es Salaam, and Charles Wani and Olaka David in Entebbe helped my work in the National Archives, whose holdings are described in the bibliography, along with other archival sources. In Uganda the Permanent Secretary to the Ministry of Health kindly allowed me to consult records and use the Ministry Library, where Mr Moses Doka was especially welcoming. I also made much use of the MacMillan Library in Nairobi, Makerere University Library, and the Medical Libraries at Nairobi, Dar es Salaam, and Mulago. Mrs Eunice Sendikadiwa of the Albert Cook Library at Mulago kindly enabled me to use the cover photograph and Mr A. Kiwanuka copied it. John Waliggo in Uganda and Mr H.M. Nguli in Tanzania helped to arrange research clearance. I had hoped to conduct a programme of interviews, but it became clear in the course of research that this would be better left to an African, preferably with medical training.

In Britain I am indebted to many institutions and their officers: the African Studies Centre Library, Cambridge (especially Sarah Irons); Birmingham University Library; British Newspaper Library; Edinburgh University Library (with thanks to the Revd James L. Wilkie of the Church of Scotland World Mission); General Medical Council (by courtesy of Dr Kate Horne); Institute of Commonwealth Studies, London; London School of Hygiene and Tropical Medicine; National Library of Scotland; Public Record Office; Rhodes House Library, Oxford; St Joseph's College, Mill Hill (by courtesy of Fr W.J. Mol); University Library, Cambridge (with special thanks to Terry Barringer); Wellcome Institute for the History of Medicine, London; and Westminster College, Cambridge. Shane Doyle, Tim Harper, Michael Redley, David Throup, and Megan Vaughan helped with materials. The book has been written during sabbatical leave granted by my university and college, while John Lonsdale has done much of my work. Gilbert Lewis and Megan Vaughan have given expert advice on the typescript. I am grateful to Richard Rathbone for his encouragement over many years. Jessica Kuper has been a most supportive editor. I thank all those who have helped me.

John Iliffe
October 1997

Abbreviations

AAMO	African Assistant Medical Officer
ACP	AIDS Control Programme
AER	*Annual Education Report*
AMR	*Annual Medical Report*
ANMC	African Native Medical Corps
BMA	British Medical Association
BW	Inter-University Council (records in PRO)
CMO	Chief Medical Officer
CMS	Church Missionary Society (records in Birmingham University Library)
CO	Colonial Office (records in PRO)
CS	Chief Secretary
DC	District Commissioner
DDMS	Deputy Director of Medical Services
DMS	Director of Medical Services
EAMJ	*East African Medical Journal*
EUL	Edinburgh University Library
FCB	Fabian Colonial Bureau
FCO	Foreign and Commonwealth Office
GMC	General Medical Council
IUC	Inter-University Council
JAH	*Journal of African History*
KEMRI	Kenya Medical Research Institute
KMA	Kenya Medical Association
KNA	Kenya National Archives
KNH	Kenyatta National Hospital
MMGA	Makerere Medical Graduates Association
MOH	Minister/Ministry of Health
MP	Mengo Papers (Albert Cook Library, Mulago)
MS	Medical Superintendent
MUL	Makerere University Library
NCPA	National Committee for the Prevention of AIDS

NRA	National Resistance Army
NRM	National Resistance Movement
PHC	Primary Health Care
PRO	Public Record Office
PS	Permanent Secretary
RAMC	Royal Army Medical Corps
RCS	Royal Commonwealth Society
RH	Rhodes House, Oxford
SAMA	Senior African Medical Assistant
SMO	Senior Medical Officer
SMP	Secretariat Minute Paper
S. of S.	Secretary of State
SSM	*Social Science and Medicine*
T	Treasury (records in PRO)
TANU	Tanganyika African National Union
TNA	Tanzania National Archives
TNR	*Tanganyika/Tanzania Notes and Records*
UMOH	Uganda Ministry of Health
UNA	Uganda National Archives
UNC	Uganda National Congress
UNMC	Uganda Native Medical Corps
UNMS	University of Nairobi Medical School
UP	Unofficial Papers
UPC	Uganda People's Congress
WHO	World Health Organisation

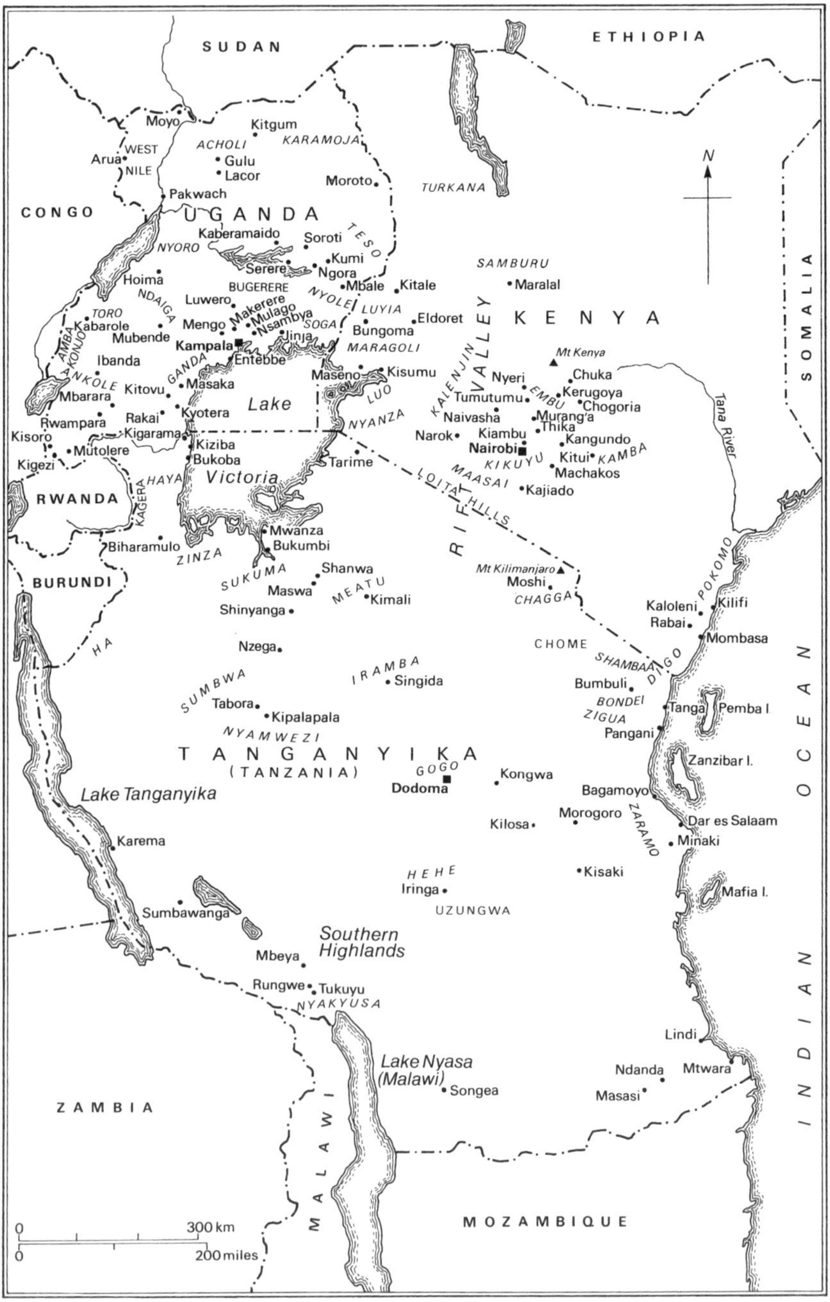
SUDAN
ETHIOPIA
CONGO
UGANDA
KENYA
SOMALIA
RWANDA
BURUNDI
TANGANYIKA
(TANZANIA)
ZAMBIA
MALAWI
MOZAMBIQUE
INDIAN OCEAN
N
Moyo
Kitgum
ACHOLI
KARAMOJA
WEST NILE
Arua
Gulu
Lacor
Moroto
TURKANA
Pakwach
Kaberamaido
Soroti
TESO
NYORO
Serere
Kumi
Ngora
SAMBURU
Hoima
BUGERERE
Mbale
Kitale
Maralal
NDAIGA
Luwero
Makerere
Mulago
Nsambya
NYOLE
LUYIA
Eldoret
TORO
Kabarole
Mubende
Mengo
SOGA
Jinja
Bungoma
AMBA
KONJO
Kampala
MARAGOLI
Mt Kenya
Ibanda
Entebbe
KALENJIN
RIFT VALLEY
ANKOLE
GANDA
Maseno
Kisumu
Nyeri
Chuka
Mbarara
Kitovu
Masaka
Tumutumu
EMBU
Kerugoya
Chogoria
Lake Victoria
LUO
Naivasha
Murang'a
Thika
Rwampara
Rakai
Kyotera
NYANZA
Kisoro
Kigarama
Narok
Kiambu
Kangundo
Mutolere
Kiziba
Nairobi
Kigezi
Bukoba
Tarime
KIKUYU
Kitui
KAMBA
Machakos
MAASAI
HAYA
LOITA HILLS
Kajiado
KAGERA
Tana River
Mwanza
Bukumbi
Biharamulo
ZINZA
POKOMO
Shanwa
Mt Kilimanjaro
SUKUMA
Moshi
Maswa
MEATU
Kimali
CHAGGA
Kaloleni
Kilifi
Shinyanga
Rabai
Mombasa
HA
Nzega
CHOME
SHAMBAA
DIGO
IRAMBA
Singida
Bumbuli
SUMBWA
Tabora
BONDEI
Tanga
Pemba I.
Kipalapala
ZIGUA
Pangani
NYAMWEZI
Zanzibar I.
GOGO
Kongwa
Dodoma
Bagamoyo
Lake Tanganyika
Morogoro
Kilosa
ZARAMO
Dar es Salaam
Karema
Minaki
HEHE
Kisaki
Iringa
Mafia I.
Sumbawanga
UZUNGWA
Southern Highlands
Mbeya
Rungwe
Tukuyu
NYAKYUSA
Lindi
Lake Nyasa (Malawi)
Ndanda
Mtwara
Songea
Masasi
0 300 km
0 200 miles

East Africa

1 The argument

Not since the origins of mankind has East Africa been so important to the world as it is today. The special importance comes from the AIDS epidemic, and particularly from the role of East African doctors in charting the epidemiology of heterosexually transmitted AIDS and devising control strategies adopted in many others parts of the world. Yet we know almost nothing about these doctors[1] and the relationship between their response to AIDS and their historical experience, the crises affecting medical systems in all three East African countries in the late twentieth century, or the parallel crises within the medical profession there. East African doctors have not only fought AIDS; they also carried out, in Kenya in 1994, one of the longest doctors' strikes the world has seen.

This book is not a contemporary sociology of the East African medical profession, much as that is needed. It is a collective biography of East African doctors, covering many aspects of their experience since Africans first practised modern medicine in the region during the 1870s. These doctors were a picked group of gifted people in whose lives many of the main trends of modern East African history intersected. Their training drew the region's education upwards to university level. Their contribution to research and intellectual life was the most important by any group in the region. They were long the 'cream of the cream', the core of East Africa's modern educated elite. They were prominent in politics, especially in Uganda. They were among the first East Africans to enter international affairs as equals. Their experience after independence displayed many of Africa's dilemmas in the quest for stability and prosperity. To write their collective biography offers a much-needed fresh perspective on modern East African history. It also offers an opportunity to explore what Africans of great skill and responsibility have tried to do with political freedom.[2] A collective biography, however, is not the same as a history of medicine. The book deals only with black Africans. It neglects many specialities, notably psychiatry, dentistry, ophthalmology, and leprology. It goes beyond qualified doctors to include the first generation of dressers and auxiliaries who pioneered the African practice of modern medicine before Makerere

College began formal medical training in 1924, but thereafter it neglects auxiliaries and nurses, which is particularly unfortunate because doctors have been so predominantly male. The emphasis on African doctors may appear to depreciate the role in research and treatment of other races and cadres, but that is not the intention; rather, only separate studies could do justice to them.[3] Even within its limits, the book is no more than a first sketch of its subject, written without specialist medical knowledge and based on sources which are often incomplete, although they are enough, it is hoped, to show that a more definitive history will be possible when East Africans themselves have carried out the necessary further research.

The chief aims are, therefore, to chart the main lines of the doctors' history and to provide background understanding of their role in the late twentieth century. The story divides into four stages. The first concerns the initial entry of East Africans into modern medical practice between the 1870s and the 1920s. A few were trained as auxiliaries, but most were allocated purely menial functions and learned by practical apprenticeship. The earliest were freed slaves and the great majority were of low social status. But they inherited an indigenous medical tradition by which young apprentices could qualify as independent practitioners. As they struggled to gather modern skills, some auxiliaries enlarged their role into an honourable career. This attracted men of higher social status into medical employment. It also encouraged European governments and missionaries to supplement practical apprenticeship by formal schooling. That combination of practice and theory was the key to effective medical education.[4] It was institutionalised from 1924 at Makerere College, whose medical school became the nursery of a medical profession, as was the normal pattern of professionalisation in the Third World.[5]

Once the Makerere Medical School existed, the history of East African doctors entered a second stage: the struggle to achieve professional status. The notion of a profession is central to this book, which argues that professionalisation has been seriously misunderstood in East Africa, much to the disadvantage of medical practice there. The idea of a profession first emerged in Britain and the United States, where the major professions of medicine and law grew up outside the universities or state employment.[6] Early analyses argued that the essence of a profession was a body of specialised knowledge which justified its holders in claiming to monopolise and regulate their occupation in return for observance of an ethical code of competence and altruistic service.[7] During the 1960s, however, sociologists pointed out that many groups possessing specialised knowledge – social workers, schoolteachers, nurses, airline pilots – had not achieved institutionalised self-regulation. The true definition of a profession, the sociologists claimed, was not knowledge but power: the power to control both its members' own occupation and everything else within their sphere, as doctors controlled not only their own work but the duties of nurses, the behaviour of patients, and even the definition of disease.[8] Such power could be socially pernicious. This view of professionalism as power was applied in the 1970s to the Third World, where Terence Johnson, in particular, argued that, except perhaps in colonies of white settlement, no true professions had come into being in former colonies, because the occupations concerned had not grown up and organised themselves from below, as they had in Britain and America, but had been created and controlled by colonial states and their successors. Third World 'professionals' possessed only the powerless trappings of professionalism.[9]

This book contests such an analysis, for four reasons. First, the wider discussion of professions has moved beyond the dispute between a first generation of triumphalists and a second generation of cynics. The third generation, as so often, consists of social historians who have studied professionalisation in other parts of the world and stressed its complexity.[10] It is no longer helpful to see the essence of professionalism as either knowledge or power or something else. The essence of professionalism is ambiguity. It embraces specialised knowledge, altruistic service, thirst for power, and blatant self-interest. That is why it has been such a potent idea in East Africa, attracting the professionals by the promise of power and profit while attracting the poor by the promise of altruism and trustworthy care. That is why all sides in the strike of 1994 appealed to it. Second, the Anglo-American model of a profession never truly existed even in Britain or America, and certainly does not exist today. Most professionals in both countries – including some doctors but almost all engineers and many other groups – have been employees and therefore not truly autonomous.[11] Many of their 'self-regulating' organisations have depended on state support. As Eliot Freidson put it, 'The profession's privileged position is given by, not seized from, society, and it may be allowed to lapse or may even be taken away.'[12] The notion that relations between professions and the state must be a zero-sum struggle in which one must lose anything the other gains is precisely the myth that has had such damaging effects in East Africa. In reality, professions and the state are in large measure symbiotic. That leads to the third point. The model of a profession which Johnson applied to the Third World was extraordinarily Anglocentric. In so far as it was true of Britain and America, it was – like so much else about those countries – an exceptional case with little relevance elsewhere. In Continental Europe, for example, professions generally grew up under the control of the state or state-dominated universities. The French medical profession, perhaps the first to secure a legal monopoly of practice, was given it in 1803 by the Napoleonic state, which claimed exclusive power to license practitioners.[13]

In Germany the higher state bureaucracy was itself one of the first professional groups, while both law and medicine were strictly regulated for much of the nineteenth century. As Charles McClelland has written, 'The German experience of professionalization, with its complicated tangle of private sphere and bureaucratically controlled dimensions, may prove more typical of professionalization throughout the twentieth-century world than the Anglo-American "model" from which much of the social-science theory of professions has been derived.'[14] Japanese experience reinforces that, for there the modern medical profession was under substantial state control until 1945.[15] So the fourth objection to Johnson's analysis is that in colonial East Africa medical professionalisation took place through this uneasy symbiosis with the state, rather than failing to follow an idealised Anglo-American model of conflict with it. It is true that colonial states created medical services and some professional institutions. But not only did the colonial medical profession include many Asian private practitioners in all East African countries and European private practitioners in Kenya, but even the medical services were far from pure bureaucracies. In particular, the Director of Medical Services (DMS), the state's senior medical officer in each colony, was to a large extent the doctors' representative in government, often writing of making proposals to 'the Government' as though he did not belong to it, sometimes violently at odds with the political administration, and periodically engaged in bizarre negotiations between the state and its medical staff via their trade union, the British Medical Association, in London. This ambivalent symbiosis with the colonial state applied also to emerging African doctors. They saw themselves as locked in struggle with the government for professional recognition and equality, as indeed they were; professionalisation was in this sense an aspect of African nationalism. Yet African doctors also depended on the state not only for their training and employment but for their protection, both against rival practitioners and against popular disorder, as Uganda's doctors learned during disturbances in 1949.

This symbiosis between profession and state continued into the third stage of the doctors' history. At independence East Africa's doctors interpenetrated with the state, although their power over medical policy varied from country to country. During the next thirty years, however, their power and status certainly declined. It would be easy to see this, as Roger Jeffery saw it in India,[16] as a process of deprofessionalisation, which he attributed to the failure of India's modern doctors either to monopolise medical treatment, much of which remained with practitioners of indigenous Indian medicine, or to prevent the state rather than the profession from regulating medical practice. Deprofessionalisation is how many East African doctors see their experience since independence, but they are probably wrong because, like Jeffery, they have a misleading Anglo-American notion of a profession. It will be argued that modern doctors in East Africa have not been seriously threatened by competition from indigenous medicine, largely because in East Africa, unlike India or China, that medicine lacked a literate tradition to provide a basis for its modernisation. The real threat to professional medicine has come from the illicit sale of modern drugs for self-medication, an outgrowth of the dominant position which chemotherapy has gained within modern medicine.[17] More importantly, what chiefly damaged the power and status of East African doctors after independence was not the *power* of the state but the *weakening* of the state in the face of population growth, economic crisis, commercialisation, and (in Uganda) political collapse. It was the states' inability to preserve free public-health systems, pay doctors a living wage, give them acceptable working conditions, or protect their monopoly privileges against lay practitioners that most seriously threatened the medical profession. This is the crucial reason why notions of deprofessionalisation and Anglo-American models are inapplicable to East Africa. Nevertheless, although the modern profession was weakened after independence, it remained the chief component of East Africa's late twentieth-century medical systems. These consisted of five main, often discordant, elements. First, the modern doctors who controlled state medical services dominated public health, preventive medicine, and the most sophisticated forms of curative care; thanks to modern communications and international bodies like the World Health Organisation (WHO) they held quite strictly to orthodox modern medicine, without the syncretism which had taken place in the past when Greek medicine was exported to the Islamic world or Buddhist medicine to China,[18] which was one reason to follow the modern doctors in seeing their medicine as distinctive and calling it modern.[19] Second, the bulk of doctors in public service had entered a trade union relationship with the state and were beginning to rethink the very notion of a profession. Third, most modern doctors were private practitioners, either openly or covertly, in response to urbanisation, social differentiation, and the decline of state services. Fourth, much routine medication came from drug-sellers and medical auxiliaries in private practice. Fifth, indigenous medicine was largely a residual activity, with some efforts towards self-modernisation. These five elements jostled one another, revealing as yet no clear trajectory for East African medicine as a whole.

The fourth stage in the modern doctors' history was the AIDS epidemic. Their historical experience profoundly shaped their responses. First, East Africa's doctors played a major part in uncovering the epidemiology of heterosexually transmitted AIDS, drawing on a tradition of epidemiological research first developed at Makerere in the 1940s. Second, they had substantial responsibility for devising strategies to control the epidemic in Third World countries; here they were hampered by the weakening of East Africa's states and medical systems, but the doctors' blend of rationalism and nationalism enabled them to counsel openness and to encourage experiment without sacrificing national dignity. Third, the doctors shared in the burden of care for AIDS patients, protected to some degree by the detachment which they had cultivated in the face of East Africa's disease environment, but nevertheless at their best showing the compassion which had moved those who first pioneered modern medicine in the region.

2 Pioneers

Africans began to practise modern medicine in East Africa from the 1870s. They owed little in a direct sense to the region's indigenous medicine, but they inherited its entrepreneurial character as a career open to talent and most learned their modern medicine through an apprenticeship not unlike that of indigenous healers. As apprentices in a menial task, the modern African pioneers had ambition but little status. Most were of lowly birth, initially indeed former slaves, and they generally lacked compensating modern education. But by their own efforts they converted menial work into a respectable career, while a few, through talent and long service at mission stations, gained positions of medical responsibility which Africans would not achieve again until the late 1920s. The majority, however, remained menials, especially in government employment. It was only on the eve of the First World War that practical medical training began to be linked to formal education in the way needed to lay the foundations of a medical profession.

Disease and medicine in nineteenth-century East Africa

Although the first East African practitioners of modern medicine seldom came from families with an indigenous medical tradition, and although the professional structures they entered could scarcely have been less like indigenous structures, there were nevertheless more subtle legacies from the old medicine to the new. The most obvious was the disease environment. It is difficult today to imagine the extent of ill-health and suffering endured in the nineteenth century, as everywhere in the world during the 'age of agony' which preceded modern medicine. Early European doctors occasionally described it:

> The Teso turned up in large force for medicine, and I saw nearly four hundred cases in the two days . . . Amongst others there were over forty lepers, with fingers and toes dropping off, some blind, alas! and others just starting the fell disease, including one a child of only eight or nine. Many had huge ulcers, with a lump of

> cow-dung clapped on by way of medicine. There were babies with malarial spleens. Enormous hydroceles, which in many cases reached the size of a child's head, or even bigger, were common. On Saturday we operated on thirty-one of these, on Sunday afternoon on forty-seven.[1]

One thing that modern doctors were to share with their indigenous predecessors was their value to a world of suffering.

Most of this ill-health was due to endemic complaints arising from environment and poverty. Broadly speaking, East Africa divided into damp lowlands (especially on the Indian Ocean coast and around the Great Lakes), arid savanna covering most of modern Tanzania and the north of Kenya and Uganda, and damp highland blocks thrusting out of the savanna (notably the homelands of the Kikuyu and Kalenjin of Kenya, the Chagga and Shambaa of northern Tanzania, and the mountain peoples of western Uganda).[2] The dominant endemic disease of the damp lowlands and the savanna, especially among children, was malaria, which African mosquitos transmitted with unique efficiency to peoples living below 1,000–1,500 metres. It accounted for one-quarter of all the early cases at Mengo Hospital in Buganda, on the northern shore of Lake Victoria.[3] Damp lowlands also fostered diarrhoea (especially in infants), dysentery, helminthic conditions which caused widespread anaemia, leprosy, trachoma (an eye complaint), the hideous tropical ulcers whose victims occupied so many beds in early colonial hospitals, the equally horrible and widespread sores due to yaws, and (especially on the coast) the water-transmitted urinary complaint of bilharzia.[4] These diseases were somewhat less prevalent in the savanna, where yaws might give place to the closely related endemic (non-venereal) syphilis.[5] Diarrhoea, yaws, ulcers, helminthic conditions, and leprosy were also common in many damp highlands, but here the absence of malaria was balanced by special susceptibility to pneumonia and other respiratory complaints, including a tuberculosis which was less fatal than that introduced under European rule.[6] Nor were East Africans spared diseases often thought peculiar to industrial countries. Within five years of arriving in Uganda in 1897, Dr Albert Cook had diagnosed cancer and leukemia, benign tumours, and several heart conditions. Epilepsy was greatly feared, often thought to be contagious, and brutally treated, as were other mental illnesses with frightening symptoms.[7]

Among epidemic diseases, the strain of bubonic plague which had caused Justinian's Plague in North Africa in AD 541–2 survived in East Africa's wild rodents and bred sporadic human epidemics, especially in Buganda, where people fled their homes at its appearance.[8] Smallpox, although common, was less feared in its relatively mild indigenous form, but long-distance trade introduced more virulent Asian or European strains which caused terrible epidemics during the last thirty years of the nineteenth century.[9] Trade also brought four major cholera epidemics from India during the nineteenth century, with especially dreadful mortality in Zanzibar.[10] Traders probably also introduced gonorrhoea and venereal syphilis, although the similarity between their symptoms and those of yaws and endemic syphilis makes these diseases especially puzzling.[11]

Not only did East Africa's first modern doctors inherit a disease environment from their indigenous predecessors, but they also inherited their patients and the patients' expectations, which were for a largely curative (rather than preventive) therapy chiefly in the form of medicines, an emphasis which was to survive throughout the twentieth century. Adults probably ignored much minor illness. 'Most people in Kenya regard a certain amount of abdominal worms as a natural, indeed necessary, condition to normal health', a Kenyan medical anthropologist has written.[12] Illness in children probably caused more alarm, for their vulnerability was widely recognised – 'one who wants to bring up a child needs medicine', said a Luganda proverb – but modern study suggests that children, like adults, were generally treated first with home remedies.[13] 'The patient first tries out all the medicines known to him before he calls the healer', a well-informed observer of the Shambaa explained.[14] When domestic remedies failed, the next recourse was probably to an elderly neighbour or relative with a purely local reputation for treating a particular complaint.[15] Only when these options were exhausted did the patient turn to an expert, an *mganga* (in Swahili) or *omusawo* (in Luganda).

East Africa's indigenous healers were diverse and did not form a coherent profession. There was generally a broad distinction between divination (or diagnosis) and treatment. In some areas, as in Buganda, the same expert often performed both functions, but elsewhere they were frequently separated.[16] Both types of practitioners were mostly male, but there were women diviners (generally using spiritual techniques) and women who specialised in midwifery or in treating women's and children's complaints.[17] Although expertise often ran in families, the diviner also generally needed a spiritual calling, through dreams, sickness, spirit possession, or solitary wandering in the bush.[18] Like pre-modern doctors elsewhere, diviners relied less on examination than on observation, shrewd questioning, and psychological insight. They might also seek spiritual guidance or manipulate material objects: the patterns formed by powder sprinkled on water or seeds scattered from a basket, for example, or the flow of blood and condition of the organs of a slaughtered beast or fowl, to quote common techniques used in the Bunyoro kingdom bordering Buganda.[19] The diviners' role was to diagnose the deeper causes of misfortune – for illness was only one of the many misfortunes on which they were consulted – and to prescribe a course of action, which might be not a medical treatment but a ritual or countermeasures against a sorcerer. In the last resort, the only test of a divination was whether the course of action worked.[20]

By contrast, the most common medical practitioner, the herbalist, generally learned his trade through apprenticeship, which appears to have provided a model and set of expectations for many of the first young people who studied modern medicine. Only two accounts of formal apprenticeship exist. One, for the Shambaa, describes a young man apprenticing himself to an expert by a blood oath promising mutual support and secrecy regarding the master's medicines. After initial instruction, the apprentice spent a year practising alone among neighbouring peoples, paid a fee, assisted his master for a period, made a second itineration, paid a final fee, and qualified.[21] The second account, for the Nyamwezi of western Tanzania, describes formal initiation into a secret society of healers, followed by a period of close service and observation with a master before receiving the gnu's tail of office.[22] Normally, however, apprenticeship was less formal. Most herbalists appear to have specialised in certain conditions or medicines and to have worked part time, mainly at their homesteads, but there were also itinerant specialists.[23] Herbs were applied to external injuries or drunk for internal conditions. Most herbalists claimed magical as well as chemical efficacy for their potions, which often had genuine, if mild, medicinal properties.[24] In addition to herbal remedies, practitioners treated fever by stimulating perspiration, countered mental and other complaints by inducing trance, and used the cupping-horn to encourage bleeding or cautery to stop it. Experts treated snake-bite, set bones, or healed wounds.[25] There is evidence, especially in the Great Lakes region, of surgical skill in repairing mutilations and in such agonising emergency surgery as trepanning and perhaps caesarean delivery, although – as in other pre-modern cultures – surgery was practised only in emergencies.[26]

Although indigenous medicine was chiefly curative, healers also had protective and preventive functions. For protection they supplied amulets, medicines, and potions, especially for children. Nyoro also inoculated their children with endemic syphilis, while inoculation with pus from an active smallpox case was known in the eighteenth century and spread widely in the nineteenth.[27] Healers also had important public-health functions which they were to lose under colonial rule. Kamba diviners in modern Kenya were expected to foresee approaching epidemics and place charms against them on paths approaching villages. In Buganda the priest of the plague god, Kawumpuli, sent agents to cleanse areas attacked by plague, distribute amulets, and treat and nurse the sick.[28] In important kingdoms the royal doctors were powerful men at court. During the 1880s the King of Bunyoro deputed a renowned healer to find a cure for plague, supplying victims for experimental purposes. Other rulers intervened more directly. The Hehe chief Mkwawa in the Southern Highlands of Tanzania, for example, ordered the isolation of plague victims.[29]

Yet such institutionalised measures were exceptional. Most indigenous medical practice was highly personalised. 'The *Mganga* is expected to take a very solicitous interest in the patient and to be understanding and friendly', a later anthropologist wrote.[30] The healer treated his patient's entire condition, social and psychological as well as medical, seeking to restore the wholeness, *uzima*, which was the word for health in the Swahili language of the coast, just as the Luganda world for health, *obulamu*, meant well-being in a more general sense. These expectations were to breed resentment of busy modern doctors who treated diseases rather than patients. Characteristically, too, indigenous healing was entrepreneurial, competitive, and often mercenary, especially among full-time specialists with wide reputations. 'All healers draw blood', said a Shambaa proverb, and they would otherwise scarcely have been respected, for in these honour cultures poverty and menial service were generally considered ignoble.[31] Unlike Chinese, East Africans did not expect doctors to disdain financial gain[32] and consequently did not expect pioneer modern doctors to do so either, so that patients were all the more impressed by altruism when it was practised. Indigenous healers often demanded an initial payment 'to open the bag' and some expected full payment in advance, but normally most of the fee was paid only if the treatment succeeded.[33] Early accounts suggest that healers were comfortably off rather than rich,[34] for the intense competition would probably have eroded excessive profits. In a world where social status owed much to birth, medicine was one career open to talent, which is how it was also seen by the first modern African practitioners. The apprentice carrying his master's medicine-bag hoped eventually to settle in a homestead replete with patients, wives, children, and social honour. This career ambition culminating in ownership of a private nursing home and enjoyment of community respect was to be another powerful legacy.

Where diseases were widespread, healers numerous, and failures common, practitioners were the targets of much scepticism, which their modern successors inherited. 'Deception, deception, that's medicine', said a Shambaa proverb.[35] Patients and their kin tried one specialist after another in search of cure. Healers, likewise, were pragmatic. 'I became a doctor to cure people', a twentieth-century herbalist explained. 'Medicines cure, nothing else works. I have some very strong medicines, but I always hope to find better ones.'[36] Medical innovation was common. Aliens with novel skills often enjoyed high reputations. Shambaa apprentices tested themselves on credulous neighbouring peoples before venturing to practise at home. Late nineteenth-century coastal medicine made much use of imported materials like copper sulphate and petroleum. In 1853 the

Shambaa ruler had a resident Muslim healer.[37] Such innovativeness would encourage receptivity to modern medicine. But at all stages it was the patient or his kinsmen and neighbours who selected the treatment. No Ganda doctor would treat a patient who arrived alone, doubtless for fear of retribution if the patient died.[38] Here the contrast between indigenous expectations and the norms of modern medicine was to be especially sharp.

Such a competitive free-for-all, pragmatic, eclectic, and dominated by patient power, characterised all pre-modern medical systems.[39] It contrasted with the closed, regulated, authoritarian medical profession which emerged in Europe during the nineteenth century, when technological advances made all earlier medical systems outdated, including that of Europe itself. In this respect, East Africa shared a universal experience. But the region had one peculiarity. It had known only an unstructured folk-medicine, whereas European and Asian societies had also possessed literate medical cultures. The lack of a literate tradition meant that indigenous East African medicine received little respect from modern doctors and was ill equipped to contest their claims to exclusive knowledge. Instead the colonial authorities forbade indigenous practitioners to adopt modern techniques, thereby reducing indigenous medicine to a residual craft which was expected to disappear. Consequently, modern doctors felt little need to adapt their methods to East African circumstances, because those patients who rejected their methods could exercise their patient power by resorting to indigenous healers. By the late twentieth century East African medicine was coming to resemble its pre-colonial pattern as a competitive, pragmatic, and mercenary free-for-all. The difference was that it now also had a literate – and modern – component. The insertion of that component is the central subject of this book.

The freedmen

The first East African known to have practised modern medicine extensively was James Ainsworth, who was first recorded in 1875 as an assistant to E.W. Forster, a Church Missionary Society (CMS) doctor at Mombasa. A mission had been established there in 1844, but it had been so unfruitful that, when it was revitalised in 1875, medicine was thought to be one of the few chances of success among the surrounding coastal Muslims.[40] Revitalisation was needed because Britain had in 1873 imposed on the Sultanate of Zanzibar a treaty ending slave exports. Slaves intercepted and freed by the British navy would be settled near Mombasa. Hitherto most had gone to a CMS settlement in the Bombay Presidency of western India. The intention had always been that these freedmen should return as

Christians to evangelise eastern Africa. Now the CMS seized the opportunity. During 1874 and 1875 some 150 'Bombay Africans' joined their superintendent, W.S. Price, in establishing a Christian settlement at Freretown, near Mombasa, to receive the expected influx of liberated slaves.[41] Forster joined them from England on 7 July 1875 and opened a free dispensary in Mombasa town. A frail man of 'morbidly nervous temperament',[42] he anxiously sought assistants. Two young Bombay Africans 'failed thro' bad morals', leaving him at the end of 1875 with only James Assura, who must at this time have been about fifteen or sixteen and had apparently arrived from India somewhat earlier through a connection with freedmen working for the previous missionaries near Mombasa.[43] By the time Forster returned to England in April 1876, Assura had become the mainstay of the medical work, which was concentrated on a sixteen-bed hospital at Freretown 'full of ulcerated legs' belonging to freed slaves.[44] Although Assura had little education and an imperfect command of either English or Swahili, Forster wrote, 'He has proved a faithful friend, a conscientious Christian, and an intelligent learner: he seems to have been sent in the Providence of God to supply a place which probably could not otherwise have been filled.'[45] By September 1876 James Assura had become known to the missionaries as James Ainsworth, probably in honour of some supporter in Britain who sponsored him. For most of the next five years he ran the mission's medical work largely single-handed.

Forster recommended that Ainsworth should have a proper medical training: 'Two or three years of sound medical education in India or England would make him a very useful man.'[46] There were already qualified West African doctors, often sons of freed slaves whom the CMS had trained in Sierra Leone to evangelise their own peoples.[47] These doctors contested European control of the West African medical profession and ensured that its training took place chiefly in Britain rather than in West Africa. But in East Africa the profession took a different course. By the late 1870s missionary relations with educated Africans on both sides of the continent were deteriorating. In 1881 Ainsworth himself signed a protest by the leading Bombay Africans of Freretown complaining that one of Price's successors had described them publicly as 'idle and slovenly'. 'Why should the missionaries be ever murmuring against the Bombay Africans', they demanded, 'and not leaving them and forming another station for himself, among the different tribes of uncivilized Africans without the Bombay Africans for a help and flourish'.[48] This protest further embittered relations at Freretown, and although missionary hostility does not seem to have focused on Ainsworth – whose practical skills and personal humility probably deflected antagonism – he was nevertheless one of its victims. In 1883 another missionary with some medical knowledge, the Swahili scholar W.E. Taylor, revived Forster's proposal that Ainsworth should receive further training:

The Society is in want of Medical Missionaries: and I suppose that native ones, inured as they are to the climate, are as likely to be useful as Europeans in that department of the Mission field. I suppose the great objection to Africans is their national indolence, and the facility with which they are spoiled by success. However I believe that in James Ainsworth the Society would find a man free from these objections. For he is one of the most active and satisfactory servants in the settlement. He is very neat; and is businesslike too for an African. He has a great attachment to his work and a natural bias for it: as is shewn in the shrewdness which he often exhibits in diagnosis and in his retentive memory for the quantities of doses and for modes of treatment. He is generally very accurate: but his great misfortune lies in having had but an imperfect elementary education. However he has a great thirst for knowledge and by his energy may eventually overcome the obstacle I have mentioned. Indeed I think if he were sent to one of the Indian Med[ica]l Schools or to some English one, he w[oul]d repay a hundredfold any expenses bestowed upon him, by using that knowledge to the higher end of bringing his benighted fellow-countrymen the light of the Gospel. This he would I am sure desire to do.[49]

Perhaps wisely, Taylor sent this letter direct to London, not, as procedure required, through the committee of Mombasa missionaries. But headquarters replied that 'unless there sh[oul]d be *very* special circumstances, they entirely disapprove of bringing the natives of India and other countries to England for training. There are exceptions but, in general, they consider the practice fraught with danger to the individual and therefore to his work on his return to his native country.'[50] The mission secretary in Mombasa agreed and doubted if Taylor had been serious: 'James Ainsworth is a steady man and is very useful in his sphere, but even if he were to obtain the sanction of the Committee for a medical training in England, I have very little hesitation in saying he would prove a failure.'[51] Two years later the bishop confessed that he had failed to persuade the missionaries to do anything 'for the first-class boys to bring up to a higher grade of education, and prepare them for the ministry, and for schoolteaching or the medical profession'.[52]

Ainsworth responded by trying to gather as much medical knowledge as he could within the confines of Mombasa. During 1887 he read 'a small book on Medicine' with a newly arrived mission doctor, who also explained cases to him and to three younger assistants.[53] 'My plan', the doctor explained,

is, first to see any of the sick brethren here, then the sick natives, and if any spare time comes between for it, give instruction to Simeon Livingston and James Ainsworth, the dispenser and assistant . . . You will be glad to hear that every fortnight, James Ainsworth goes up to Rabai; to see patients there and at Kya Fimboni.

After the Medical Mission is over, on Tuesday afternoon he starts; then after a sleep, on Wednesday morning he sees patients, Thursday also; then on Friday with Nathaniel the catechist of that place, he visits Kya Fimboni, a Wa-Nyika village. On Saturday again he sees folk at Rabai and returns to Frere Town in the evening. The last time he went 167 patients were treated at Rabai and Fimboni.[54]

Not surprisingly, this schedule left little time for instruction and the doctor was soon 'waiting anxiously for the arrival of skeleton or the anatomical plates I wrote about. James Ainsworth does not make much progress through merely reading.'[55] Shortly afterwards this doctor too left East Africa. His successor showed little interest in training his staff and Ainsworth's formal instruction ended. By now, however, he was sometimes given the courtesy title of doctor and was competent to handle routine work on his own. 'James Ainsworth has taken all the hard work in the medical line this year and has been of the greatest service and comfort to me', the next mission doctor reported in 1892, 'he is so trustworthy and patient and does not lie up for trifling ailments as most natives do'.[56] In 1894 and again in 1899 Ainsworth stood in while the doctor was on leave for several months, 'to the complete satisfaction of the Finance Committee and the Doctor'.[57] Invited to congratulate him, however, London headquarters resolved to 'correspond with Dr Edwards, not direct with Mr Ainsworth'.[58] His status and pay at this time were those of a village pastor and less than half what he could have earned in other employment, according to Edwards.[59] But this does not seem to have troubled him. On the eve of the First World War, after thirty-eight years in mission service, he had charge of two dispensaries at Freretown and Mombasa and also acted as anaesthetist in the Mombasa Hospital.[60] 'He has no qualification except that of experience', the mission doctor wrote:

but on the medical side he has had a good deal of this, and it is remarkable how much he knows, especially with regard to prescribing; he is also our anaesthetist. He knows English and Hindustani, which is of great use in the town dispensary, where a large proportion of our patients are Indians from Bombay and Karachi.[61]

James Ainsworth last appears in the records in 1928. His daughter had by then married the son of a local clergyman in 'a grand native wedding'.[62] His son, a former mission teacher, was dead. The old man himself was living with his wife just outside the Freretown settlement where he had worked for fifty years.[63]

James Ainsworth had entered modern medicine through the normal route of apprenticeship. But there was another possible route which was later to supplant apprenticeship, that of formal medical education. That this route was also available to a handful of pioneer freedmen was due to Charles Lavigerie, Cardinal-Archbishop of Carthage and founder in 1868 of the

White Fathers. Lavigerie's experience in the Islamic environment of North Africa had taught him to seek his initial converts among young men uprooted from their societies. In 1872 his missionaries in Algeria began to buy and liberate black slave children brought across the Sahara from West Africa. Disappointed in attempts to train priests, and sharing the widespread Catholic view that the most effective initial approach to non-Christian peoples was through works of mercy, Lavigerie planned in 1877 to train 'very intelligent and very young' freedmen as medical catechists who could return to tropical Africa, support themselves by medical practice, and exercise influence through their skills. For his training institution Lavigerie chose Malta, where a Catholic medical college had existed since 1674. It taught a six-year course, but Lavigerie's students did not complete it or graduate, lest they should choose to practise outside the mission. Much of their training was in fact private, for the missionaries feared the corrupting influence of the other medical students. Only nine students underwent extensive medical training before the scheme was abandoned in 1896.[64] Seven travelled to East Africa with parties of White Fathers during the late 1880s and early 1890s. Two posted to Buganda met hostility from the local missionaries; one, Michel Abdou, joined the British medical service, while the other, François Gogé, died in 1892 at the Battle of Mengo between Catholics and Protestants. A third, Joseph Gatchi, was intended for a mission south of Lake Victoria at Kipalapala or Bukumbi, but both refused him and he was welcomed instead on the western shore of Lake Tanganyika, where he died of sleeping sickness contracted from his patients. His colleague there, Charles Farraghi, spent twenty years in mission service and later worked for the Belgian government before dying as a small trader. Augustin Mechire and Louis Coro joined the White Fathers mission at the south-eastern end of Lake Tanganyika in what was becoming German East Africa. Mechire eventually entered German service and was killed during the First World War, while Coro served the British in Tanganyika after 1918 and died as a successful farmer.[65] That left only one: Adrien Atiman.

Atiman was the most remarkable of the East Africans who pioneered modern medicine, not only because he served the Catholic mission at Karema on Lake Tanganyika for sixty-seven years from his arrival in 1889 to his death in 1956, but because he was the only East African medical man who has ever (by 1997) written his autobiography, whereas not a single word by James Ainsworth appears to have survived.[66] Atiman was born in about 1863 as the son of a fisherman in a village on the Niger to the west of Timbuktu. He was kidnapped by a Tuareg, sold to an Arab, and marched across the desert – he later wrote that he was treated kindly – to Mitlile in Algeria, where a White Father bought and liberated him in 1876. Four years later he was one of the first students sent to Malta, where he spent seven years and passed through that experience of mortality and responsibility which separates young doctors from their contemporaries:

> During my first few days in the dissecting room I was much impressed by all I saw, as also by the human body in front of the professor in the lecture theatre . . .
>
> I was never ill, and could not believe that one day I must die.
>
> When a student died I thought he had only gone away for a time and would return. It was only in the theatre when I had to see and dissect a dead body that I learnt to believe really in death.[67]

Later, he recalled, a patient died in his care: 'For thirty years this death haunted me.'[68] Like other medical students, too, he struggled to master the vast body of knowledge necessary to his profession:

> Our lectures in midwifery were at first especially difficult, because we had no contact with the other students, still less with the women. Also we had nothing to read except our notes that we were continually taking. I was, however, able to obtain a French text-book of midwifery, and one in two volumes on surgery.[69]

'At the end of our studies', he claimed,'we were as good as the average of the Maltese students',[70] but he did not formally qualify, receiving instead only a certificate saying he had given 'evident proofs of intelligence and thorough application'.[71] His missionary party reached the East African coast in August 1888 and began the seven-month walk to Karema, suffering repeatedly from malaria and passing terrible caravans of slaves, 'almost walking corpses, weakened by smallpox and dysentery'.[72]

'On the day after my arrival I began my medical service', Atiman later recalled:

> Cases of tropical ulcers, dysentery, fevers, and children with yaws and scabies were all lying together.
>
> My medicines comprised 20 kilos of camphor, a little carbolic acid, and ipecacuanha. For instruments, a thermometer, an irrigator, and nothing else. There were very many ticks, which we swept up each morning, before they had finished their meals of blood for the day.
>
> Each morning I visited the orphans and treated those who were ill. Persistent fevers were prevalent owing to lack of quinine. Since this cost 1,000 francs a kilo, it is obvious that it could not be given to everyone, and it took a year to obtain fresh supplies of medicines. Bandages were made from clothes used by the orphans. Although washed they looked more like khaki than white material.
>
> I did not approve of treating the ulcers with camphor. With 40 francs that had been given to me by Sister Spiridion, my godmother, one kilo of iodoform was purchased, and when received in the following year the treatment of ulcers improved greatly, and many were healed.
>
> In addition to medical treatment I gave religious instruction, taught in classes, and prepared the dying for baptism.[73]

Atiman was as much a catechist as a doctor. As a young man he frequently visited the sick in their homes and toured the countryside, carrying a portable medicine-chest and sometimes the patients themselves. Later in his life, like an indigenous healer, 'he has gained the confidence of his patients who come to him instead'.[74] Near the dispensary he built a settlement for chronic elderly patients, ulcer cases, and sufferers from leprosy and sleeping sickness. He trained African nurses, although this responsibility soon passed to European sisters. With a missionary as anaesthetist, he performed amputations and caesarean sections, set fractures, and treated haematuria, although it was not until 1938 that the mission built the hospital of which he dreamed. In addition, like many later African doctors, he served as a pioneer of rationality, successfully opposing the poison ordeal used locally to detect malefactors. The missionaries tried to make him a point of access to local society by marrying him to a relative of the chief, a marriage which brought him fifty years of unhappiness concealed beneath a habitual gaiety. Unlike other freedmen trained in Malta, he rejected invitations to enter government service, including one to teach at a medical school the Belgians planned in Burundi.[75] Instead he accepted the deprivation of a remote mission and a salary which a domestic servant would have refused,[76] a remarkable sacrifice for one born in poverty and then brutally uprooted. He venerated the missionaries, visiting their cemetery at Karema daily, and the greatest delight of his life was that his son became one of Karema's first African priests. Atiman clearly valued this well above his own medical profession.

Although Atiman's practical training was considerable, the medical school at Malta was old-fashioned and he was never a modern doctor to compare with the German physicians reaching East Africa at this time. Like the missionaries, he believed fervently in the Belgian Black Stone (actually charcoal) as a remedy for snake-bite, he was convinced of the healing property of water from Lourdes, and he was fascinated by extraordinary phenomena of all kinds. His approach to treatment was as experimental as a herbalist's, and like indigenous healers he was consulted on many non-medical issues. Yet he also remained alert to medical advances. 'Even in Africa one must keep pace with the times', he wrote in 1940.[77] Twenty-one years earlier he had for the first time acquired a microscope and delighted to show patients the micro-organisms responsible for their complaints. He was also fascinated by the X-ray equipment which missionary sisters introduced when the new hospital was built. He was then about seventy-five and remained eager to learn until he died eighteen years later.

With their different training and their contrasting cultural backgrounds, James Ainsworth and Adrien Atiman were both remarkable pioneers. But that was all they were. Atiman's son became a priest, Ainsworth's a schoolteacher. Lavigerie's experiment evaporated, the Bombay Africans lost their identity in a wider Kenya. Neither established an enduring *medical* tradition. That would happen at Mengo.

Mission work

Until the 1920s medical care and training for East Africans remained largely in missionary hands. Both Protestants and Roman Catholics had begun work on the coast in the mid-nineteenth century and had penetrated far inland to Buganda and the Great Lakes during the late 1870s. But their work expanded chiefly during the first twenty-five years of colonial rule before 1914. On the Protestant side, the Church Missionary Society created a pioneer hospital at Mengo, the capital of Buganda, expanded its work throughout Uganda, and entered both the Nyanza region and the central highlands of Kenya, where it worked alongside the Church of Scotland Mission and two American organisations, the Society of Friends and the non-denominational Africa Inland Mission. Further south, German Lutheran societies occupied many of the more populous areas of German East Africa, leaving Anglican enclaves for the CMS in the centre and the Anglo-Catholic Universities Mission in the north and south. The Roman Catholic missionary orders were equally diverse. The whole western half of East Africa, around the Great Lakes, was occupied by the French-speaking White Fathers, supplemented in Uganda by the English-speaking Mill Hill Fathers in the east and the Italian-speaking Verona Fathers in the north. The Holy Ghost Fathers, long established on the coast, moved cautiously into the hinterland of German East Africa and more dramatically into the Kikuyu highlands of Kenya, which they shared with the Consolata Fathers, another Italian order. This left the south of German East Africa to German-speaking Benedictines.[78]

Although their converts' demands led all missionaries to adopt broadly similar practices, there were differences in the importance they attached to medical work. At one extreme, the Church of Scotland Mission among the Kikuyu and neighbouring peoples insisted that every station must have a resident doctor,[79] so that the few stations it opened were dominated by graduates of the famous medical schools at Edinburgh and Glasgow, notably J.W. Arthur, who pioneered medical work at Kikuyu. These doctors not only established hospitals needing African assistants, to whom they gave a training equalled in quality only at Mengo, but they left a uniquely detailed record of their work.[80] At the other extreme, the unworldly gentlemen of the Universities Mission, although pioneers in the training of African priests, took little interest in health (including their own) until well into the 1920s.[81] Most missionaries stood between these extremes. The

White Fathers and some other Catholic orders included hospital service in their training, so that most could operate the elementary dispensaries at their stations. One compared his practice to that of a charlatan at a French country fair.[82] Anything more elaborate was generally left to the sisters who soon accompanied each Catholic mission. Some specialised in nursing, notably the Franciscan Sisters in Uganda who began to build a hospital at Nsambya in 1906 before they even built themselves a convent.[83] But sisters were nurses, not doctors – no Catholic sister was allowed to study medicine until 1936[84] – and they did their works of mercy themselves, so that such medical training as they gave was quite elementary and their African staff remain even more anonymous in the records than the sisters, even when, as in the case of Peter Sabakaki, they worked at Nsambya Hospital for sixty years.[85] By contrast, Dr Maynard of the Africa Inland Mission in the Shinyanga area of German East Africa worked on the principle that a missionary must do nothing that an African could do. 'We are here', she explained, 'not so much to do the work, as to get it done'.[86]

Among these early missions, the CMS hospital which Albert Cook founded at Mengo in 1897 was distinctive because it was not a work of charity designed to break through the indifference of a virgin mission field but was introduced into the most successful mission in the world. This was one reason why it became so influential and why interaction between events in Buganda and in the rest of East Africa became a central theme in the medical history of the region. At the same time, however, the Buganda kingdom, which had been a British Protectorate since 1894, had a complex, stratified social order in which work in a mission hospital was a relatively lowly occupation. Cook soon learned this. The Ganda chiefs eagerly built him a hospital and asked to send him young men for medical training,[87] but nothing came of it, partly because hospital work was repugnant to a culture emphasising honour and cleanliness:

> For the first few years it was difficult to get anyone to do even the humblest work, and we had to fall back on convalescent patients, a few of whom having experienced the benefits of medical and surgical treatment were willing to stay on and help their fellow sufferers. As in many heathen countries, there was often real affection shown for relatives who were sick, but a callous indifference to the sufferings of others. Moreover the nature of the work required often repelled them. A patient rotten with syphilis or covered with loathsome sores, a new arrival with a compound fracture perhaps untreated for days, loudly proclaiming its advent to the nasal organ, a native of an inferior race with discharging wounds, or a helpless paralytic needing everything to be done for him were not attractive to the natural man or boy.[88]

Early Ganda hospital workers reported that when visiting their homes they were considered defiled and were not allowed to help themselves to food, which was instead handed to them.[89] This fear of pollution was shared by other East Africans, notably the Kikuyu and neighbouring peoples, who on occasion deserted a hospital en masse when an inmate died.[90] The first medical worker at the Kikuyu station, Samson Njoroge, later described his experience:

'Around 1907 [actually 1910]', he says, 'I was working as a houseboy for a missionary doctor. I was asked if I wanted to join medical work . . . and I accepted it . . .

'One of my jobs during the training was to help the doctor dispose of the dead bodies.' Both he and the doctor carried bodies of dead patients up to the ridge, dug the graves, and buried them.

If a person touched a dead body he was required to undergo a cleansing ceremony carried out by a witchdoctor. But did Mr Njoroge agree to this procedure every time he touched a dead body? No! Not him. He was a Christian and that made him clean, he says.

'I used to accompany the doctor', he continues, 'to the villages to assist him during the delivery of babies – a type of domiciliary midwifery. Doing this sort of thing was, again, contrary to jobs traditionally meant for men. It was only specialised women who conducted deliveries in my tribe. I was, therefore, treated as an outcast.' He didn't mind a bit.[91]

The final comment was doubtless bravado. 'These difficulties were real and formidable', Cook wrote of Mengo:

. . . But they were overcome by force of example, love in activity. They saw the doctors, the matron, the nurses, and best of all their own native friends, doing quietly and as a matter of course just what repelled or frightened them most. It was enough. As St Augustine said: '. . . One loving spirit sets another on fire.' . . . It was heart-breaking work at times, and the result was a few, very few, who survived the test of time and trial . . .

Three stand out above the others as pre-eminent.[92]

The first of the three was Semei Kasaja, who epitomised those – 'quite one half of our native boys and girls who are helping us in the wards'[93] – who entered medical work through their own experience of its benefits. Semei Kasaja had intercepted Cook while still on the road to Mengo. The side of his face was swollen by a slow-growing cancer which had penetrated the bones of his skull. He survived four operations and in gratitude begged to care for other patients.[94] 'He is very intelligent and quick at catching anything up. He takes the temperatures, night and morning marking off the decimal point quite correctly, and I have just taught him to give the hypodermic injections', Cook wrote in 1899.[95] This route to medical work through personal healing was common among the first hospital assistants at other missions, again notably in Kikuyuland. Samson Njoroge first went to the Kikuyu mission with an eye complaint. Luke Gicimu at Tumutumu was healed of yaws and remained, 'doing any work, however menial, if only to help the other sick folks', eventually taking charge of a dispensary.[96] One consequence, there as in Buganda, was that many early hospital staff were of low social origin and often entered mission service in purely menial roles. At the CMS hospital at Kabarole in the Toro kingdom of Uganda, for example, the two senior assistants in 1924 had begun work nineteen years earlier as gardener and washerman. In the Shambaa kingdom the key helper at the mission leprosarium, Jonathan Panduka, had been a pawn in the service of the neighbouring chief. Equally marginal, although in a different sense, was Charles Kasaja Stokes, the son of a Ganda woman and the executed missionary-turned-gun-runner Charles Stokes; partly educated in Scotland and trained in East Africa as a dresser, he had a long career as a laboratory technician in Kenya and Uganda.[97]

When Semei Kasaja left Mengo Hospital in 1910 for higher pay and lighter work at a government dispensary, his place as Cook's chief assistant fell to Yusufu Musajawaza, who had entered mission service in 1899 and was described two years later as 'a quiet, faithful Christian lad . . . always ready at a moment's notice, day or night, to come on duty'.[98] Musajawaza became chiefly responsible for the operating theatre, where he performed his own first operation in 1902 – 'cir[cumcisio]n quite by himself, tying 6 arteries and stitching the wound'[99] – and subsequently performed much of the minor surgery. In 1919, for example, the hospital's operations book shows that he performed 26 of the 627 operations and gave the anaesthetic in 129 more, while other African staff did 38 operations and gave 84 anaesthetics. (Of the 64 operations, 57 were circumcisions, a curious fact given that Ganda, unless Muslim, did not circumcise and reportedly had a horror of it.) Nine years later, Musajawaza performed 56 of the hospital's 616 operations but gave only 2 anaesthetics, while other Africans did only 3 operations but gave 43 anaesthetics. Of Musajawaza's 56 operations in 1928, only 26 were circumcisions and his surgical skill appears to have diversified, for he also undertook 4 skin grafts, incised several abscesses, inserted stitches, and performed several other procedures.[100] Such wide responsibility was commonly and necessarily given to trusted African assistants at this time and was probably important in attracting them to the work. 'These lads today are *thoroughly efficient*', Arthur wrote from Kikuyu in 1913:

> They have been trained to nurse cases, give medicines, attend to proper feeding, take temperatures, apply poultices, give enemas, inject stimulants hypodermically, and go through all the regular *régime* of a nurse's work at home. In addition, they have had their training in outdoor dispensary work, dressings, teeth pulling, and the treatment of eyes, ears, &c. They are able efficiently to sterilise dressings for operations, prepare basins, instruments, operating-table, and the patient himself. At the operation they can give chloroform, assist me in the actual operation, or even do it

themselves in minor cases. They are sent from time to time to see cases in the villages and return to report to me the seriousness or otherwise of them. They know to a certain extent weights and measures, and can make up medicines and ointments from simple prescriptions.[101]

In a more remote area like Kabarole the dressers ran the mission dispensary alone for weeks at a time when the solitary doctor was away. Dressers and teachers from Kikuyu established the Tumutumu mission before any white personnel arrived, and Tumutumu men later did the same at Chuka.[102] Samson Njoroge at Kikuyu was not only 'one of the best administrators of chloroform I have ever seen' and 'had an extensive ear-repairing and circumcision practice, which made him famous far and wide among his people', but in an emergency he could deliver a baby with instruments under chloroform or perform spinal punctures to test for cerebro-spinal meningitis. 'Really his knowledge, his ways of working, his particularity in everything he did, made one almost afraid to do anything in his presence', a visiting Scottish nurse reported.[103] Like early African catechists and evangelists, these first medical assistants enjoyed a social space within which to create their own roles. Only slowly did the growth of medical professionalism reduce them to mere auxiliaries. 'At that time', Samson Njoroge's interviewer reflected, '. . . there seemed to be no division between nursing and doctor's work'.[104]

Soon after Cook himself retired in 1934, Yusufu Musajawaza also withdrew, leaving his son, pledged to the mission in return for education, to take his place in the hospital. By then the third member of Mengo's pioneer trio, Kosiya Tabula, who had shared the minor surgery and anaesthetics, was already dead at the age of thirty-eight, poisoned by pricking his finger during an operation in 1921, after seventeen years of service which he had initially been obliged to conceal from his parents.[105] His death brought home the danger of early medical work. In 1917 five of Mengo Hospital's ninety African workers died in a smallpox epidemic. 'Save us from sudden death and heal us from the pain of sleeping-sickness, smallpox, and every other kind of illness', said a prayer composed by Semei Kasaja.[106] Nor was hospital work materially rewarding. 'These dear lads . . . lead a most self-denying life', Cook reported in 1899. 'With hard work and no wages, but just the clothes and food they need, they work on cheerfully, doing nearly all the rough work.'[107] The unmarried male staff long shared a crowded room six metres square within Mengo Hospital. The early wage-books have not survived, but in 1916 Mengo's worst-paid, newly engaged menial worker earned two rupees a month, rather less than half the government's unskilled wage, and the average wage of all hospital workers was about six rupees, although by then Yusufu Musajawaza earned twenty-nine rupees a month and could save nearly half his wages.[108] Discipline was severe. Cook had no inhibition about beating his servants. Those found with women in their quarters were taken to Buganda's *Katikiro* (Chief Minister), who put them in the stocks or set them to hard labour. Sunday evenings were often spent in religious meetings under Cook's leadership, while trained staff were expected to conduct regular services in their wards. Mengo Hospital's matron was Cook's domineering wife, who could reduce European nurses to nervous prostration and must have been deeply resented by African men.[109] The monthly wage-book shows that seven hospital staff were sacked during 1922–3 alone, the reasons recorded being 'very dense', 'disobedience', 'so lazy', 'left ward until 4 a.m. when on night duty', 'very lazy', 'disobedience', and 'immoral'.[110] Similar conditions reigned at other mission stations. Church of Scotland missionaries formally apprenticed their medical staff in order to exert greater discipline over them.[111] These workers had to adjust themselves to the rigorous time-discipline of a hospital (in 1921 Samson Njoroge expressed anxiety for a watch so that 'I may not be late at the house of work'[112]), respect the doctors' often seemingly pointless obsession with hygiene, observe the requirement to preach as well as nurse, and suffer the patronising contempt of Europeans.

Amid all these deterrents, one wonders why anyone undertook hospital work. One reason was certainly gratitude for healing and admiration for the doctors' skill and charity. Another was probably fascination with the new. In 1912 the locally trained dressers at Kabarole 'asked for classes in elementary anatomy, physiology, and medicine, so that they might be the better able to take an intelligent interest in the diseases of the patients'.[113] A student from the CMS high school at Budo who toured Mengo Hospital in 1911 recorded the excitement of learning that disease was caused by bacteria which 'cannot be seen with naked eyes, but with a microscope', that X-ray equipment could reveal the human skeleton, that skin could be grafted, and that 'the doctors know the human body from the head to the toes, every capillary where it starts and ends!' 'Whatever they do is amazing', he concluded.[114] Young people probably hoped that by apprenticing themselves to a doctor they would themselves in due course become doctors, as had been the practice with indigenous healers. Soon after Arthur reached Kikuyu a Chagga youth from a Lutheran mission 300 kilometres away at Kilimanjaro arrived seeking to become a doctor.[115] At Maragoli in western Kenya,

> A small boy soon learnt to do the simple dressings – usually nothing more than cuts and sores – and became my surgical assistant. He amused me very much one day by his budding ambition, coming up after the patients had gone to know if he might not also learn to dispense the medicines besides doing dressings! I explained that *that* was a 'very big work indeed'; that first of all he would have to learn to read, then learn 'many words' about medicine which even English people took years to

do, or else he would very soon kill the patients instead of curing them. This presented the matter in a new light, and he appeared satisfied.[116]

It seem unlikely that the satisfaction lasted long, but European medical professionalism ruled out the former possibility of becoming a doctor purely by apprenticeship. Apprentices did gain some of their masters' prestige. They were generally known by the same title as *mganga*, *omusawo*, or (in Kenya) *dakitari*. By 1914 several Kikuyu medical workers were becoming modestly prosperous householders,[117] while Samson Njoroge, who came from an important local family, had acquired a considerable reputation. Generally, however, those whose skills were learned by apprenticeship rather than schooling ranked low in the eyes of the best-educated Africans of the time, none of whom is known to have sought a career in medicine, whereas one able Kikuyu dresser, Muteithia, abandoned his work to train for the ministry.[118] Medical workers of this period seem also to have been less self-aware and articulate than their interwar successors. Letters to the Swahili press in German East Africa, for example, told at this time of witchcraft and death rather than healing. Yet there was one exception to this lowly standing in the status-conscious but eagerly modernising society of Buganda, where modern medicine could become a means of advancement within indigenous society.

In 1901, for example, Buganda's chiefs expressed pleasure that hospital assistants had learned to vaccinate. In the same year Cook treated the five-year-old Kabaka (King) of Buganda for pneumonia and then sent Semei Kasaja to nurse him. Delighted 'at their king being nursed by a trained native', the Katikiro promised Semei a 'garden'.[119] Cook deprecated this. Through their medical training, he explained,

these boys thus acquire a good deal of 'kitibwa' (glory) in the eyes of the people and sometimes get valuable presents. Also our head boys have taken advantage of their confidential positions with chiefs to ask for themselves gardens or land which they readily get, thus turning themselves into chiefs – as I explained both to the chiefs and to them they lay themselves open to the charge of doing their work for filthy lucre's sake and not from love of the Lord. I reminded them of their humble origin and how they really had acquired their 'kitibwa' owing to the training we gave them. Finally I announced my intention of writing to the Katikiro and asking him only to confer plantations on them on condition that if they left off doing the work of the sick the gardens should be taken away from them, for as I pointed out, otherwise they were in a position, if reproved, to grow huffy and snapping their fingers in our faces to retire to their gardens and live as chiefs.[120]

Yusufu Musajawaza, who was also expecting a garden, did grow huffy in response to this, for a time, but he did not abandon his quest for *ekitibwa* through medicine. When he wrote his letter of resignation to the Hospital Superintendent thirty-three years later, he copied it to the Kabaka, Cook, and the DMS, in that order, pointing out that not only had he served the mission with devotion, but 'I bore in mind every good and bad for the honour of the shield of my mother country Buganda.'[121] Desire for social honour in indigenous terms was an important motive among the first generation of Ganda to practise modern medicine.[122]

Despite continuing attachment to indigenous values, there is little evidence that early medical assistants tried to combine modern and indigenous medical practices. A renowned Christian healer at Freretown near Mombasa, brother and father of teachers, was said in 1910 to treat anaemia and debility with infusions of iron and a special diet combined with observance of various taboos, but there was no indication that he had modern medical training.[123] East African Christians of this period who recorded an opinion shared the view that 'indigenous doctors (*waganga*) are enemies of education and work',[124] and although the first published account by an East African of his people's customs, published in 1918, distinguished fraudulent diviners from 'real doctors who cured diseases through the administration of medicines', the author, Apolo Kaggwa, was also remembered for arresting indigenous practitioners while Katikiro of Buganda, a practice also followed in Toro where the Christian king ordered the imprisonment of all 'native doctors'.[125] Missionaries applauded this draconian measure, although several also showed considerable interest in indigenous herbalism.

It was at Mengo that modern medical training was carried further. As early as 1900 Cook had lamented his lack of time to give 'systematic lectures' in physiology and anatomy.[126] When the Medical Sub-Conference for the Diocese of Uganda met for the first time in 1908 it regretted that no true 'native assistant' had yet been trained. 'None knew English, no regular lectures in anatomy, physiology, materia medical [sic], medicine, surgery or midwifery had been given nor could they be entrusted with the dispensing of any but the simplest drugs.'[127] One reason was that educated young men knowing English, who were beginning to emerge from King's School, Budo, and other mission institutions, had other career opportunities than medical work. Lecturing at Budo, Cook claimed to have been asked, 'How many rupees will you give us to come and be taught?' while one student said, 'We would not mind being trained medically, if you would send us the books to Budo, so that we might not have to attend cases in Hospital.'[128] Nevertheless, the Sub-Conference suggested that a three-year medical course might be started at Budo. Cook envisaged a time when 'a medical faculty will be established in the future Mengo University',[129] but when he discussed the matter again with his colleagues in 1909 they found that 'the scheme bristles with difficulties': inadequate staff and facilities, the lack of educated volunteers, and, as 'a more serious danger the creation of a class of inferior medical practitioners with "swelled heads" possessed of an easy confidence in their own powers, to whom the natives would eagerly resort in preference to the hospital, firstly because there would be, or might be, no Christian teaching attached to their work, secondly because their promises of cure, etc, would be far in excess of their ability'. For the next five years, they suggested, only 'preparation for the training of native doctors at Mengo' was possible.[130] By 1911 there was even less optimism: 'as a result of further experience gained during the last 2½ years it was decided that the time had not come for systematic instruction of indentured boys'.[131] Cook's younger relatives were more enthusiastic, as increasingly were CMS headquarters, missionaries engaged in education, government doctors who urged the Cooks in 1913 to collaborate in a training scheme, the Ganda chiefs, and a handful of educated young Ganda, one of whom, a Budo graduate named Isaka Mukibi, stated in 1914 'that he would greatly like to train in Medicine as the 1st Muganda Dr. to his own people'. But Cook and his formidable wife questioned whether such training was properly mission work.[132] It was only in January 1916 that a Medical Sub-Conference at Mengo agreed that, provided it did not interfere with missionary or medical work, an experimental class of medical students could be formed at Mengo Central School. They were to be aged about sixteen and to undertake a two-year course at the hospital in elementary science, laboratory work, and dispensary and ward practice, the object being 'to train efficient "clinical assistants" and "dispensary boys" for supplying the Base Hospital, the branch dispensaries, and the Government'.[133] Opposition continued, however, while staff shortages and wartime needs also interfered. Only in February 1917 did seventeen students attend the first classes at Mengo Medical School.[134] Like the hospital itself, it was to give Buganda a lasting advantage in the training of modern African medical staff.

Government service

Before the First World War, Africans found less opportunity for modern medical training and employment in government than in mission service. Whereas the French in West Africa began to train African *aides-médecins* in 1905,[135] no East African government had a coherent training system before the war, confining themselves to employing Africans in menial roles or preparing small numbers for specific tasks. In either case the employees remained virtually anonymous.

Colonial medical departments were created to care for white soldiers and officials, to protect them against epidemics arising from the African population, and generally 'to make the tropics fit for the white man to inhabit'.[136] Only later did the departments concern themselves directly with

African health, and then chiefly in response to epidemics threatening population levels and labour supplies. Urgent necessity seemed to compel these priorities, for not only did colonial doctors enter a disease-ridden environment but Europeans added to it their own complaints – notably new strains of smallpox, tuberculosis, and venereal diseases – and caused social disruption and population movements which brought East Africa its first known epidemics of sleeping sickness and cerebro-spinal meningitis. The early colonial period was an exceptionally unhealthy time. Populations probably fell in most regions.[137] The few modern doctors concentrated on diseases which they believed they could treat, notably malaria and spectacular epidemics like smallpox, sleeping sickness, and syphilis, rather than the insidious spread of tuberculosis, intractable helminthic complaints, or diseases of women and children.[138]

Yet although young Africans entered merely embryonic medical services, they also entered a profession at one of its most creative moments. Modern medicine had come into being in nineteenth-century Europe through a series of technical advances which included anaesthetics, antiseptics, professional nursing, state-directed public health, devices like the stethoscope for detecting internal conditions, and above all the perfection of the microscope which enabled researchers to see the cell structure of the body (during the 1850s) and the micro-organisms causing specific diseases (from the 1870s) – advances which in turn led to synthetic drugs and the chemotherapy which dominated twentieth-century medicine.[139] Among colonial doctors working in East Africa before the First World War were several pioneers of this new medicine, notably Robert Koch who studied malaria in German East Africa in 1897–8 and sleeping sickness in the Lake Victoria region during 1906–7.[140] The combination of medical crisis and scientific innovation made this an exciting time and place for young Africans to touch even the fringe of modern medicine. It is sad that only faint traces of their experience survive.

The Germans created East Africa's first medical service during their invasion in 1888. It still retained its military character in 1914, when it employed forty-three military doctors, eleven civilian doctors, and sixty-four medical NCOs.[141] By contrast, the British services established in Uganda in 1897 and in Kenya in 1901 were predominantly civilian, with fewer European doctors – twenty-four in Uganda in 1912 and twenty-five in Kenya in 1914 – supplemented respectively by seventeen and forty-one Indian Assistant or Sub-Assistant Surgeons. There was a handful of private practitioners, chiefly Indians and chiefly in Kenya.[142] Registration of doctors began in Kenya in 1910 and extended to Uganda in 1913 and Tanganyika in 1920. The legislation restricted medical practice to those with qualifications recognised by the General Medical Council in Britain, but it also provided for the licensing of Sub-Assistant Surgeons and contained an important proviso:

> Nothing contained in this Ordinance shall be construed so as to prohibit or prevent the practice of systems of therapeutics according to Native, Indian or other Asiatic method by persons recognised by the community to which they belong to be duly trained in such practice; provided that nothing in this section shall be construed to authorise any person to practise any native, Indian or other Asiatic system of therapeutics except amongst the community to which he belongs, or the performance of an act on the part of any persons practising any such system which is dangerous to life.[143]

This proviso defined the official status of indigenous African medicine until the end of the twentieth century. There was to be no synthesis of indigenous and modern medicine, such as had been contemplated at times in India and in West and South Africa,[144] for the colonial doctors who reached East Africa in the late 1880s no longer thought any other medical system worth serious attention. Yet indigenous practitioners were not to be banned or persecuted, as was suggested at the time[145] and as happened in some other parts of Africa.[146] Rather, they were to be confined to their own communities and prohibited from borrowing modern medicine's powerful new drugs and techniques. Indigenous practitioners became a residual category, 'best ignored', as the Governor of German East Africa put it in 1910,[147] and expected to die out as modern doctors multiplied. Early colonial governments were interested in indigenous medicine – in 1895 the chief medical officer in German East Africa instructed his doctors to report on the subject and collect samples 'in the interests of science'[148] – but the interest was only in whether its drugs were worth appropriating.

The main field in which Africans could enter government medical service was hospital work, chiefly of a menial kind. The Germans opened military hospitals in Bagamoyo and Pangani in 1889. Three years later an Indian merchant, Sewa Haji, donated Rs.12,400 for a hospital and school in Dar es Salaam for Africans, Indians, and Arabs. Located on the foreshore close to the docks, the hospital opened in 1893 and served the capital for nearly seventy years, giving the territory's doctors, black and white, their basic training in care for the poor. In 1905 its staff included five or six illiterate African attendants earning an average of Rs.14 (nearly £1) a month, from two to four menial servants to fetch and carry, and two women cooks. The doctor in charge pointed to the need for educated African nurses.[149] By 1914 German East Africa had some twelve general hospitals in the main towns, plus smaller institutions and two fine European hospitals at Dar es Salaam and Tanga where European nurses gave some instruction to African attendants, whom British doctors found after the war to be often admirably trained but illiterate.[150]

Hospital development in the British territories was similar but cruder. In 1907 the African medical staff in Kenya and Uganda were described as '200 native attendants as dressers, ward servants, sweepers, &c', working at three European hospitals and some fifty African hospitals and dispensaries.[151] Some were appalling, notably the Native Civil Hospital in Nairobi, established for the workers who built the Uganda Railway, condemned in 1904, but not replaced until 1922 owing to dispute over where to locate the town's African quarter. In 1913 the governor called this hospital 'the filthiest sight he had seen since he came'.[152] Apart from old and unsuitable buildings, disgusting bedding, no hot water, its use as the municipal morgue, and a staff who worked only during office hours, 'The Nursing of the hospital is performed by likely boys engaged off the street in the same way one engages a house boy and teaches him his duties.'[153] Uganda, too, recruited its hospital staff chiefly as menials and gave some of them elementary on-the-job instruction, but by 1910 its standards were slightly better:

> Some of the senior ones have attained to a fair proficiency as dressers and clinical assistants, and the few who have some knowledge of reading and writing are able to help to some extent in keeping books and records and occasionally to give some slight assistance in compounding. Very few understand any English. The general standard of education is, however, improving and with it the class of native attendant improves also.
>
> The great majority of senior attendants are attached to the station in which they are employed by local ties and they are therefore practically not transferable, while the great majority of the juniors embrace the calling, or indeed any calling, only for a short time. So long as these conditions persist no scheme for the central training of native attendants is likely to be of any use. Each learns his work at the hospital or dispensary to which he is attached.[154]

As will be seen later, this situation changed on the eve of the war. Until then, however, the most skilled attendants in British service worked in Zanzibar, where Sewa Haji had financed another hospital whose staff included African women nurses in the female ward and skilled male staff drawn from the Bombay African community and other mission followings, notably Simeon Livingstone, a freed slave who had studied alongside James Ainsworth at Mombasa. By 1913 he was the compounder at Zanzibar Native Hospital. Fifteen years later a list accorded him the courtesy title of Doctor. Moreover, because Zanzibar was densely populated, small, and relatively wealthy, it established from 1909 East Africa's first system of government rural dispensaries, initially staffed by Indian or Goan compounders.[155]

Somewhat larger opportunities lay outside the hospitals. The dominant institutions of the new bacteriological medicine were laboratories. Without a microscope, so a German physician observed, a tropical doctor was 'a blindfolded man hunting for pins'.[156] The Germans opened their government laboratory in 1897–8, when Koch himself worked there. One of his assistants, Hassani Selemani, remained in its employment until 1941, but neither he nor its other African staff seems to have had any technical functions.[157] Those arose elsewhere. The first evidence of East Africans trained to use a microscope came from Tanga, where an attempt in 1905 to eradicate malaria by mass administration of quinine required microscopic examination of numerous blood samples, for which Dr Otto Panse trained Africans from the town's excellent government school.[158] The campaign failed, but in 1909 it provided a model for an attack on the helminthic diseases which disabled labourers in the plantation area inland of Tanga:

> For assistance I was given three pupils of the Government School in Tanga who had been trained for several months in the Government Hospital at Tanga to recognise the eggs of Ankylostomiasis . . .
>
> I used the native assistants only to examine the faeces preparations under my supervision. I had the slides recognised as Ankylostomiasis eggs submitted to me for confirmation and I re-examined the preparations designated as negative. The diagnoses submitted were mostly correct, but they frequently overlooked eggs. The assistants' lack of enthusiasm for their task and seriousness in their work clearly argued against using them independently. Yet in time the assistants became a considerable help to the doctor in the microscopic examinations, if they worked under continuous supervision.[159]

Another doctor was more impressed by the microscopists, who 'were diligent and worked conscientiously and reliably under supervision'.[160]

This campaign in the Tanga hinterland was part of a new engagement with problems of African rural health. Hitherto German medical work outside hospitals had been limited to hasty annual tours, chiefly to vaccinate against smallpox. In 1909, however, German doctors began to produce their own lymph for vaccination. They claimed, perhaps with exaggeration, that during the next five years nearly four million people were vaccinated, or over half the colony's population, a proportion matched only in Zanzibar.[161] In both cases success owed much to training Africans as vaccinators. The same principle was applied in the campaign against sleeping sickness, which offered Africans a wider range of paramedical roles. Whether this disease had existed in East Africa before colonial rule is uncertain, but an epidemic began in the mid-1890s in Busoga, to the east of Buganda, killed an estimated 200,000 or more people on the northern shore of Lake Victoria, expanded into areas of Kenya and German East Africa bordering the lake, infected also the shores of Lake Tanganyika, and subsequently appeared in small outbreaks in savanna areas.[162] The Uganda Government relied upon the chiefs' authority to evacuate the lakeshore population and segregate sufferers into camps. The Germans also created camps in Bukoba District to the west of the lake, but found that chiefs elsewhere lacked the necessary authority.[163] Africans were employed to catch the tsetse-fly vectors for research, to care for victims in the terrible segregation camps, to ensure that people did not return to evacuated areas – an operation which lasted well into the 1920s – and especially as 'gland-feelers', a task for which, as for all their sleeping-sickness work, the Germans employed mission-educated men from Bukoba District:

> The Medical Officer sent young men all over the villages to go and press the necks of the people to see those who had signs of Botongo disease. If they found any, they would send the person to [the segregation camp at] Kigarama for treatment.
>
> They captured a lot of people, but when some saw how the Doctor pierced their shoulders injecting them, they feared and migrated to other areas.[164]

Of all the medical campaigns on the eve of the First World War, the one with the most lasting impact on medical training was the attack on venereal disease in Uganda. Albert Cook had detected 'rampant' syphilis as soon as he arrived there,[165] but it was only a decade later that fear of depopulation led the government to seek an inquiry. Syphilis was news at this time. The Wassermann test (which detected venereal syphilis but could not distinguish it from yaws, endemic syphilis, or consequences of some other diseases) was discovered in 1906. New methods of injecting mercury were also devised, and in 1907 experimental chemotherapy had its first dramatic success with Salvarsan as a remedy for syphilis.[166] Colonel Lambkin, who conducted the Ugandan enquiry, was misled by Cook's statistics, unreliable tests, and his own exaggerations into reporting that over half of all Ugandans were infected with syphilis and stood 'a good chance of being exterminated in a very few years'.[167] He recommended that the chiefs should compel their syphilitic subjects to undergo mercury injections by Indian assistants. However, Captain G.F. Keane, who chiefly implemented the recommendations, had exceptional sympathy for Africans, was impressed by Mengo Hospital's African staff, and decided to train his own African assistants from the pupils with elementary English now emerging from mission schools:

> In 1912 a nucleus of five well-educated English speaking boys was asked for from the high-schools at Kampala and were eventually obtained with the greatest difficulty. The difficulties were two-fold. There existed a very strong prejudice amongst the Chiefs and educated classes against allowing their sons to embark on a medical career. The idea of such an occupation was entirely new to them and the handling of sick was regarded as degrading. The Chiefs had a horror of sick people and shrank from them. It is the custom of the Baganda to eat with their hands from a common dish, and they are most scrupulous about washing their hands before joining at meals. Any person who had touched a sick person was expected to eat alone.

> The Mission Schools again, keenly alive to the native objections, were in no way anxious to send their best pupils into a hitherto untried avenue of occupation whilst the Administration and commercial pursuits seemed to offer so much better and more immediate prospects. At this time every educated boy was eagerly snapped up either by Government offices or by the commercial houses in Kampala, and the demand for English speaking boys as clerks, interpreters, and Chief's assistants was far in excess of the supply.
>
> However the five boys were at length obtained and proved most satisfactory.[168]

In 1913 these young men moved with Keane to a temporary hospital on Mulago Hill, near Kampala, which was to become the medical centre for the entire East African region. They learned laboratory techniques, to recognise and classify venereal diseases, to record the observations on cards, and to perform intramuscular injections of mercury. 'They were deft, intelligent, patient', it was recalled.[169] Keane was eager to expand this class into a broader medical training scheme and won the chiefs' support. But Government lacked money[170] and Keane lacked the time to run a training school himself. It was this that led him in 1913 to encourage the Cooks to develop their medical training at Mengo. The two streams of modern medicine, mission and government, were at last joining to launch systematic medical training.

3 The age of the tribal dresser

The First World War enlarged the modern medical training and employment available to East Africans. During the 1920s government medical services first penetrated the countryside, recruiting numerous 'tribal dressers' to staff dispensaries. Some came from locally privileged families, extending the social spectrum from which medical workers were drawn. Higher levels of training also expanded, drawing together the practical skills and formal education whose combination was essential to the emergence of a medical profession. Between the wars, moreover, the thinking of African medical workers can to some extent be discerned, chiefly from their contributions to the vernacular press. They showed a special concern with the relationship between modern and indigenous medicine, most seeing it as necessarily antagonistic, but some as complex and a few as potentially cooperative.

War

The First World War made a positive contribution to the emergence of an East African medical profession because war caused such appalling suffering. While the allied British, Belgians, Portuguese, and South Africans sought a quick conquest of German East Africa, a small, mobile German force tried to commit as many enemy troops as possible by a fighting withdrawal from north to south which left it still undefeated when the war ended. Fought in a hostile physical environment, with little but human transport, at a time when military communications and tropical medicine were embryonic, the campaign caused fearful losses, more from disease than from combat. The Allies employed between 210,000 and 240,000 troops, losing at least 4,100 in action and 7,800 dead of disease. The Germans began with 15,017 men and lost 2,532 dead. However, these figures were dwarfed by the African civilians, perhaps up to a million, pressed into porterage and other labour. Of these, the British admitted losing 44,911 dead of disease, but the real losses may have been up to five or six times that number.[1] Malaria, dysentery, undernutrition, exhaustion, and sheer neglect were the chief killers. 'The Chief chose women and men to carry the loads', an old woman recalled. 'This work was dusty and heavy and tooth-grinding on account of those soldiers. Blows, slaps, and kicks were the food we ate, morning and evening, but no-one spoke if he was ill or tired. It was all the same: work was work until nightfall. We paused only to sleep.'[2]

Moreover, the war was a medical disaster even for those Africans who escaped the recruiters, because mobility bred epidemics. Cerebro-spinal meningitis penetrated the region, with especially devastating effects among the porters and in northern Uganda. Tuberculosis, bilharzia, malaria, and venereal diseases spread. The worst crises came in 1918, when a severe famine coincided first with widespread smallpox and then with an influenza pandemic which may have killed between two and five per cent of the entire population.[3] Medical services were neglected. Over half of Uganda's medical officers joined the forces, for example, and the anti-venereal campaign was abandoned for the duration.[4]

Not only did lack of European staff augment the responsibilities of some African subordinates,[5] but war created other medical opportunities. The small German force had highly trained medical orderlies (*Sanitätsaskari*) under severe discipline who sadly remain anonymous.[6] The Allied troops employed regular medical staff at their huge base hospitals or recruited untrained attendants from the Carrier Corps who were treated as menials and paid less than cooks or domestic servants.[7] But they also created three elite units. Keane abandoned his venereal work at Mulago and formed his African assistants into the nucleus of a Uganda Native Medical Corps, who after much negotiation gained the status of 'troops' rather than the menial role of 'followers' and served with the Ugandan forces which reached Tabora in 1916. Most were then paid off and partly replaced by German-trained dressers.[8] But the campaign was still expanding and the former UNMC men began to lose their identity in the larger forces:

> The native from Uganda was dismayed at his new circumstances. The uniform in which he had taken pride was denied him; any attempt to display technical knowledge, such as the reading of the thermometer or keeping of temperature charts, or any medical skill, was unexpected and often looked upon as a species of impertinence. On more than one occasion an officer, after asking who they were and to what tribe they belonged and what they were capable of, sent them to work with porters at grass and wood-cutting as a disciplinary measure.[9]

Pressed by Keane, the authorities agreed in April 1917 to absorb the UNMC into a second elite force, the African Native Medical Corps, which eventually contained 10 British and 1,500 African personnel, some 60 per cent of them Ganda. A few had medical training at Mengo, but most came from the mission schools, where young heirs to a military tradition volunteered en masse, making a remarkable sacrifice of educational prospects.[10]

They left Kampala to the beat of the royal drums, 'because the job we were going for was to honour Buganda'.[11]

The ANMC reached Dar es Salaam by sea in July 1917. They provided trained staff for its huge carrier hospital, the Sewa Haji hospital, many other centres on the coast and inland transport routes, and occasionally frontline units. Standing orders defined their elite status:

> Enlistments into this Corps have been voluntary and for the performance of skilled medical work, not for that of Stretcher Bearers, or sweepers, waterboys and other menials for whom application will be made to the proper quarter.
>
> ANMC are attested soldiers and are on the same footing as other African Troops . . . *Corporal punishment cannot be awarded to NCOs*, and generally is only to be awarded for offences of a disgraceful nature and for offences for which repeated previous convictions *have been recorded*. The men have been specially selected in recruitment and Os.C. are asked to view the punishment of flogging as a most serious matter.[12]

Only one member of the Corps died in action, although several were decorated for gallantry. Some 111 died of disease, to which their work continuously exposed them. At one point one-third of the Corps were themselves in hospital.[13] Senior NCOs often bore heavy responsibility. At Lindi in June 1918, for example, Staff-Sergeant Samusoni Bazongere, formerly a master at King's School, Budo, had charge under European doctors of a hospital with 45 ANMC servicemen, numerous sweepers and attendants, and nearly 2,000 patients.[14] 'We are very glad to know', a member of the Corps wrote, 'that ever since we started this job, the mortality rate in hospitals has declined. So you should also acknowledge us because if we perform well, Buganda also is known.' They sang:

> We left with joy,
> But more so:
> Among the countries we saw
> Buganda was the best.[15]

The third elite force, the Kikuyu Mission Volunteers, was not a medical corps but a body of carriers, formed in April 1917 by Protestant missionaries in order to protect their converts against conscription into the regular Carrier Corps. They were commanded by Arthur and chiefly carried supplies and wounded men up and down the precipitous Uzungwa escarpment south-east of Iringa. It was a dreadful task, somewhat ameliorated by relatively humane treatment, a high morale which led men returning from carrying duties to congregate in self-education groups, and the special medical care provided by the Scottish missionaries and their assistants at a field hospital headed by Samson Njoroge.[16] 'There were about 20 dressers working under me', he recalled, 'and they did the nursing care work. They were supposed to observe the patients and report their observations to me. I also saw to it that the patients were bathed and that all their daily care was meticulously carried out.'[17] About 100 of the 1,800 Kikuyu Mission Volunteers died, a much lower proportion than the Carrier Corps average.

The ANMC was expected to provide postwar East Africa with the trained medical attendants hitherto lacking. That did not happen immediately. Most hastened home to rest, while the Kikuyu Mission Volunteers dispersed so quickly that their demobilisation parade had to be cancelled. Trained dressers would not accept prevailing pay levels in government hospitals.[18] They expected the fruits of victory and the Buganda government did allocate many freehold (*mailo*) land.[19] Eventually, however, a large number entered government or mission service. Yusufu Mukasa, already in medical employment and one of the first students at Mengo Medical School, joined the UNMC in 1916, spent fifteen years after the war as an assistant dispenser, and retired in 1935 to open Uganda's first modern, African-owned drugstore at Wandegeya, outside Kampala.[20] Erisa Mutyaba returned from the ANMC to Mengo Hospital and then volunteered for fifteen years of missionary medicine in Kigezi.[21] Rawson Watts, educated by the Universities Mission in Zanzibar, went to Dar es Salaam as a sergeant in the ANMC and became the first African to work in the British Secretariat, 'thanks to the character he secured from the head of the ANMC, Major Keane'.[22] He helped to pioneer Tanganyika's elite politics, as did Erica Fiah, a Ganda interpreter and medical assistant at the Carrier Corps Hospital in Dar es Salaam who later launched Tanganyika's first African-owned newspaper, *Kwetu*.[23] Nor was the ANMC the only source of skills for the new British regime in Tanganyika. Many of its early African medical staff had been trained at the Blantyre Mission Hospital and served with troops from Nyasaland. Others made the delicate transition from German service. Swedi Abdullah, who spent thirty-six years in the sleeping-sickness service and won the British Empire Medal, had been a British prisoner. The senior hospital attendant at Morogoro was in chains when the British arrived, for having attacked a German. 'I struck off his chains', the British doctor recalled, 'feeling that he very probably had good excuse for his offence'.[24]

Wartime medical service left a deep imprint on African minds. For some it was ambiguous, as for the *beni* and *bati* dancers whose satires of military drill included sick parades and nursing sisters.[25] For others it evoked pride, especially for the ANMC Old Comrades Association, which existed as a football club by May 1919 but claimed to have been formally 'written down' in 1924[26] and held reunions on Remembrance Day and other imperial occasions until at least 1943, when it is last mentioned, appropriately, holding a memorial service for Keane in Rubaga Cathedral.[27] Members called themselves *bakawonawo*, veterans. Whereas the Carrier Corps 'did not like to discuss what they had seen because so many of their friends had died',[28] *bakawonawo* liked nothing better. With their former European officers as guests of honour, they would share a meal, criticise the current secretary, perhaps discuss the origins of the war, and then settle to the serious business of recounting their wartime experiences, each speaker being limited to twenty minutes. Their accounts laid much stress on deaths and recoveries, on comradeship and mutual aid and its divine rewards. 'In between the children of Mengo Central [School] sang a song of the fighters and it was right to be there in person and hear for yourself.'[29]

For Europeans the impact was equally emotional. 'We can never forget these days together', Arthur wrote,

> and what they meant for us and for the boys we love: iron bands of love were being forged which no hammer of worldly force will ever break. We have received a vision of a new Kingdom and a new earth and have by faith entered it. If we ever go back on what God has revealed to us or allow other men to sway us on the backward track, may we be anathema.[30]

Without this comradeship, the subsequent medical history of East Africa, and especially of medical education there, would be incomprehensible. All the Europeans most deeply engaged in training East African medical staff during the 1920s had learned to do so in the ANMC. Keane, 'who went to war with many Ugandans and made them acquire ranks',[31] became the chief architect of medical training in Uganda. D.G. Tomblings, his Adjutant, became the long-serving Principal of Makerere College, where he 'would be on the same level with his students', as one said, 'at a time when Government officials behaved like small "gods" in the company of Africans'.[32] H.B. Owen, in charge of ANMC training, became Makerere's first medical tutor. R.Y. Stones, his wartime assistant, took charge of Mengo Medical School. In addition, several of the most progressive inter-war colonial doctors, notably W.H. Kauntze in Uganda and A.R. Paterson in Kenya, came to East Africa during or immediately after the war, often from West Africa.[33] Most shared a sense of guilt. Keane responded to it by renewing in 1919 his plan to create a medical school. Others, shocked by the ill-health revealed by mass examination of potential carriers, sought to extend medical institutions into the countryside. It was, wrote Kenya's DMS, 'a realisation . . . of the debt that was due . . . for services rendered during the war'.[34]

Expansion into the countryside

The vernacular press reveals the growth of modern medical practice by Africans between the wars. Before the 1920s it said little about medicine.

From about 1924–5, however, the government-controlled Swahili press in Kenya and Tanganyika contained numerous articles by Africans, mainly from up-country districts, describing the opening of hospitals and dispensaries or their own experiences as paramedics. During the 1930s and 1940s these articles came from increasingly remote areas and – especially in the only privately owned Swahili newspaper, *Kwetu* – sometimes expressed greater scepticism about modern medicine. By the 1950s the genre had largely disappeared. Throughout the period, moreover, there were markedly fewer articles about disease and medicine in Luganda newspapers, whether controlled by Africans or Europeans. The implications are that modern medicine was an exciting novelty in rural Kenya and Tanganyika from the mid-1920s, although less so as time passed, but was more familiar and less noteworthy in Buganda.

Rural Africans had first had access to state-run dispensaries in Zanzibar, from 1909. They atrophied during the war, but by 1926 there were twelve in Zanzibar and nine in Pemba, supervised by a European medical officer who trained the staff at a central dispensary in Zanzibar town. Known as 'little doctors' and not necessarily Africans, the dispensers 'must be able to read, write, and speak English [and] are taught the elements of anatomy and physiology and given a general outline of common diseases and their treatment'.[35] They were to be available day or night, to inspect sanitary conditions in surrounding villages, and to give intramuscular but not intravenous injections. Standing orders decreed:

> A notice stating that all treatment (including medicines, Dressings, etc.) is free to all races will be posted in the verandah of each Dispensary. Any Dispenser demanding or accepting any payment or presents for treatment supplied, will be immediately dismissed for [sic] the service.[36]

Despite many criticisms, medical officers remained convinced throughout the colonial period that these dispensers were the core of Zanzibar's medical provision.[37]

Kenya, by contrast, had left rural medicine to missionaries and continued to look to them when war revealed the scale of disease in the African reserves. Government subsidies then enabled the Scottish mission at Tumutumu to expand its medical attendances from 3,959 in 1918 to 75,000 in 1920, while unspent funds donated by Africans for the comfort of troops were allocated to missions to build medical training schools at Maseno and Kikuyu, the latter aiming at 'an education evolving eventually into a University course'. During 1919–20, however, government decided to provide its own rural medical facilities, apparently in order to justify and palliate large increases in African taxation.[38] The medical college at Maseno remained uncompleted, that at Kikuyu became the Alliance High

School, but the Medical Department gained an orientation towards rural Africans which was surprising in colonial Kenya and was accentuated by the European settlers' reliance on private practitioners. By 1932 government controlled seventeen permanent and ten temporary hospitals and seventy-seven permanent and thirty temporary dispensaries in African reserves, the dispensaries having generally been financed by Local Native Councils.[39] Dressers for the dispensaries were trained at district hospitals 'to dress ulcers and local injuries, to diagnose to the best of his ability the complaints of the people, to treat those which he can treat with the means at his disposal, and to transfer the seriously ill to hospital or to persuade them to come again on the day of the doctor's visit'.[40] Dressers also gave intramuscular injections to patients suffering from the widespread, contagious, but seldom fatal disease of yaws which could reduce victims to 'pictures of sheer horror . . . confluent sores literally from head to foot, sometimes a gaping hole where the face had been, or a leg hanging by the skin only'.[41] A cheap, apparently effective, and easily injected remedy for yaws, bismuth sodium tartrate, had been discovered during 1921–2 by Tanganyika's Chief Medical Officer, J.O. Shircore, and had been adopted quickly in Kenya, where it gave the government and its African dressers the opportunity to popularise their free rural service. During 1930 they treated a peak of 103,711 cases.[42] In reality one or two bismuth injections only suppressed yaws while removing the cross-immunity it had given against venereal syphilis, but immense suffering was relieved:

> We are grateful to Government for sending doctors for us to every small hamlet which is any distance from Mombasa. Any man who is ill with yaws or any other bodily sickness, or sore, can go to the doctor to get medicine or to be injected without the trouble of going all the way to Mombasa. Already in this part of Digo, yaws and sores have greatly decreased.[43]

In Tanganyika the relationship between the yaws campaign and the rural medical system was more complicated. Shircore was eager to train rural dispensers to administer injections.[44] The rural response was generally enthusiastic:

> Sumbwa, Ha, and Suwi [Zinza] greatly like injection medicine. Every injection day very many people attend, because they have seen that the medicine is much better than herbal medicine for diseases of yaws, syphilis, gonorrhoea, sores [*mti*], and others. Countless numbers have been cured.[45]

By 1930, when a peak of 137,112 yaws cases presented, roughly one Tanganyikan in every seven had been treated.[46] But the government had not amalgamated yaws treatment with another and chiefly political priority: a network of dispensaries and tribal dressers controlled by the native administrations established throughout the country under the policy of indirect rule introduced by Governor Cameron in 1925. Somewhat like the 'barefoot doctors' of the 1980s, tribal dressers were young local men chosen by native authorities, trained for three months at a hospital, and then sent home with a box of equipment, a box of drugs, an instruction pamphlet, and orders to improve public health, provide first aid, and treat routine complaints like hookworm. The target was to train 1,000 dressers, but in 1930 there were 288 dispensaries, treating 352,423 cases during the year.[47] Political rather than medical officers controlled this network. Supervision was difficult and the medical authorities banned most dressers from performing injections, although many appear initially to have done so.[48] The result was a worse rural medical system than Kenya's,[49] but remarkably widespread and popular, chiefly because it met the demand for *local* institutions, for, in a proverb much quoted in the vernacular press, 'A distant shroud does not bury the corpse.' 'In this country, subject to Morogoro District Office, there were only two hospitals, Morogoro and Kisaki', a correspondent explained, 'but last year the chief's people were taught medical work until they knew it. Now they have been returned to their towns to heal, and each has got medicine to use in his locality [*kipande*].'[50] Letters also suggest that the system met its political goal. As one put it simply, 'Europeans do not come to harm black people but to help them.'[51]

No such excitement marked the Luganda newspapers of the 1920s. This was not for lack of rural dispensaries. Uganda's rulers also planned a countrywide network during 1919. By 1932 there were eighty-five and their attendances – said to be about two million a year – far exceeded those in neighbouring territories.[52] But in Buganda, where the newspapers were written, both the missions and the anti-venereal campaign had made dispensaries familiar before 1914. Moreover, yaws was rare in Buganda, if common elsewhere, and the Medical Department did not adopt bismuth treatment until the 1930s, possibly because it was accustomed to using Salvarsan against syphilis. In 1930 Uganda treated only 38,066 yaws cases. Its yaws campaign did not peak until 1939.[53]

Training

For Africans the expansion of rural medical services created many opportunities for training and employment. Hitherto most African medical staff had been confined to menial work and had learned on the job any skills they possessed. 'Bwana Pumps' (from the bicycle pump which was his only equipment) had learned his medicine as office boy and sweeper before he ran a dispensary in the South Nyanza region of Kenya throughout the influenza epidemic of 1918, dispensing chiefly quinine and Epsom Salts. Tanganyika's tribal dressers, with a three-month course under a busy

District Medical Officer, were not much improvement; by the 1930s it was 'not uncommon to find a Tribal Dressing Station in charge of a "promoted sweeper"'.[54] But both Tanganyika's Medical Department and other territories aimed higher.

At first they naturally turned to the missions. These continued to train medical workers throughout the interwar years. In Tanganyika, for example, three missions – Lutherans at Bumbuli, Anglicans at Minaki, and Roman Catholics at Ndanda – trained hospital assistants and dispensers to the same level as the best government institution.[55] But the numbers were small, for all interwar missions suffered acute financial stringency and concentrated on producing staff for their own needs, especially those who could cover the cost of their training by their work in the hospital, which increasingly meant female nurses. The fate of the Mengo Medical School illustrates this vividly. After years of discussion it opened in February 1917 with seventeen students, eight of them existing hospital staff and others from mission schools attended largely by the sons of chiefs and other notables. Only four of these completed the course, which was repeatedly interrupted in the early years by lack of staff. By 1929 some twenty-six had graduated,[56] each receiving a certificate stating that he

> has been trained as a Clinical Assistant in Mengo Hospital for the space of three years, and has passed an examination qualifying him to take temperatures, and chart them, record pulses, give enemata, pass catheters and bougies, prepare patients for operations, read and make up simple prescriptions, give medicines at stated times in measured doses, dress wounds, wash patients, and generally to carry out intelligently medical orders.[57]

'They learn to diagnose diseases and identify causes by using a microscope which has the capacity to magnify small things', wrote Yoswa Mukasa Naluma, one of the first students. 'They learn English to enable them to read medical books.'[58] The course also included injections, circumcisions, extracting teeth, and using a stethoscope (issued to each of the first students). The training was 'severely practical', with only two hours of lectures each day but a strong emphasis on nursing skills.[59] According to Stones, the normally perceptive doctor in charge, 'African students are great believers in theory, and would like to be in the classroom all day long hearing lectures; they care little for the practical part of the work.' But the first students asked to participate in ward work rather than take their vacation, suggesting that they really wanted both kinds of training.[60] 'Our students certainly are keen', Stones reported:

> It is not usual for an African to be willing to pay for learning but some of these students have left well-paid work to take up this study, receiving but small wages and having themselves to find the money for their uniforms. When recently asked if they

wished for a course extending to three years or for one year only, they unanimously decided for the former.

They were said to have taken turns through the night to read the only available book on biology.[61] Although obstetrics, gynaecology, and treatment of female patients were explicitly excluded by resolution of the female missionaries,[62] the syllabus did include 'General instruction in disciplinary matters':

Relations and behaviour with Europeans. Obedience. Punctuality. Willingness. Replying by question. Ready acceptance of reproof. Sulking. Responsibility for Patients in charge and any accidents that may occur to them also for all articles in charge. Stealing food and comforts provided for the sick. Striking and ill-treating the sick. Malpraxis. Liability of medical attendant to the charge of Manslaughter owing to neglecting to follow instructions. Varying medical treatment prescribed by Medical Officers. Bribes. Selling medicines etc. Extorting money from sick or quarantined persons.[63]

The students fought a long struggle against paternalism, winning a reversal of the ban on wearing boots in the wards – one of their earliest demands – securing the right to wear khaki clothes rather than white kanzus, and petitioning Albert Cook in 1929 to protest against their hours of work, their pocket-money, and their treatment by a new superintendent who 'does not recognise us as human beings'.[64]

The Mengo Medical School trained forty-nine students[65] to a somewhat lower level than that later attained by medical assistants, the best-trained medical sub-professionals in East Africa. For the first eight years all appear to have been Ganda, but from 1928 onwards, when the level of training seems to have fallen somewhat, sixteen of the last twenty admitted were from other parts of Uganda and caused more trouble to the school authorities. These data come from the register of students, which also shows that of fifty-four admitted between 1916 and 1932, at least twenty-five were still engaged in medical work in 1939, fourteen with goverment, nine with the mission, and two in 'private practice'. Yoswa Mukasa Naluma became medical tutor at Mulago Medical School. Other early students included Erisa Mutyaba, the pioneer dispenser-evangelist in Kigezi. Among later alumni were the saintly Onesimo Busimo, who for many years taught the children at the Ngora leprosarium, and Erica Lutwama, who had charge of its hospital.[66] After 1922, however, the government withdrew its subsidy in order to start its own medical school. Mengo struggled for another ten years until the government refused to employ any more of its graduates. Cook concluded that its chief importance had been to prepare the way for the first government training scheme on the East African mainland at Mulago.[67]

Keane had trained African assistants for the venereal disease campaign at Mulago before the war. After postwar delay, Mulago was converted into a general African hospital, Keane was made responsible for all African medical services, and two training schemes began in 1923. One, designed to produce African medical assistants equivalent to the Indian Sub-Assistant Surgeons who headed small rural hospitals, will be examined in the next chapter. The other, at a lower level, sought to train medical attendants for subordinate hospital posts and rural dispensaries.[68] It initially handled large numbers of attendants – ninety-three during 1924 alone – but was of poor quality until the early 1930s, when improved schooling enabled teaching to switch to English and the course became more popular.[69] Meanwhile, in 1925 Keane divided the male African staff into three grades of medical attendants, earning between 20 and 79 shillings a month, and two grades of medical assistants, earning from 80 shillings upwards. A year later 'there are over 500 native employees in the medical department, all of whom can read and write and many of whom are English-speaking. This occupation is now one of the most popular and sought-after forms of native employment.'[70] Probably at least 80 per cent were Ganda.

The Tanganyika Government began to train African medical staff from a different angle because, as a new colonial invader, it was chiefly concerned with the health of towns where white people lived. From 1919 it concentrated on training urban sanitary inspectors, employing in 1926 some 207, which gave its Medical Department a greater preventive emphasis than at any time before the immunisation campaigns of the 1980s.[71] This emphasis, and that on tribal dressers, retarded the training of medical assistants for hospital and dispensary work. A course for this purpose began at the Sewa Haji Hospital in 1924, taking about a dozen students a year, but plans to enlarge it into a proper medical school were aborted in 1931 by the depression, so that although it continued into the 1940s to provide the best training available in Tanganyika, the scale was small and teaching hampered by the archaic state of the hospital.[72]

This did little to help the tribal dressers. By the 1930s they were targets for criticism by both doctors who thought they tried to do too much and political officers who thought they were capable of doing too little.[73] The main attempt to produce a better-qualified rural practitioner began in 1935 at a training centre attached to the Mwanza Native Hospital and financed by the local native administration. The course, mainly in Swahili, lasted eighteen or twenty-four months and ranged from practical work and elementary anatomy to the use of the microscope, with which graduates were issued.[74] Initial reports on their work were good, but by the early 1940s the officer in charge believed that 'probably at least 90% of them are useless from the medical point of view, having quite naturally degenerated from the effect of their surroundings into dishonest and incapable practitioners'.[75] The remark became ammunition in a campaign which the DMS, P.A.T. Sneath, launched against the entire system of tribal dressers soon after his arrival in 1944, a 'battle with my government'[76] which illustrates how much a DMS was a spokesman for the medical profession rather than an agent of the political administration. Sneath saw tribal dressers as an offence against medical probity, 'a medicine racket', 'an appeasing sop to primitive opinion (European and other) . . . a substitute to the witch-doctor, with a garnishing of "western" respectability . . . as an element of barter for good-will to a populace who have been raised in the tradition that our profession deals in magic, surgical miracles, psychoneuroses and the relief of pain', leading 'to the degradation and permanent discredit of European medicine'.[77] By contrast, the provincial administration, which controlled the dispensaries, insisted on their popularity, their usefulness in training Africans to manage their affairs, and their value as centres of enlightenment in an otherwise neglected countryside, blaming the lack of supervision on the idleness of medical officers.[78] The dispute was fought with exceptional venom until the Secretary of State's Medical Adviser ruled in favour of the provincial administration on the grounds that 'as so often in medical work in Africa, the better is the enemy of the good'. Sneath was curtly told to retire.[79]

The last East African government to undertake medical education was Kenya. Small numbers of dispensers and laboratory assistants were trained during the 1920s,[80] but otherwise the situation there was recalled by Hugh Trowell, who was posted to the Nairobi African Hospital in 1930: 'It had two water taps, several barely literate male nursing orderlies, but no female nurses. Four British nursing sisters were doing their best; they knew "Kitchen Swahili" and "trained" the African staff just as British housewives "trained" their cooks on the "do it like me" principle.'[81] Plans for more systematic training on quasi-military lines had been drawn up during the 1920s but were long delayed by dispute over where to locate Nairobi's projected new hospitals.[82] A Medical Training Depot linked to the African Hospital there was finally opened in 1929, taking well-educated students, mainly from the Alliance High School, for a three-year course which had a strong nursing emphasis rather than the aim of preparing African counterparts of Indian Sub-Assistant Surgeons, a goal which had been contemplated in 1926 but abandoned in response to European (and possibly Indian[83]) opposition.[84] When Trowell became principal of the Training Depot in the early 1930s,

> the trouble was that none of the doctors at the main native hospital, and particularly none of the nursing sisters wanted these mission boys. They were quite keen on the old illiterate type of African . . . They all feared that semi-educated schoolboys,

coming largely from the more numerous mission schools, would be too big for their boots. Indeed they would probably wear sandals and not walk barefoot . . . It was feared, and not without reason, that the new semi-baked Hospital Assistants would pose as embryo doctors.[85]

Although Trowell broke down some of this hostility, he could not shake the decision to produce nursing orderlies rather than sub-assistant surgeons. The medical authorities had decided that any African seeking that career would have to do so at Makerere College in Uganda. When the first did, in 1936, Trowell followed him there.[86]

The world of the tribal dresser

The dressers, hospital attendants, and other paramedics of the interwar period came from a wider social spectrum than nineteenth-century pioneers. Many were still former patients, especially at remote mission hospitals. Tumutumu had to turn away many aspiring apprentices because they had physical disabilities. The idea that medical work was for educational failures remained strong, but entrance standards at the better training centres were rising quickly. The first entrant to Mengo Medical School, Ezekieri Walusimbi, had graduated in third place from the elite King's School, Budo.[87] Moreover, medicine had always attracted individualists. Of the two main African assistants at Ndolage Lutheran Hospital in north-western Tanganyika during the 1930s, one was a former patient who had started as gardener but the other, who called himself Mfisi (Hyena), claimed to be a dispossessed Rwandan chief and friend of King Musinga. After the normal hospital apprenticeship of menial tasks – performed inconspicuously before dawn with the comment, 'If you force the lion to eat grass he will do so eventually if he has no alternative' – his literate skills and strong personality eventually made him supervisor of the entire institution.[88] Tanganyika's tribal dresser system brought into medical work members of chiefly families favoured in selection for training. Moreover, many regions now had a local educated elite whose numerous progeny sought medical work. The leading teacher at Kongwa in central Tanganyika, Eliezer Kiduo, trained one son as a teacher, another as a court clerk, and two as tribal dressers. And medicine was becoming hereditary. Samson Njoroge's son Simeon was educated at Alliance High School and the Medical Training Depot in Nairobi before working in the Central Dispensary there and marrying a student nurse.[89]

Medical training remained a severe discipline. The initial period of menial work was a deliberate test, for the European authorities were determined to break what they saw as young Africans' pride and callousness, although in reality it was their notion of honour. A battle of the bedpans was fought in hospital wards for half a century until the authorities won a temporary victory during the 1950s. Many mission hospitals had insisted from the first that sanitary duties belonged to an attendant's normal work, but government institutions had employed sweepers. Attempts to generalise the mission practice led in the late 1940s and early 1950s to a series of strikes and mass dismissals in Uganda and Kenya.[90] The next hurdle for the trainee was to dress the 'great, loathsome, dirty ulcers' which were among the most common complaints taken to hospitals. 'They turn me all round inside so that I don't want to eat', one dresser complained, and many found that such work made others unwilling to eat with them. Medical assistants in training in south-western Tanganyika during the mid-1940s refused to undertake dressings, claiming that those too were the work of sweepers, and it was alleged that 'the sweeper at each dispensary did the dressings – the "doctor" could not be expected to soil his hands'. At a more advanced stage, the trainees also had to condition themselves to attend operations – '*I* wasn't afraid, but my middle was once or twice!' one explained – and, if women, to the maternity ward. 'I was always nauseous', one remembered. 'Smelling blood all day long.'[91]

Trainees were helped through these experiences by the excitement of learning so much that was new and remarkable. This included the new European theory that many diseases were caused by invisible germs, translated into Swahili as *vijidudu*, 'tiny insects':

> Sarro was for years a dresser here. He learned to recognise pulmonary tuberculosis when severe. He often saw the germs under the microscope, and once saw the post mortem findings on a fatal case. One day his good friend John came to me in concern. John was the microscope boy, and on his own he had examined Sarro's sputum and found that he had T.B. . . . John told Sarro, showing him the slide. His progress was quite rapid when he was told. After it was evident to the family that Sarro was very ill, a diviner was consulted who convinced them that Dora, an aunt of Sarro's, had bewitched him, and that he was dying because of the spell she had cast upon him. He died a few weeks later firmly convinced that he had died of witchcraft.[92]

Microscopes were the chief wonders of the new medicine, as exciting to the medical trainee as to Adrien Atiman. The experts were the laboratory assistants, whose training was pioneered in Kenya by W.H. Kauntze, a doctor of strong humanitarian principles – he had nearly become a missionary – who had come to Kenya with West African troops during the First World War, taken charge of the Nairobi Carrier Hospital, and then in 1919 moved to the Medical Research Laboratory in Nairobi, which he directed for the next fourteen years. He launched a training scheme for African laboratory assistants in 1922. 'At the present time', he reported in 1930, 'the two best assistants we have are drawing respectively Sh.120 and

Sh.100 [a month]; as one is capable of carrying out Wassermann, Sigma and Kahn tests, equally as well as a European assistant, and the other can take complete charge of a small laboratory without supervision, it will be realized that some of these Africans are capable of quite advanced instruction'. These two men were probably Elisha Nyalondo and Gideon Otieno, the only Africans mentioned by name in the Medical Department's staff list at that time.[93] Three years later Kauntze moved to Uganda as DMS and revitalised laboratory training there by bringing in Charles Stokes, the man of mixed blood from the Kikuyu Mission whom Kauntze had trained in Nairobi and now used to instruct Ugandans.[94] Some became valued assistants in early medical research at Makerere and Mulago, although the best-known worker in this field was Fabian Mzoo, who spent over thirty years with Tanganyika's Malaria Research Unit and published several articles on the disease.[95] He had been trained in the Dar es Salaam Laboratory, which produced several other prominent men of the 1930s, notably Alexander Kanyamala, who ran a laboratory at Tanga Hospital which in 1938 examined 12,372 specimens, and Yohana Mnkande, a leading figure in the African Association.[96]

For local communities, the training and return of a tribal dresser was cause for rejoicing:

> Chome is a cold country, so that it has had to coax doctors, for they came from very hot countries. Three dressers have all begged for transfers, and they have been listened to. But on account of the local resentment, Chief K. Herieli Makange selected his child [*mdogo*] M. Francis Makange to study medicine. In August 1944 he completed his studies and returned. Now we are delighted because we have our own man. And we are pleased at how the chief put his child into the examination so that he might know how to help the people here in future.[97]

Fifteen years earlier a visitor had described a dresser at Shinyanga who 'was trained at his own wish and at his own expense, has returned to his tribe and, as there is not enough money, he works practically without pay'.[98] Other dressers, as Tanganyika's DMS put it, 'carried Western ideas of medicine and hygiene into the farthest corners of the territory' – men like the Gogo students from central Tanganyika who helped Stones to open medical work at Maseno in western Kenya or the Mombasa-trained dresser who in 1920 headed a dispensary on Kenya's border with Ethiopia.[99] In either situation the dresser saw himself, and might be seen by his neighbours, as a focus of enlightenment. The vernacular press shows that the dresser was often the first person consulted in emergency: 'At dawn on 6 January we saw a youth go hurriedly to the *dispensary* to request the *medical auxiliary* to go to his place as fast as possible. When he was asked the reason, he said that there were two bodies which had died in a very wonderful way . . .'[100] Isolated dressers might perform emergency operations of great difficulty:

> So he collected the necessary instruments and dressings, and set out over the hills in the darkness of the night . . . Kneeling down on the floor he committed the case to God, and then by the light of a Dietz storm lantern applied the forceps with the woman apparently unconscious. He delivered a dead baby but saved the woman.[101]

In 1936 a sanitary inspector and a dresser in south-eastern Tanganyika diagnosed cases of sleeping sickness and smallpox, thereby checking epidemics. A tribal dresser in the Tarime area east of Lake Victoria was shown in 1947 the dead body of a child bitten by a dog, persuaded the parents to let him remove the brain for examination, and prevented a possible rabies outbreak.[102] In famine or epidemic it was to the dispensary that people turned:

> At Koromije [in Sukumaland] we hit it [cerebro-spinal meningitis]; 200 people crowding round the dispensary howling for dawa – medicine – or 'MB'.[103] About 12 cases actually there, some of them dying, some delirious, some recovering. Huts were being built pretty quickly, but it was a tough job for a boy of 20 with two years training only to tackle. But Joseph was doing pretty well . . . Came to Bungulwa – the same thing again, many patients, no accomodation, and Lewis rattled getting frantic and scared stiff of getting the disease himself.[104]

In less dramatic ways, also, the dresser could be a source of enlightenment. 'It is most important', wrote Daudi Mfuko, who taught medicine at Minaki, 'that the dispenser should be able to explain to the people amongst whom he lives and works the difference between Christian medicine and witchcraft, and wherever possible to explain the reason for any particular treatment . . . They appreciate one of their own race and they have said to me, "A European is a European, and they cannot understand all our miseries, will you explain for me?"'[105] One official noted how the patients at the local hospital increased once an African medical assistant was stationed there. In 1928 a man from over 160 kilometres away arrived at Kabarole Hospital in western Uganda shouting, 'Isaka, Isaka', to locate the dresser whose reputation had brought him.[106] Dressers were acutely aware of their duty to embody rationality and enlightenment:

> Dresser! Remember that you are bringing things of profit or health to the sick, that you may do your work with skill and absolute honesty. For you can bring injury or death if you do your work with even slight negligence. Neither must you offend by reason of changing the medicines in the bottles, nor must you forget to attach to the bottle a label with the name of the medicine. Beyond this, when you are giving someone medicine you must first read the label on the bottle before using it. For you should measure accurately every quantity as instructed, even if it is as small as a milligramme.[107]

One public area in which the dresser might be asked to display enlightenment was at communal initiation rites. Some proclaimed themselves 'converts to science' by sending their sons to hospital for circumcision.[108] Others were called upon to sanitise traditional rites, as at Singida in north-central Tanganyika:

> Senior Chief M.B. Saidi Gwao and all his headmen and people agreed together with the Government that the children entering initiation [*jando*] should receive the help of the hospital here in their camp. Now with this help the children are healing well without any defect. Senior Chief M.B. Saidi Gwao issued an order and announced to all the people that anyone who wanted his children to enter the initiation must inform the Government Dresser so that he might be ready to help. May God Almighty help our chief to continue to rule rightly.
>
> Since this arrangement began, 175 children have healed during May 1943, 120 children during June 1943, all have healed well. During July too the work is continuing satisfactorily. All the elders have recognised the value of this help from the Government medicine. And they thank God for giving us the power and intelligence to succeed in this task.[109]

Such responsibilities clearly raised the dresser above the menial status of many earlier medical workers. Indeed, a reading of the interwar Swahili press might suggest that paramedics were outpacing schoolteachers and clergymen as protagonists of enlightenment. Certainly medical workers showed greater self-awareness than their predecessors, partly because their training was no longer merely an apprenticeship but increasingly also a schooling.

Yet their status was in fact ambiguous. They were upwardly mobile. 'The Medical Service attracts applicants for training', a Ugandan newspaper noted in 1944, 'while the teaching profession is doing so less and less', chiefly because teachers were so badly paid, although better than clergymen.[110] In towns and at district headquarters, paramedics were no longer menials but belonged to the circles of educated men who met to celebrate one another's career or family ceremonies. They took a full part in Uganda's Native Civil Servants Association and in the Tanganyika African Association. Ngariuya Dedan Gethegi, senior instructor in the Kenya Medical Department, was Chairman of the Alliance High School Old Boys' Association throughout the 1930s. Gibson Mkandawire, instructor at the Medical Training Centre in Mwanza, was the dominant figure in the town's African elite during the mid-1940s, presiding over the Government Servants Association, the Mwanza Cultural Club (which brought together Africans and Indians), and the Euro-African Discussion Group.[111] But the notion that medical work needed no brains died hard. In 1939 a correspondent in *Mambo Leo* lumped together, as occupations of similar educational status, 'work like that of the dresser, domestic servant, cook, soldier, and other work'.[112] And in the countryside the old status distinctions often survived. At Masasi, a nurse wrote in 1933, 'dispensary work is still looked on as inferior sort of work for which brains and education are not needed'. Clergy and teachers there treated the mission paramedics as youngsters to be kept in their place, one formidable old clergyman being remembered 'for putting the African dispensers through their paces like a veritable sergeant-major'.[113] Both chiefs and district officers in Tanganyika sent dressers on errands, treating them as part of their staff, as indeed they were. In Buganda, similarly, paramedics were only beginning to gain respectability and penetrate the enclosures of power. Ezekieri Walusimbi, the high-flyer from Budo who was one of Mengo Medical School's first students, eventually left medical work to become chief of the royal capital at Mengo and Treasurer of the Buganda kingdom, but he was an exceptional case.[114] Interaction between medical skill and the Ganda social order was to remain complex and fascinating for decades to come.

Indeed the status of modern medicine and its African practitioners was in every way ambiguous. Some patients were astonished by the kindness of medical staff who were total strangers:

> I went to Mulago suffering from syphilis for about six people. I never thought that anyone would touch me, my whole body covered with wounds and skin rash . . . but you cannot see unkindness in the face of Nsubuga,[115] the chief Muganda doctor. When he came you could think that the love would stop at this one. When the white doctor came it seemed as though I was his brother. I never thought to be touched, but it happened that one white touched me and one black also touched me. Then I thought at this time that if God had given the world this kindness it would be peaceful.[116]

Perhaps the most sacrificial service was performed by Africans who worked at the great leprosy settlements of the period, notably Onesimo Busimo, who failed the government medical examination at Mengo and went first to teach the children and then to manage the Kumi Leprosy Centre, where he spent twenty-eight years. 'Because I have realised the meaning of the love of Jesus Christ', he explained, 'and because that knowledge has brought such love and comfort to my life and home, I long for these leper children to know the meaning of that love too'.[117] Many dressers received inspiration from the Revival movement which spread through many Protestant churches from the 1930s. 'One triumphant outcome of it', the doctor at Maseno reported,

> is that at last our dressers have come to see that the handing of bed-pans to patients is part of the common duty of any nurses, and the ones whose lives have been changed have helped to set the lead in the regular performance of this duty: it meant much opposition and ridicule from a number of their educated and pagan relatives and friends, but they have stood firm, and it is now the 'done thing' for the dressers

and nurses to perform this simple duty, though it has meant that 7 who did not agree to this have now left the hospital. Three years ago when this issue was brought up before them, the big majority of the Ward staff came in a body and threatened to leave: the miracle of Regeneration has brought about what all our persuasion and wisdom failed to do.[118]

Yet however dedicated they might be, dressers had very varying skill and resources. 'I watched one African dispenser at work for an hour', the academic Margery Perham noted in the Nyanza Province of Kenya in 1930:

He tended to accept the patient's own diagnosis but at least gave a quick glance himself. But he was very pressed for time. The ailments fall into one or two classes – yaws, syphilis and ulcers coming at the top. I saw this young dispenser give intravenous injections for syphilis, a very delicate job. He got the right spot every time, as the jet of blood proved. The doctor himself dared not do it, as the vein is so difficult to spot under a black skin.[119]

By contrast, Hugh Trowell's recollection of inspecting dispensaries in the poorer and less progressive Machakos area was more jaundiced:

A dispensary was just a mud and wattle hut. It was about three yards by three. A low-thatched house, and you got inside it, and found a rickety table, with probably only three legs surviving, and these of unequal length – all eaten by white ants and dudus [insects] – propped upon some stones. You saw some shelves across there, with some bottles on – all empty. There was an enormous book, though, for attendances, where they all had to be written down, even if they didn't get any treatment at all. There was usually a stretcher, which was full of cobwebs.[120]

Where remedies were available, they were often heroic. In Uganda it was customary to test every dispensary patient for 'syphilis' and to give all those found positive 'a rigorous course of arsenical injections regardless of whether the syphilis was active or latent and regardless of the patient's general condition'.[121]

Not only were skills and resources limited, but dressers could expect opposition and even danger. It began with their own relatives and friends:

In the year 1927 I was chosen by our chief to be Tribal Dresser of the tribe and I did not refuse the good fortune given to me by God. Then my comrades came up to advise me to abandon the work. They asked me why I agreed to this evil work of cleaning ulcers every day. Will you eat at the hearth with a skewer? Others said it would be better to choose the work of a clerk or teacher. I heard their words as though they were explaining their dreams. I did not reply. I followed my own path in the medical instruction which the doctor kindly gave me as his pupil. In the year 1928 I finished and I was given medicine to come to work in my district. I settled down in my hospital. Then those relatives who had advised me to abandon the work all came to me to beg for shillings, others to seek my friendship. I cannot say much, but people like those have no principles. They no longer remembered anything, nor knew the words the people had said, that bad work is no good game. So, my friends, do not abandon your work by listening to people's malice.[122]

Among neighbours and community leaders, too, an eager dresser or sanitary inspector might have a sour reception. Witchcraft accusations against them surfaced especially during *mumiani* panics when people feared that the taking of blood samples was cannibalism or sorcery. Dressers had to be withdrawn from the Meatu chiefdom of Sukumaland in 1923 because of fears evoked by taking blood slides. African medical staff in the Jinja area worked in fear of violence for years after a European laboratory assistant was murdered there in 1942.[123] The fear of hospitals also remained strong, especially fear of 'the room-of-splitting-people', as the operating theatre was known at Kaloleni on the Kenya coast:[124]

> Many times I have seen people made miserable by sickness, and when asked why they did not go to hospital, they replied, 'I fear to go to hospital lest I may be given bad medicine, for these hospital people have no sympathy.' Even if a man has an abscess or a swelling and you tell him to go to hospital, he will reply, 'I do not want to suffer the sharp knife [*majisu*] like a beast.'[125]

Hospitals were also seen as demeaning. Ganda agitated for years for separate wards at Mulago so that they need not mingle with their Rwandan migrant labourers. Sewa Haji – known to European doctors as 'the Sewer' – was under continuous attack from Indians, who complained that its 'intolerably over-crowded and positively disgusting . . . insanitary wards of corrugated iron sheet . . . may be likened to dog-boxes in a railway carriage', and educated Africans, whose protests filled the Swahili press.[126] Scarcely any accusation launched at public hospitals after independence, except perhaps their lack of drugs, was absent from vernacular newspapers of the 1930s and 1940s. Many were directed at European or Indian staff, but African dressers were also attacked:

> The safety of a sick person in Sewa Haji Hospital is to give the dressers cigarettes, tea, sugar, food, and the like every day. If you do not do this, you will suffer cruelty of every kind. I do not think that the dressers have authority to abuse the sick in this way, so that we hope the Government will put an end to these things.[127]

Corruption was not universal. Kaloleni reported in 1948 'a strong public opinion amongst the dressers and nurses against the stealing of hospital money and goods'. The Revival movement was influential here, as in the case of an orderly at Mulago who voluntarily confessed the theft of sulphonamide tablets, morphia, food, charcoal, syringes, rubber tubing, and 'the foolscap on which this confession is written'.[128] Yet, as this suggests, corruption and minor crime were rife: charging patients for dressings or injections, stealing their clothes, and especially stealing drugs for sale on the black market – M & B 693 tablets disappeared so quickly that some medical officers ground them up and injected them, painfully, to prevent theft.[129] The problem was worst in Uganda, where from the mid-1930s the authorities campaigned against former medical staff who sold black-market drugs or, more seriously, gave injections. Penalties ranged from three to eighteen months' imprisonment, with or without the option of a fine, with especially heavy sentences where injections caused death.[130] This campaign peaked in 1941 with the prosecution of Yusufu Mukasa – UNMC veteran and pioneer student at Mengo Medical School – for conducting an unlicensed practice at Wandegeya by selling drugs and performing injections, as he had done openly for years.[131]

The degree of autonomy which a dresser might exercise was a delicate issue, especially for the small number who performed minor operations. Pioneers like Yusufu Musajawaza had done many and given anaesthetics at more. The practice continued, as in a circumcision at Maseno in 1933:

> I received instructions to do the operation on Nyoro. At first I refused, I did not want to do it when Dr. was not there. When I was told, I did it. Henry [Olango] gave the anaesthetic that day. I told the Sister we wanted her to help us. She said 'Very well' 'you start it, I am coming.' After I started to cut, I looked round and found Sister had vanished. Henry got the anaesthetic on the box. He took it all right and then I began to operate. Saulo was also there. After I had cut the skin and had put in three stitches and was about to put in the fourth, I noticed the blood was dark. I said so. He said 'He is breathing all right' 'Go on with it.' I was about to put in the fourth stitch when I saw the blood was very dark, I said so, Henry said breathing was all right. I told him to stop chloroform. I sent for the Sister. Saulo started to go but met her coming in at the doorway. She said start artificial respiration. We did so. He did not improve, so we gave him an injection. The breathing stopped. I think we worked about ½ hour before this. It might be 10 or 12 when we were done. I have done operations for circumcision since 1928. I have no qualifications.[132]

This *cause célèbre* ended an era. Owing to a misunderstanding, the operation (on a patient with a condition which made chloroform fatal) had broken the unwritten rule that a doctor must be present in the hospital when unqualified staff performed such procedures. Now white opinion in Kenya and fear of scandal elsewhere led the authorities to ban operations by Africans, except under direct supervision, and to restrict administration of anaesthetics and potentially lethal injections to those completing training courses.[133] The paramedic's role in operating theatres was increasingly confined to preparing the instruments and assisting the surgeon. It was one example of growing tensions between different categories of medical staff. Dressers had long suffered under white paternalism, but that was at least a personal relationship with some compensations. After the First World War it gradually gave way to impersonal assertions of authority. One reason was the arrival of young white doctors, often with military experience, and white nursing sisters whose relations with male African staff were often tense. Another was a clash between European determination to uproot 'barbaric' customs and African anxiety to minimise cultural conflict, which led medical workers of both races in central Kenya to take extreme positions in the dispute of 1929 over female circumcision, when the entire medical staff of Chogoria Hospital in Embu deserted the mission.[134]

Other grievances were long-standing. One was pay. 'A Hospital dresser, who must be able to read and write Kiswahili and is in as responsible a position as a nurse at home, gets 20/- a month – and it costs him 25/- a month to feed himself and his wife here under present conditions', a medical officer in Mwanza noted in 1943. 'Then they wonder why they sometimes steal.'[135] Hospital housing was notoriously bad. Disease was an occupational hazard. But perhaps the most pervasive grievance was the limited opportunity for advancement, given the ambitions bringing young people into medical work and their unfamiliarity with promotion according to qualifications rather than experience or competence. 'These men knew little English on arrival', Trowell remembered of the Nairobi Medical Training Depot in 1933, 'but they were frantically anxious to learn and were all under the impression that they would become doctors at the end of four years' training. There was even a riot when they discovered this to be impossible for I refused to issue stethoscopes.'[136] Twelve years later Mugo Gatheru joined the institution to train as a laboratory technician. He liked the work and some of the doctors, notably one who taught them, 'Believe in science. That leads you to truth. There is no God like they tell you.'[137] But he also became aware of the squalid conditions in which Nairobi's Africans lived and the discrimination against senior African technicians, who after twenty years earned less than a European trainee:

> Every day during 1945 and 1946 I washed the test tubes and ran the blood tests at the Medical Research Laboratory. In the evenings I took my correspondence course and I read much. I was learning more and more about the troubles of my people. My blood was boiling inside me. I felt I was wasting my time doing this kind of work. I wanted to get an education as soon as possible to do something to help my people.[138]

He resigned in 1947. Sixteen years earlier a patient at Masaka Hospital had put it more tersely after watching a European doctor abuse a medical assistant who had served with the ANMC and graduated from Mengo Medical School. 'Those who do health training without going through Makerere', he wrote, 'are training for nothing'.[139]

The problem of indigenous medicine

Correspondence in the Swahili press shows that tribal dressers and other paramedics were especially troubled about their relationship to indigenous medicine. Often serving in the countryside, limited in resources and skills, and subject to patient power in the choice of therapy, paramedics were more truly in competition with indigenous practitioners than fully qualified doctors would ever be. They could not ignore indigenous medicine.

Nor could they wholly embrace it. Modern training centres were contemptuous. 'It was difficult not to comment and laugh at the way these traditional doctors dramatise when diagnosing diseases', a student at Mengo Medical School wrote in 1927 after a meeting at which the two therapies were contrasted.[140] Some native authorities, too, openly discouraged indigenous medicine.[141] Colonial governments did not generally interfere unless healers professed to practise witchcraft or accused others of doing so:

> We have not the knowledge nor the means to consider registering such people yet; if we did register we should in fact accord them Government recognition and greatly strengthen their position. Except for prosecution when they offend against the criminal law we have therefore no alternative but to leave them alone, trusting to the growing intelligence and knowledge of the people gradually to protect them from cheats and charlatans, and for this . . . the Tribal Dressers are probably the most valuable agency we have.[142]

The sting lay in the last sentence. The tribal dressers were to be the champions of modernity.

Almost all paramedics who recorded their views were hostile and contemptuous towards indigenous medicine. Their unrecorded actions may have differed, but in public they clung more closely to their training, and thought less for themselves, than some contemporary African clergymen and evangelists, perhaps because dressers were generally less educated and had before them more dramatic evidence of the power of modern skills. As a dresser wrote in 1941, 'These days our uncivilised medicine is powerless.'[143] 'In the past', another added,

> in Kangundo in Ukambani, it was just darkness, and now people are beginning to have their eyes opened a little. For they used to employ forest medicine. The sick man who might drink such bad medicine died. But now we have here among us a European doctor who is very clever and knows every sort of sickness, how to deliver the women and to give people injections and medicines . . . My friends, doctors are the servants of God and it is enough for us to pray that God may give them more skill.[144]

Injections won the greatest admiration. 'The doctor began to treat [sleeping-sickness victims] with the needle', an assistant described, 'and all those who received injections recovered, and all those who did not receive injections died, and now the sickness has decreased and all the people have been at peace until today'.[145] Yet this was only the most spectacular ground for belief in the superiority of modern medicine. Dressers were also impressed by its systematic methods of diagnosis:

While being taught medicine I came to know that every disease we catch has its cause and its vectors [*wadudu*], then its medicine to treat it and prevent it. At the hospital the sick are told to provide stools, urine, sputum, or to give blood and pus. These are to examine the truth of the disease which is troubling the person. The practice of African doctors is quite different; someone feeling pain in the chest is told that a fly has entered him by witchcraft, and it needs propitiation.

The hospital wants to know the cause, so that proper medicine may be given for the complaint, for every complaint has its medicine.[146]

Modern treatment, too, had apparent rationality and precision, especially the precision of dosage which was drilled into dressers during their training and contrasted with the lack of concern for quantity, as against quality, which was common (although not universal) in pre-modern medicine:

A woman arrived at the hospital to bring her child who had been sick for many days. The child was known to have malaria . . . We explained to the mother that she should bring the child every day to receive medicine twice a day for five days.

When the mother returned home she went to Mr Tyaile (an Iramba doctor). He took out his beads (his measuring instrument [*darubini yake ya kupimia*]) and he moved them around [*akapiga bao*] and he told the mother that her child was suffering illness on account of the bad milk which she was providing. The doctor wanted payment for his medicine and then he told the mother, If you bring a sheep I shall make medicine for you and your milk will be good and your child will get completely well. When the mother returned home, her relations brought a sheep and led the mother to the doctor. The doctor boiled medicine for more than four hours; then he presented it to the mother and she drank, even the child was given to drink. When they had just arrived back, the medicine began to make them giddy. In a short time the mother took leave of the world. By good fortune the medicine did not harm the child. By the grace of God the child is alive today.

Many of our medicines are bad because they have no measure [*kipimo*]; the patient can be given a whole basin. Hospital medicines have exact measures, nor will you see a patient being given a basin. To give a patient medicine that exceeds its measure is not to cure the patient but to harm him.[147]

Kila dawa ina kiasi chake: every medicine has its dose[148] – one can imagine it repeated endlessly to medical apprentices. Modern medicine also drew authority from its apparent universality. Warning his readers against local drugs designed to accelerate childbirth and against the risk of contracting disease from unhygienic local midwives, a dispenser wrote that the difference was that 'European medicine is all one kind; if you go to Germany it is what they use in France, and if you go to Belgium it is what they use in England.'[149] Indigenous medicine, by contrast, was depicted as parochial, irrational, fraudulent, and dangerous. 'Let us abandon the business of divination [*Ramli*] and the medicines of doctors who exorcise spirits by moving sticks [*waganga wapungao Tenga-wano*]', a correspondent urged; 'these are not medicines at all but just to take part in and enjoy dances'.[150]

'I know', wrote Daudi Mfuko of Minaki, 'that many times a Zaramo patient will not come to the dispensary unless he has tried "Madogoni", the evil spirit dance, or consulted Mwanambago or Kinyamkela the devil. Hence patients get worse and worse before they come to be helped, as they have to pay for all the above treatments and it takes a long time to collect the money.'[151] The moral was clear: 'When we are sick, let us go to the hospital at once, let us never go to native doctors, for their medicine is just trouble after trouble.'[152]

This was almost the universal view recorded at the time by paramedics and other educated East Africans. But there were rare dissident voices, seldom those of dressers, but perhaps enough to indicate that this troubled educated people, pitting their training against their racial pride, especially when new diseases seemed so threatening.[153] At a superficial level, *Mambo Leo* during the 1930s carried a desultory debate on whether indigenous medicine could properly be described as uncivilised (*kishenzi*). 'Is it only we who lack civilisation?' one correspondent asked.[154] More thoughtfully, some drew distinctions. 'European medicine is very good if a man gets yaws [but] we have some very big diseases and Europeans cannot cure them', schoolboys in the Masasi area wrote in 1928. 'They cannot cure elephantitis [sic] and they cannot cure snake bites, but African doctors can.'[155] In 1941 a dresser in north-eastern Tanganyika was convinced that he had watched an indigenous healer cure leprosy sufferers.[156] The most thoughtful analysis was written in 1943 by a member of the Tanganyika Medical Department, Cuthbert Ley, possibly a man of mixed race. He argued that much of value in the African past was being lost. Whereas the European doctor might be confident that his treatment would work, the African healer also tried to infuse his patient with that confidence. On the other hand, indigenous medicine had many defects. Its training and practice were unsystematic, as was its understanding of the causes of illness and its development in the body, while its methods of administration were less effective than injections. Yet in listing these defects, he insisted, he was not scorning indigenous medicine but pointing to what needed to be learned from Europeans:

> For the diseases of Africa are too difficult for all without distinction to be treatable with medicines from Europe. Since God has so created us that we can endure the great heat here, which we can clearly see that Europeans cannot, then it is surely possible that he has also created herbs [*miti*] which can treat us. It is therefore now our duty to search out these herbs as he has arranged them. We may come unexpectedly on what will be work of great value, for many of our people are greatly afflicted with diseases of leprosy, consumption, and the like.[157]

Ley's contribution was original chiefly because it came from a medical worker. A mission teacher had appealed for research some months earlier[158] and men with political agendas had sought to rehabilitate indigenous medicine for several years. In the early 1930s Martin Kayamba had written a respectful account for his superiors in Tanganyika's Native Affairs Department.[159] At the end of the decade two especially enthusiastic tributes were published. Erica Fiah, newspaper editor and former ANMC interpreter, insisted that pre-colonial Africans had enjoyed good health, for food had been plentiful and they had not yet been weakened by European civilisation and medicine, so that their own medicine had been sufficient for their limited needs. If Africans still ate their own food, he asked, why did they not use their own medicine?[160] At the same time Ali Ponda, a schoolteacher in Dodoma who was becoming one of Tanganyika's most active elite politicians, urged African healers to come out of hiding and publicise their skills, so that even European doctors searching for new medicines could learn from them.[161]

The political and racial sensitivities that inspired educated men with interest in indigenous medicine during the late 1930s remained their chief motives for the rest of the century. Modern medical workers, too, generally retained their caution and instinctive hostility. Between them, throughout, stood those like Cuthbert Ley who sought a balanced, mutually beneficial relationship. The lines of debate between indigenous and modern medicine were drawn in the age of the tribal dresser.

4 Makerere and its students, 1923–49

Medical professions in Third World countries have generally grown out of one or more medical schools and their graduates.[1] In East Africa, Makerere College in Uganda filled this role. It was there, between the 1920s and the late 1940s, that practical apprenticeship and formal education were fused in the training of doctors. Once this had happened, progress was remarkably swift, suggesting both that the intensive, hands-on training characteristic of medicine was an especially effective way of transferring skills and also that the medical students were in general exceptionally gifted. No longer drawn from the margins of society, but selected by talent and accident of birth from a broad social spectrum, they experienced a rigorous socialisation which left them with strong group solidarity. Within colonial society, however, they were still merely assistants, embittered by subordinate status and unrewarding conditions of work. During the 1940s, as wartime and postwar stringency retarded Makerere's development and frustrated the ambitions of its former students, they clashed for the first time with the colonial state, learning thereby much about their potential and their vulnerability.

The evolution of medical education

Although Albert Cook had envisaged a 'medical faculty . . . in the future Mengo University' as early as 1909, the first consideration of a government training college in Uganda took place in 1912, when, as an economy measure, a committee drafted plans for an African civil service and clerical training school, which some thought of enlarging into 'a Native University or Institute'.[2] Financial stringency and war intervened until 1919, when another committee urged 'the formation of Government Schools in the following branches, Medical, Clerical, Technical, Mechanical, and Agricultural'.[3] The Medical Department was eager to train young men of the type so successful in the ANMC to replace Indian Sub-Assistant Surgeons, who were difficult to recruit.[4] Moreover, Uganda Africans were seeking higher education in Britain, Ceylon, and (most undesirably) the

United States, which was a major reason for creating and subsequently upgrading Makerere.[5]

Having chosen Makerere Hill, formerly reserved for the Kabaka's blacksmiths, as an appropriate site for the Uganda Technical School, the government opened classes for carpenters and mechanics late in 1921.[6] Medical training began in 1923, when H.B. Owen, who had commanded ANMC training, was appointed medical tutor. Initially he took charge of ten students from Mengo Medical School to be trained for 'the comparatively humble part' of medical assistants.[7] Owen believed the students should aim higher, but only if they could study in English. Since the existing students could not, he replaced them in 1924 by four young Ganda men from mission schools. They were to take a four-year course, extended in 1926 to five years, following the standard sequence of European medical education from basic sciences through pre-clinical medical sciences to clinical studies.[8] 'The Medical Assistant', Owen explained, 'is intended to approach to the standard of a Sub-Assistant Surgeon. He is trained on the same lines as a doctor, though his training is pruned and simplified to suit the local educational standard and requirements.' The long-term aim was 'a course comparable to that of a European school of medicine'.[9] Initially Owen did nearly all the teaching. This ambitious programme, which even Keane thought premature, raised Makerere's goals beyond its original craft-training. During 1924 the government decided to detach the technical classes, develop literary and vocational (including medical) courses into a 'Higher College', and appoint a new Principal: D.G. Tomblings, a district commissioner and former ANMC Adjutant.[10]

In 1926 Owen's first four students moved from pre-clinical training at Makerere to clinical work at Mulago Hospital, on the neighbouring hill a kilometre away. This raised difficulties, for Owen had no status at Mulago and clinical training depended on the hospital doctors, who were often newly arrived, posted to Mulago for only a few months, uninterested in teaching, and already responsible for training medical attendants. Uganda faced a problem which had long vexed Europe and the United States: whether medical education should have a practical bias and be based in hospitals, whether it should have an academic emphasis and be based in universities, or whether some compromise was possible.[11] In 1927 a committee decided to establish a Mulago Medical School, designed for the whole of East Africa, with an academic component but a hospital-based, practical bias.[12] This decision had repercussions for the rest of the century, for it tied the Medical School to departmental control and policy, obliged the academics in the late 1940s to demand a more equal balance, meant that neither they nor their colleagues elsewhere in East Africa controlled a university teaching hospital, and ensured that medical professionalisation centred to an unusual degree on government service. More immediately, Owen moved in 1928 from Makerere to Mulago as Medical Superintendent of the Hospital and responsible for training medical students to become Senior Native (later African) Medical Assistants (SAMAs). They would be admitted initially to Makerere and take a two-year science course there before moving to Mulago for pre-clinical medical sciences and clinical studies, to which an additional year as an intern was generally added during the late 1920s. 'The system of training', Owen explained,

> is directed to the production of an assistant able to diagnose and treat with understanding the more straight-forward, and common disease conditions, to appreciate the possibilities of major Medicine and Surgery in more expert hands, and to know sufficient of the rarer and less simple conditions to realize when to call an European superior to his aid.[13]

The emphasis was curative, with little attention to surgery, which was thought beyond the students' competence, and virtually none to hygiene and sanitation – which Owen thought pointless until Uganda's sanitary conditions improved – until the mid-1930s, when preventive medicine gained a limited place. Midwifery was added in 1928.[14]

Late in 1927 three of the first four students – Antonio Bamugye, Dionysius Bamundaga, and Yakobo Baziwane – passed their final examinations and entered government service. By the end of 1936, thirty-four had completed the course successfully.[15] Output was less than at the School of Medicine in Khartoum, also opened in 1924, which had by 1935 trained fifty-three surviving medical staff to a similar level, but it was more impressive than in British West Africa, where the first medical school, at Yaba in Nigeria, graduated its first students in 1935.[16] The thirty-four who had passed through Makerere included two Arabs from Zanzibar but as yet no one from Kenya or Tanganyika, although Joseph Mutahangarwa from Tanganyika was in his fourth year and Jason Likimani from Kenya in his third. Tanganyika's school standards were low and its officials had long resisted sending young men to Kampala where 'the type of political thought prevailing among Africans tends to be of a somewhat extremist nature' likely to breed 'versatile political agitators', so that Mutahangarwa – already an experienced medical assistant – had entered Makerere only by going back to school in Uganda for a year.[17] Kenya's schooling was better, at least at the Alliance High School, but European suspicion of allowing Africans to study medicine at Makerere was strong and Likimani had done so only by switching into the medical course without seeking the government's approval.[18] From 1936 a Joint East African Examining Board conducted the Medical School's examinations. It extended clinical instruction to three years, lengthening the entire course to six.[19] Uganda's senior medical officers supported the school, but some other Europeans were sceptical, although they recognised that SAMAs were cheap and much preferred them to Indian Sub-Assistant Surgeons. Indeed, African medical training profited greatly from European hostility to Indians, as in Khartoum it profited from anxiety to replace Egyptian and Syrian doctors.[20] Makerere also gradually overcame the suspicions of Africans, who had initially seen it as an expensive and inferior substitute for education abroad. By 1927 the College was attracting the brightest students from the mission schools, especially into the medical course.[21] In Tanganyika the ambitious Martin Kayamba saw it as the best education for his son:

> I do not wish him to be trained as a dispenser or compounder and that is all. I am willing to pay the fees at Makerere, provided the course there is a complete one. This is my only son and I wish to give him the best education I can and to make him a better man than myself if I can help it.[22]

The de la Warr Commission of 1937 confirmed the Medical School's standing. Invited by the Governor, Sir Philip Mitchell, to conduct 'an educational stock taking and some rails laid down for the next few years',[23] the commission consisted of distinguished academics, including Z.K. Matthews, the African Vice-Principal of the University College at Fort Hare, chaired by the junior minister at the Colonial Office, Earl de la Warr, a young aristocrat of well-publicised left-wing views.[24] In a far-sighted and somewhat euphoric report 'proposing the establishment of a University College in the near future, and of a University at no very distant date', the commission commended especially the Medical School, where 'Higher Education in East Africa has approached nearest to degree standard' and the graduates were already better qualified than Sub-Assistant Surgeons. Within a few years, the commission suggested, the College should ask the General Medical Council in Britain to recognise its medical diploma, thereby making its holders fully fledged doctors.[25] Delighted, Mitchell began to rebuild Makerere as a university college. He was warned, however, that GMC recognition was impossible without a new teaching hospital.[26] In August 1939 the British Government announced a grant of £240,000 from the Colonial Development Fund for a medical school and hospital at Mulago with 540 beds, possibly later to be expanded to 1,020.[27] A month later the Second World War began.

Meanwhile Makerere had also contacted the GMC, which had inspected and recognised Indian medical colleges since 1892, although it could in law decide only whether those qualifying at medical institutions could be registered to practise in *Britain* – a fruitful source of future confusion. In February 1940 Sir Richard Needham, who regularly inspected Indian colleges, visited Makerere informally. He reported that its students had inadequate preparatory schooling, science teaching needed improvement, there must be an additional pre-clinical year of anatomy and physiology with full-time teachers, and the new medical school and hospital must be built. He ended his report with a carefully worded encouragement clearly designed also as a warning:

> It will, I believe, not be easy to obtain from the Council the recognition of the Uganda Diploma for Registration on the British Register. But I know of no reason why the attempt should not be made. If the arrangements outlined earlier in this note in regard to preliminary general and pre-medical education prove satisfactory, students who join Makerere College in January 1941, and enter the Medical School to commence study in October 1942, would complete the five years' curriculum in July 1947. Sometime before 1947 it would be necessary to inform the Registrar of the General Medical Council of the intention to apply for recognition and to ask for information as to procedure. But long before this I suggest that it would be in the interests of the Medical School to seek advice by means of unofficial visitations.[28]

Unwisely, the Medical Department's published account ignored Needham's warning that recognition would not be easy and claimed that he 'definitely visualized attainment of the standard of a registrable qualification at Mulago in five or six years time', provided that his conditions were met.[29] 'This report brought great hope to Makerere Medical Graduates', one remembered, 'and many of them thought that within six years their qualification would be fully recognised and their conditions of service, status and salaries would improve'.[30] It was not to be. On 10 May 1940, only days after Needham completed his report, Germany invaded France.

Makerere and Mulago decayed during the war. Mitchell, who had supplied much of their dynamism, moved to Nairobi. A new Principal, G.C. Turner, transformed the students from schoolboys into undergraduates but envisaged a liberal education tailored to African conditions in which students would 'regard the medical profession as one among several professional channels to social service . . . rather than as the apex of professional glory'.[31] He raised Makerere's entrance requirements towards school certificate (i.e. four years of secondary education) but East Africa's schools, starved of staff and money by depression and war, could not keep pace. In 1945 all Tanganyika's candidates failed the entrance examination and a year later the territory had no more students at Makerere than in 1940.[32] Kenya's settler-influenced government deliberately reduced its entry by requiring school certificate. Even Uganda's entrants declined in the middle years of the war, so that Makerere's student body fell between 1939 and 1943 from well over 200 to only 141. Between 1940 and 1946 only thirty-four students completed the medical course successfully.[33] At first their quality held up well. In 1943 experienced external examiners borrowed from the military reported enthusiastically that most candidates in surgery and some in medicine, gynaecology, and obstetrics would probably have passed the conjoint examinations (the minimum British medical qualification). 'What we have seen here', the examiners added, 'has filled us with enthusiasm for what you are trying to do'.[34] Kenyan medical specialists who also examined the students, however, were critical, especially in 1945, when 'in some subjects teaching had been completed with the utmost difficulty because of shortages of staff'.[35] The medical certificate was converted into a diploma in 1944, giving the graduates a long-sought set of letters to put after their names. Two years later the extra year of physiology recommended by Needham was added. In 1945 Makerere for the first time admitted women.[36] But impatience with the college was growing among both Africans and Europeans. In 1945 only three students completed the medical course, all Ugandans. By then, after twenty years, Kenya had only three African Assistant Medical Officers (AAMOs) – as they were now known – in service, while Tanganyika had only five in 1947, out of twenty-one who had started the course.[37]

Planning for postwar development began in 1943 when Uganda's DMS proposed to enlarge Mulago Hospital, upgrade the Medical School, expand its output to twenty a year, and appoint full-time staff.[38] This hardened into a plan for a 1,000-bed hospital costing £477,500, exclusive of the new medical school. Late in 1944 the British Government approved this, but the architect prepared plans costing three times as much.[39] The ensuing debate raised two important questions about the Medical School's future: whether it should be controlled by the government or Makerere, and whether its students should take a local diploma seeking GMC recognition or should be external candidates for the London degree of Bachelor of Medicine (MB).[40] In 1945 a very influential British commission chaired by Justice Asquith recommended that colonial universities should follow the British model – selective, residential, and autonomous – by first entering a special relationship with the University of London and taking its external degrees until each university was mature enough to award its own. Medical schools should be integral parts of universities and controlled by academics, but, exceptionally, they should aim first at local qualifications:

> The first step to be taken is to raise the standards of teaching so that the local medical diploma obtains recognition by the General Medical Council. The final stage would be reached when the centre of which the medical school is part becomes a university awarding its own degrees. Between the first and final stages there will a period in which we hope that the more able of the students would be afforded opportunities for taking the degree of a home or Dominion university; we would in particular support the proposal that arrangements should be made available for such students to become candidates for degrees of the University of London.[41]

Makerere's non-medical staff were suspicious of the proposed special relationship, which was not accepted until 1949. The medical teachers, however, welcomed the priority given to their diploma, for several reasons: London might not permit Makerere courses to be adapted to local medical conditions; the London degree was unusually difficult, so that some East African students would probably have to take an inferior local qualification; and experience in West Africa and the Caribbean had shown the difficulty of creating a successful medical school if the ablest students did part or all of their training abroad.[42] Moreover, although this was not stated, pursuit of GMC recognition gave the medical staff leverage in demanding development funds, a consideration especially important to the very able group of teachers who took over the leadership of the Medical School at the end of the war, notably Alexander Galloway (the Dean), Eric Holmes (a physiologist), Jack Davies (a government pathologist and brilliant research worker), and the long-serving Hugh Trowell.

The teachers' preference for the Makerere diploma rather than the London degree eventually won the day, partly because it followed the Asquith Commission's recommendation and partly because London University rejected the Makerere Medical School as insufficiently advanced to warrant special relationship – a judgment which was not wholly concealed[43] but was overlooked by medical students when they later agitated for London degrees. The Uganda Government, however, would have preferred the London degree as politically more acceptable in Uganda,[44] and this was one element in a bitter conflict during the later 1940s between the academic leaders of the Medical School and the East African medical departments. In 1946, when Galloway became Dean, control of the Medical School was transferred back from the Uganda Medical Department to Makerere, but it remained utterly dependent on the Department for clinical teaching and the use of Mulago.[45] Moreover, Uganda's new DMS, T.A. Austin, unlike all his predecessors, 'loathes the A.M.O.', as Holmes put it – a hostility towards the training of Africans as doctors shared by Austin's counterparts in Kenya and Tanganyika at that time and by many Europeans within and outside the medical service who, as an external examiner reported in 1948, regarded and described Makerere's staff as 'white trash'.[46] Austin did not want a university medical school, but he did want a new Mulago Hospital at the British Government's expense. He therefore resisted the appointment of university clinical teachers at Mulago until the new hospital was built.[47] 'I am convinced', Galloway complained in November 1947,

> that there is strong opposition in some higher places here to African University Education. The DMS has stated quite openly his dislike of Africans being given a medical education approaching a University standard. Again, I feel that much of

the opposition of the Uganda Government to higher medical education lies in its unwillingness to hand over its control of the hospital and the Medical School.[48]

In reality, however, inflation was putting a new hospital out of reach. In May 1948 the Uganda Government decided instead to renovate the existing hospital and spend any additional funds outside Kampala. The Colonial Office agreed, provided that the renovated Mulago could be made an acceptable teaching hospital.[49] By 1951 it had grown to 630 beds. A modest new Medical School costing £60,000 and a small number of university clinical posts were approved in 1949. At the same time Makerere invited its first official GMC visitation.[50]

The Asquith strategy had prevailed. Makerere controlled its medical school. The students were to read for its diploma. Everything now waited on the GMC visitation.

Medical students

The first East Africans to practise modern medicine had generally been of low status. Makerere's medical students, by contrast, often came from privileged strata within colonial society. By the late 1940s they were the leading element in East Africa's educated elite. Apprenticeship had carried menial connotations, but the Medical School was declared by de la Warr to be East Africa's closest approximation to university education. In reality, however, much of the Medical School's work was a 'hands-on' training in practical skills under direct supervision by a qualified doctor. Ironically, that probably made it particularly effective. A medical education at Makerere acquired its high reputation precisely because it successfully combined the academic and the practical.

Few medical students came from families with indigenous medical traditions. Diane Zeller, who investigated this in Buganda, found only two, A. Lubega and J.Y. Musitwa, who both came from Buganda's specialised and hereditary bone-setters.[51] Of the two East African regions most renowned for their medical specialists, Kamba country in Kenya sent few students to Makerere, while the Shambaa-Bondei-Zigua region of north-eastern Tanganyika sent numerous students but from schools run by the Universities Mission which rated teaching and the ministry higher than medicine.[52] Occasional cases can be identified later, such as the psychiatrist Joseph Muhangi, who 'continued to be fascinated by stories of his grandfather's exploits as a traditional doctor',[53] but generally the children of indigenous healers lacked the chief characteristic of early medical students: an educated father, for medicine was predominantly a career for the second-generation educated, perhaps because a literate home gave a head-start in the educational race and the moral and financial backing to complete an immensely demanding course. This point emerges clearly from the relatively few students of high indigenous status. The most prominent among them, Joseph Mutahangarwa – the first Tanganyikan to complete the course, in 1940 – came from a chiefly family in Kiziba, on the border with Uganda, which had been unusually quick to adopt European culture and favour missionary work.[54] Raymond Kafamba, the third successful Tanganyikan student, was from the same family.[55] Ivan Majugo was a nephew of the Omukama of Bunyoro,[56] but none of the Ganda students appears to have come from the core of the royal family, although Sam Mukasa was related to Kabaka Mutesa II, Solomon Matovu married a princess,[57] several came from families entrenched in the chiefly hierarchy,[58] and others were sons of lower-level chiefs.[59] Rather, where educational background was vital, the most important single origin of medical students was naturally from within the emergent elite. Benjamin Kipkorir's tart comment on Kenya's leadership at independence – 'Its origins are traceable to the first generation of colonial collaborators'[60] – was also largely true of its first doctors. The archetype was the first Kenyan to enter the Medical School, Jason Likimani, whose father was an early and wealthy evangelist among the Maasai who sent at least three of his sons to Alliance High School.[61] Another early Kenyan doctor, James Ang'awa, was born to a district commissioner's clerk, while a later but striking example was the surgeon Nelson Awori – the first East African to perform a kidney transplant – whose father was Canon Jeremiah Awori, a pioneer pastor in western Kenya whose seventeen children became prominent among the educated elites of both Kenya and Uganda.[62] A.K. Kibaya, a leading early Ugandan doctor, was also a son of the manse, as were Barnaba Kununka, Godfrey Binaisa (future President of Uganda and one-time medical student), and two early Tanganyikan doctors, John Omari and W.B.K. Mwanjisi.[63] Yet men of lower status in the colonial system also fathered medical students. David Kiremerwa, in Uganda, was the son of a cook and interpreter. In Tanganyika, Charles Mtawali's father was a policeman and Swedi Mwankemwa's a carpenter, while Francis Mwaisela, perhaps the most impressive early student from Tanganyika, was born to a hospital orderly, as was Justin Gesa, a future Ugandan Minister of Health.[64] By 1941 Makerere had its first student, C.W. Sewanywa, who was the son of a previous medical student.[65]

Of all Makerere's students before 1954, only about 15 per cent came from entirely illiterate homes,[66] but entry to the medical course was so competitive that there was room for some brilliant young men of humble origin. The most academically successful of all the early medical students was Arthur Okwemba, who passed in 1941 with distinctions in anatomy, physiology, pathology, pharmacology, and surgery. He came from the prestigious Alliance High School but was described by its headmaster as 'a Church of God boy' from a very poor family.[67] Raphael Onyango, who became a distinguished specialist on trypanosomiasis, had no known parents and was regarded as a dependant of Namilyango Mission.[68] 'A considerable percentage of successful students here are the sons of poor parents, and have been in receipt of private assistance from missionaries and others', Uganda's Director of Education wrote in 1927.[69] The silence of the vernacular press about the very first medical students to qualify in the late 1920s suggests that they too may have been of modest origin.

In 1936 exactly half Makerere's students were from Buganda. They were even more dominant in the Medical School, where the first two classes to complete the course were all Ganda, the only other entrant, from Acholi in northern Uganda, having dropped out.[70] The first successful Soga student from south-eastern Uganda, Ivan Kadama, later Uganda's first African DMS, qualified in 1937 and the first northerner, Alexander Odonga, later a leading surgeon, in 1948.[71] Medical students from Kenya and Tanganyika were still too few for ethnic origins to mean much; there was a broad correlation with educational advantage – Kikuyu (especially from Kiambu), Luo, and Luyia from Kenya, Haya and Nyakyusa from Tanganyika – but it was not complete: Bondei and Chagga were prominent among Tanganyikan students but not in the Medical School.[72] More striking was that six of the first seven successful students, and many of their successors, were Roman Catholics, who were only 29 per cent of Makerere's students in 1938.[73] One possible reason in Buganda may have been that Catholics chose medicine because they had fewer opportunities for political and administrative careers than members of the Protestant establishment. Another reason, with wider relevance, may have been the ethos of Catholic schooling, especially the sisters' influence on young children. But this is speculation.

The motives of this first generation are hard to identify, especially because few were still alive in the late 1990s. Probably the most important motive was simply that medicine was the longest, most difficult, and most prestigious course, for although this deterred some students,[74] it challenged others who had already tasted success in a fiercely competitive school system.[75] As in the past, a medical training was an exercise in entrepreneurship. To these men from honour cultures, what mattered most was relative status, *vis-à-vis* other students, Indian Sub-Assistant Surgeons, nursing sisters, graduates in other fields, and above all the registered British doctors who never fully understood the compulsion to excel which would lead men in their fifties and sixties to travel half-way across the world in pursuit of qualifications. 'In all undertakings, Man seeks and strives for nothing else but success and glory', a Makerere student wrote sententiously in 1938.

'... Wealth and social advancement at this stage in life are often given much more consideration than they really deserve.'[76] The material motive was certainly there, although it was probably less compelling than colonial officials thought. The motive of service was also there, as Dionysius Bamundaga, one of the first to qualify, explained in old age: 'During that time there were no African doctors so I thought I'd better be a doctor in order to help my people.'[77] The paediatrician Nimrod Bwibo had watched his father, a village pastor, treat ulcers and other complaints as he travelled the countryside and 'was determined to be able to do more for the sick than his father was doing'.[78] Some scarcely made the decision for themselves. They might, like Godfrey Kayamba, be driven into the medical course by an ambitious father. More fortunately, like Charles Mtawali, their headmaster might put them down for Makerere rather than let them leave school for immediate employment.[79] Childhood experiences could be formative. 'Another thing that made me interested in medicine', Swedi Mwankemwa recalled:

> When I, myself, I had a small abscess in my foot, and during those days anaesthesia was not available. The way I was handled by the nurses and the doctor who incised the abscess and relieved me from the pain – I was very struck and said that oh, it is a very good job done, and since then I developed an interest in medical care.

Another influence in his case was a role model, Mtawali, who examined his school in 1943, 'and I was very much impressed by the way he addressed us'.[80] The first three Makerere practitioners were especially influential as models,[81] as probably was Francis Mwaisela during his service at Nzega. The model might be a European. George Sembeguya once borrowed Albert Cook's clothes to act in a play and was told sternly, 'Do not end here, you must one day put this stethoscope round your neck as a full doctor and not as an actor.'[82] Some dealings with Europeans provided more bitter incentives. Samson Kisekka, who was to become both a doctor and Vice-President of Uganda, professed to recall that his dying father had been neglected by a European doctor: 'I said I'd rather do something better. I didn't like the way this doctor treated my father. But he didn't belong to my group, my people.'[83] A more common experience was probably that of a later medical student:

> It had been a dream of mine to work my way to the position of a District Medical Officer . . . like that young, cheerful, British doctor who once or twice a year used to visit the small dispensary near my home during my primary school days. The dispensary would be tidied up before his visit, and patients would be informed about his coming and would be instructed to come with clean dresses. Cleanliness was so much a part of him that his presence and actions seemed to personify it. Dignity seemed to be an inherent quality of his office. He was as unperturbed by the respect and fear with which people regarded him just as those with royal blood naturally accept the cheer and pomp with which they are received.[84]

Makerere was as far from Dar es Salaam as London was from Vienna. The new student's first impression of the College was probably the sheer diversity of people. It was a small place – in 1938 only 169 students were in residence, including 36 reading medicine – but a year later they were said to come from thirty tribes.[85] In 1940 a medical student from Toro, Hosea Banura, made a sensation by donating blood for a patient, the sensation being that the patient was from Buganda. 'Racial [meaning tribal] distinction', Mwaisela commented, 'is the first thing to be eradicated from the head of students entering Makerere College'.[86] Yet diverse as the students were, the new arrival was unlikely to be lonely, for almost all came from a handful of schools. Of 153 students at Makerere in 1936, no fewer than 62 were from Budo, 38 from Kisubi (Uganda's leading Roman Catholic school) and 24 from the Alliance High School, which produced 13 of the 17 Kenyans who qualified in medicine by 1958.[87] Loyalty to Budo was strong – Samson Kisekka was to cite it as a model for Ugandan patriotism – and students from newer schools like Tabora in Tanganyika confessed to an 'inferiority feeling'. Turner recalled that one of his tasks on taking charge of Makerere was to break Budo's domination.[88]

For many students the chief problem was money. Makerere's interwar fees were Shs.300 a year, all included – less than Budo's Shs.430 and nothing to a senior Ugandan chief, but beyond the reach of a village chief on Shs.80 a year or a labourer earning Shs.5 a month.[89] Tanganyika, Zanzibar, and Kenya (through its Local Native Councils) gave bursaries to all their students who could not afford the fees, while Uganda awarded between ten and twenty part-cost scholarships each year and made loans to needy students.[90] Almost all medical students held scholarships and their last two clinical years were free – the first students had indeed been paid during their course.[91] But scholarships covered only fees, plus, in Tanganyika's case, pocket-money of ten shillings a term, repayable from future wages, so that some Tanganyikan students had to work as labourers during vacations.[92] Tanganyika bonded medical students to work for the Medical Department for four years, although Uganda found no legal way to do this.[93] Most students appear to have depended in part on relatives or local communities. When Jason Likimani became the first Maasai to enter Makerere, his Local Native Council awarded him a railway fare exceeding the annual fees.[94] 'Some people think we are too high for them', students complained. '. . . They are always looking for faults.'[95] Return to the village became a stock theme of East African novels and a matter for self-congratulation by students at the end of vacations. Many, especially in the senior medical classes, were full adults in their twenties and a few, such as Joseph Mutahangarwa, in their thirties. These older men faced special financial difficulty, especially if married. When Hamza Mwapachu left his post as instructor at Mwanza Medical Training School to undertake the medical course at Makerere, for example, he had to send his family home to Tanga and withdraw all his Shs.2,543 savings from the provident fund to support them.[96]

The other bane of student life was examinations. Makerere tried – prematurely, some thought – to teach in a university manner, in contrast to the didactic character of East African schooling:

> There was a time when our teachers exercised parental care towards us; there was a time when lessons were hammered in until they had made an everlasting impression on the brain. But at Makerere the horse needs only to be taken to the water and it is its duty to drink.[97]

Most students found the transition difficult, especially the strain of attention during lectures, and blamed themselves for it. 'Our teachers experienced great difficulty in the beginning', one recalled. 'Everything was very new and mysterious to us but obstacles were overcome and they got used to the limits of our ability to understand.'[98] Examinations were taken almost every year. In addition to written papers, medical students took oral and clinical examinations, which some probably found especially stressful. They also had to pass every paper taken. Any paper they failed had to be retaken and passed the following year. If they failed more than one paper they might have to repeat the whole year, initially at their own expense, or discontinue entirely – a practice which caused much discontent when introduced in 1933.[99] Even the cleverest students often failed at some stage. Okwemba, for example, repeated his entire third year before passing his final examinations brilliantly.

Makerere in the 1930s was a spartan place. The food was worse than at some boarding schools.[100] Students slept in dormitories. There was no proper library. Electricity was installed in 1938. Tomblings's regime included uniforms (with caps) 'worn *at all times*', prefects (known to students as police), fagging, compulsory games, physical training at 6.30 a.m. under the Principal's leadership, and a daily schedule ordered from reveille at 6.15 a.m. to lights-out at 10.15 p.m. 'Breaches of discipline are usually punished by defaulters' drills or some form of extra "fatigue" in connection with food distribution or clearing-up of the dining-hall. Corporal punishment is in the hands of the Principal only and is used seldom and only in cases where example is needed.'[101] There was delight when Turner decided 'to help our students to live less as schoolboys and more as self-directing young men':[102] '"No Prefects, no roll-calls, no Prep. bells, P.T. voluntary, to choose our own rulers, why, gentlemen we are in for a heaven on earth!" And the students danced late into the night on the strumming of Guitars and Banjos.'[103] The revolution affected medical students less than others, not only because the

Medical School was a more adult environment but also because its students were notoriously dedicated to 'digging', as private study was known, and took a relatively small part in social life once their pre-clinical course began. There were exceptions. Samson Kisekka was Head Prefect of Makerere and played football for Uganda at a time when Makerere dominated sporting life. But medics were generally noted for studiousness.

They were indeed a picked group. If entering Makerere was difficult, entering the medical course after two years of basic science was even harder. 'To get in you had to be a genius or very lucky', one recalled.[104] Students could choose the course they preferred, a right which the College defended vigilantly against authoritarian officials. But admissions to medicine were limited. Only about half the applicants were generally admitted, and only about 80 per cent of those completed the course successfully.[105] The School naturally tried to pick the best, relegating the rest to train as teachers or agricultural or veterinary officers. Failure to enter medicine embittered some men for life and led one to commit suicide after telling a friend 'that he had no other alternative in life and that he did not think he would go home this time . . . and that his being refused entry into the medical school was the greatest blow he had ever met'.[106]

East African medical students were, first, medical students, and a modern medical education is an extraordinarily rigorous socialisation which doctors often see as a *rite de passage*, a shared, unique experience separating them from laymen. 'A properly and fully qualified doctor', the elderly Samson Kisekka later told a student gathering, 'has a kind of bondage with the medical profession which is also similar to the bondage that is declared by a clergy at a marriage ceremony'.[107] The first thing to learn was how to be a medical student. This meant, first, mastering a potentially limitless quantity of factual information and technical terms amounting almost to a new language. (Medical students are said to learn at least 10,000 new words.[108]) 'Reviewing our medical training', Simon Senkubuge recalled,

> I must say that colleagues and I wrestled often very sorrowfully with the hard subjects. We found the subjects often boring and the work a very disagreeable necessity; our minds were sometimes in distress and we expected nothing in particular from the future.[109]

At Mulago, moreover, much learning took place in what was almost a pauper hospital, where patients were washed and their heads shaved on admission, bedsteads were flamed with blowlamps once a week, 'the confusion and noise are such as to make the task of diagnosis most difficult, while clinical instruction to students has become almost impossible', and dishonesty and corruption were not only common among the nursing and menial staff[110] but might tempt the student himself: in 1947 one was expelled during his final year for giving illegal injections and prescriptions,[111] following which a course in medical ethics was instituted. Learning to be a medical student meant a new intensity of work, with only two weeks' holiday a year during the clinical period. It meant a new weight of responsibility, as in the practice of summoning the student on night duty to make an initial examination and diagnosis before the Medical Officer arrived.[112] It meant a continuous struggle to gather the information and experience without which the student knew that he could not handle his future cases. 'As a medical student advances in his studies', one wrote in 1940:

> he gradually comes to realise, partly from practical experience, but mainly from instruction by his tutors, that although Medicine is a profession on which much has been written in books, a person can never become a doctor however much he reads his books. A student of Medicine has to see patients with his own eyes and touch them with his own hands if ever he is going to be a doctor.[113]

One Mulago teacher was remembered for dragging students out of the library to learn 'properly' in the wards. This was the British tradition of medical education, especially among surgeons: 'What I read – I forget; what I see – I remember; what I do – I know.' They quoted the dictum repeatedly.[114]

In other continents, the most traumatic parts of the medical *rite de passage* were witnessing grave injury and disease, attending autopsies, operating on living animals, and especially dissecting a cadaver in the anatomy laboratory. Not only did this bring home the reality of death, as Adrien Atiman had found, but it revealed to students the immense intricacy of the human body, it taught them to separate their objectivity from their emotions, and, because only medical professionals could legally perform such actions, it set them apart from other people.[115] Unfortunately, there is no record of student response to this experience at Mulago during this period. There is evidence that anatomy was the 'make or break' subject it has been elsewhere. Until the late 1920s it was taught from models, including one female model thoughtfully painted black, but facilities for dissection were available from 1929 and there were plenty of unclaimed bodies to dissect, although precautions were needed against suspicions of cannibalism and sorcery.[116] By the early 1950s the medical course required each student to attend and perform post-mortems and to 'have dissected the whole body at least once to the satisfaction of his teacher'.[117] It is clear also, as Owen wrote in 1933, that

> Students enjoy greater opportunities for acquiring practical experience than do those in Great Britain. Both before and after qualification, in the field of surgery

alone, they perform a great many operations such as circumcisions, curettage of ulcers, skin grafts, passing of bougies and catheters and give many anaesthetics. They also assist at major operations and even perform a few under supervision. In emergencies and when a Medical Officer is not available, they should be able to undertake such surgical work as amputations of limbs, operations for the relief of impassable stricture and extravasation of urine, the application of obstetric forceps and should make a good attempt to deal with cases of strangulated hernia.[118]

This may have reduced the trauma surrounding dissection and autopsy, as also may the fact that most students came from rural homes where both human death and the slaughter and butchering of animals were commonplace. The sources do not dramatise the anatomy laboratory,[119] but there is one later account:

One cannot forget his or her first few days in a medical school when he had to among other things come into contact with dead bodies or what we call cadaver in medical terms. I will not forget my first day in the Nairobi Medical School. We were a big class of 105 students dressed in our white coats and I felt great to have joined a medical school and I already felt like a doctor. But this feeling was not to last long. That morning we were given a lecture by our anatomy Professor. At 2 p.m. we were asked to go to the dissection room the site [sic] of cadavers rapped [sic] in polythene bags sent us cold. There were some people who were seeing cadavers for the first time. The lecturer who was taking us that day was so gentle that he said no word except simply asked us to open the first page of our dissection manual which read 'incise the skin over the gluteous maximus and . . .' What a start it was.[120]

An additional problem for medical students was that their work brought them into closer relationship with Europeans than other East Africans of the time. The relationship was not very close. 'Social intimacy between students and lecturers is neither encouraged nor discouraged', the Principal of the Medical School, J.P. Mitchell, explained in 1939. 'Excepting on occasions of festivity and celebration they do not usually mix. It is embarrassing to both, not because of either social or racial distinctions but purely because of their different interests in life.'[121] When the Parliamentary Secretary for the Colonies visited Mulago in 1946, he found tea served in separate rooms for Europeans and Africans, and took his with the latter.[122] In the wards and lecture rooms, however, interaction was inevitably close. Arthur Williams, later Dean of the Medical School, recalled that dealings with students and assistants during the 1930s 'were friendly enough — how different from the 50s and 60s!'[123] At best the relationship was probably paternalistic. Mitchell himself, who was much respected, was said never to have passed on a negative report about a former student and gave each a set of medical textbooks for reference during his future career, expecting them to repay him in instalments, which by his own account they always did.[124] Yet some Mulago doctors openly loathed medical students,[125] and there were contested relationships with

European sisters and Indian Sub-Assistant Surgeons, all jostling for authority within the wards. By the later 1940s relations were bad. The medical student, one wrote in 1946,

> is not on good terms with his European and Asian master. They control everything. They are at every road and path to wealth, health and happiness. They have him at a distance . . . He is black and that is enough to seal his fate.[126]

The surviving records suggest an intellectual, political, and racial awakening among Makerere's students, including its medical students, during the later 1930s. This may be an optical illusion, for College magazines began at that time, and if there was an awakening, the reasons for it are unclear. The de la Warr report may have been one. Another may have been international events, especially the Italian invasion of Ethiopia, which received great prominence in the Luganda press. Continuing discontent that the government obstructed study abroad was a third possible reason, while a fourth may have been the return of Ugandans educated in America, notably Balamu Mukasa, who had studied at Yale and took a teaching post at Makerere, Ernest Kalibala, who in 1935 opened the independent Aggrey Memorial School as a seedbed of radical ideas, and the arrogant and clever Akiki Nyabongo, who returned from Lincoln and Oxford Universities in December 1937 in the company of a Trinidadian doctor, H.A. Beckford, who set up private practice in Kampala.[127] In April 1938 Nyabongo published a bitter attack on the Medical School:

> There are two pseudo-Medical Schools. Yaba in Nigeria and Mulago in Uganda. These two places are a disgrace to the medical profession, and an insult to the intelligence of the civilised world. It is criminal to foist such places upon the African people. Three hundred years ago the training given there might have been considered adequate. No one could consider them adequate to-day. The men turned out therefrom are not permitted to prescribe for Europeans. That would be too dangerous. They are only allowed to experiment on their fellow.[128]

This denunciation may have expressed views circulating among students, but it came too late to awaken them.

The published evidence shows that student thinking in the later 1930s included much interest in 'the once-African Negroes now in the New World' and rejection of the ideal of racial collaboration fostered by liberal Europeans. Christianity retained a powerful hold, although the Protestant Chaplain noted in 1948 that students tended to abandon chapel attendance when they entered professional courses like medicine.[129] The importance of education remained a central conviction, along with the duty of educated men to provide leadership: 'The populace, backward as they are, are looking forward for leaders from Makerere.'[130] But there was also a new social awareness. In April 1938, for example, a medical student, Sam

Mukasa, published a remarkable study of the Wandegeya slum at the foot of Makerere Hill:

The houses were in a pitiful condition; some were at such an angle that they seemed to defy the learned Newton . . . The inside of them was dark and the floor full of holes. The rubbish was thrown away just anywhere and in advanced stages of decomposition smelt horribly . . . Altogether life, in these places, seemed hard indeed. He knew that it must look more cruel to them because they were so near the people that were far better off; and yet these people, with all their learning, never even took a step to help their wretched neighbours by teaching them even the simple principles of Hygiene . . .

After he had thought out that plan he put on his cap and went out to see how these people spent their leisure time after work. He found most of them sitting glumly by the doors of their huts . . . Others . . . indulged in drink . . . Thc urchins were dirty, ill-clothed and not cared for . . .

The women represented their sex at its lowest . . . They submit to the unquestioned lordship of their husbands . . . They submit as many as four of them to have one husband and to be treated like properties.[131]

The most striking feature of the medical students' thinking at this time was interest in indigenous medicine. It coincided with sympathetic articles in the Swahili press, but they were written by politicians rather than modern medical workers. The sympathy certainly did not reach the students from their teachers, who were unrelievedly hostile. Yet in 1936 Richard Kafamba and M.M. Wabunoha read papers describing indigenous surgical methods to the Makerere Scientific Society,[132] while the most interesting contribution was a talk on indigenous medicine by the clergyman's son, A.K. Kibaya, in which he saw it as a distinctive African contribution to world medicine:

I am told that long ago people used to cure many diseases and I quite agree. Then one might ask, 'Are those people still curing diseases by the same methods as they used a long time ago?' The answer is in the negative. As far as I know the native doctors seem to have lost the ambition to improve in native medicine. There is stagnation in that branch of science and the doctors are rare . . . When a man has no children then there is the end of everything. The theory he had perishes . . .

So I put it before you young men to try and advise your relatives about this subject. Science does not become old when there are young men who always spend their time in seeking for the unknown and that is what we should do at Makerere. Native medicine ought to be revised and improved so that it may suit the changing circumstances

If any of you happens to know a man with a collection of drugs it is time for you to advise him to pass the knowledge on to other native doctors who will record the list. That is how science has been built up by people who started at the very bottom. If you do so, I am sure that the time will come when we shall have Committee meetings of native doctors and chemists and perhaps we shall take part in the medical science of the world.[133]

African Assistant Medical Officers

Triumphant in his final examination, the medical student still faced a year or two of apprenticeship as a hospital intern. By tradition this was an especially stressful period when the young practitioner lived in or close to the hospital, sometimes slept in the wards, was almost permanently on call, and was at everyone's disposal, although he might come to look back on it as invaluable experience. In East Africa internship was the more demanding because it was served in an overcrowded, frenetic, and sometimes filthy hospital like Sewa Haji.[134] At the same time interns often faced a second challenge: marriage. Few seem to have married while at Makerere – they were probably too busy and too poor – but many took wives within two or three years of qualifying: generally, it would appear, former schoolgirls – by the 1950s it would be nurses – for whom, as Samson Kisekka's wife remembered, 'getting married to a man who was a doctor by profession was prestigious'.[135] Probably most practitioners married within their ethnic group, although there were exceptions: Francis Mwaisela married a girl brought up in Jamaica. The classic pattern was perhaps A.K. Kibaya's marriage in Namirembe Cathedral in January 1942: the bride in white, a matron of honour, six flower girls, a colleague (Kisekka) as witness, a reception filling Makerere's main hall, four days' honeymoon in a friend's house, and then to Kibaya's distant station at Gulu.[136] Large families were common: Kisekka had fifteen children, Y.M.K. Musoke nineteen, E.S. Lubulwa fourteen, Peter Muganwa at least thirteen.[137] Ivan Kadama had twenty-three by three wives,[138] but polygyny seems to have been rare. Within a few years of marriage the practitioner might also care for children of relatives and probably support aging parents. Not surprisingly, therefore, his other pressing problems were pay and status. The first Makerere-trained practitioners to qualify, in 1927, became Senior Native Medical Assistants, renamed Senior African Medical Assistants in 1931 and African Assistant Medical Officers in 1939. They were not registered doctors and resented some Europeans' refusal to address them by that title, although Africans commonly used it (and for many less qualified medical workers) and the vernacular press adopted it during the 1940s.[139] The first SNMAs received a certificate, but their successors in the early 1940s refused it 'because we think it does not connote the real Medical Educational Status we have reached',[140] so that a diploma was substituted. The khaki uniform and helmet issued to SNMAs survived until 1949. Starting pay in 1928 was Shs.130 a month, increasing each year by Shs.10 a month. By 1942 the starting level had risen to Shs.180, but there was no major change until 1946, when pay roughly doubled. Indian Sub-Assistant Surgeons earned between two and three times as much during the 1930s and European Medical Officers about six times as much.[141] SNMAs appear initially to have accepted these differentials quietly, but after 1937, when de la Warr declared them better qualified than Sub-Assistant Surgeons, discontent mounted.

Of the first three SNMAs to enter service in 1928, one remained at Mulago to teach medical attendants and the others replaced Sub-Assistant Surgeons in charge of small dispensaries. Such was the authorities' lack of confidence that each was required, when treating a non-African, to show the patient a circular absolving the government from any liability for the treatment.[142] This nervousness was soon justified. During 1929 Yakobo Baziwane was sentenced to two years' imprisonment and dismissed from the service for breach of trust and acceptance of illicit fees. He was reinstated on release from prison to continue a long and chequered career, retiring in 1950 on grounds of old age but still working at Masaka Hospital twenty-four years later.[143] Dionysius Bamundaga avoided trouble for another year until he was severely reprimanded in 1930 for illicit sale of drugs, overcharging for injections, and extortion. After further repeated conflict he resigned in 1952, was twice convicted of failing to record the issue of dangerous drugs, was refused employment in 1962 'due to old age and debility', and died sixteen years later while still in private practice.[144] The third of the '3 Bs', Antonio Bamugye, had a briefer and smoother career, despite or because of a fondness for alcohol, and spent twenty-four years of honourable service at almost every medical institution in the country before retiring in 1952 and dying in 1964.[145]

If race presented difficulties in employing SNMAs in Uganda, the problem was more acute in Tanganyika and even worse in Kenya. The solution was to post them to remote medical facilities, preferably financed by native authorities, where there were virtually no Europeans or Indians. When Jason Likimani was sent to care for his own people at Narok in the Maasai Reserve in 1950, both the European sister and the Goan clerk were first removed from the hospital.[146] Tanganyika largely rotated its Makerere trained staff around a circuit of small hospitals like Nzega, Maswa, Biharamulo, Sumbawanga, and Songea. Uganda's problem was less acute, but its practitioners spent their first ten or fifteen years of service shuttling between small outlying hospitals. Between 1946 and 1950 N.O.P. Edyegu – the first Itesot to qualify in medicine – served in Karamoja, Soroti, Kaberamaido, Serere, Moroto, Gulu, and Arua.[147]

The joys and sorrows of the new practitioner are best followed in the career of Joseph Mutahangarwa, the first Tanganyikan to complete Makerere's medical course. When he arrived in Dar es Salaam in 1940 to serve his internship at Sewa Haji, Mutahangarwa was already thirty-five years old, having joined the Medical Department as a dispenser in 1928 and won golden opinions. He had experienced great difficulty in passing

Makerere's examinations and rumour had it that he would have failed if the Tanganyika Government had not insisted on a return for its money.[148] Nevertheless, he was feted by the Medical Department and the African community, for whom his gazetting as AAMO 'will be recorded indelibly in white and black in our history'.[149] His work at Sewa Haji was highly regarded; in 1942 he performed the hospital's first major all-African operation.[150] But Mutahangarwa was in financial trouble. He was naturally anxious to marry, he was both a professional man and a Haya prince who felt obliged to return European hospitality, and he was being paid exactly Shs.40 a month more than he had earned as a dispenser seven years earlier. He was soon heavily in debt.[151] Mutahangarwa himself and the Swahili press protested bitterly:

> In the draft estimates, the first African Assistant Medical Officer appears after the Sub-Assistant Surgeons. Who is senior: the SUB or the ASSISTANT? It would be interesting to know. If on the side of pay, this Assistant is contained twice in a Sub-Assistant Surgeon, then the more appropriate title for him would appear to be 3rd Grade African Dispenser.[152]

In 1942 Mutahangarwa was posted to Shanwa, a remote station south of Lake Victoria with no railway or telegraph and often cut off during the rains. 'This is one of those unfortunate "hybrid" hospitals', it was explained, 'with wards in temporary materials provided by the generosity of the local authority'.[153] Mutahangarwa, however, was understandably proud. 'I took over the administration of this department from Dr Y.A. Haidri M.B.B.S. on the 26th April 1943', he wrote. 'This is the first appointment of African Assistant Medical Officer to be in charge of a station in the Territory. The hospital is now being run by African Staff only.'[154] He found, however, that he had inherited a crisis. An epidemic of cerebro-spinal meningitis, one of the most acute and fatal of East African diseases, had broken out during 1942. 'The peak of the heights is in September where the figure reached 152 patients', Mutahangarwa reported at the end of 1943:

> A temporary C.S.M. Camp was elected at Kidema about 15 miles from Shanwa. Quarantine measures have been vigorously applied . . .
>
> I visited all the dispensaries, with the exception of Kimali, each at least twice and the work of combating the scourge was everywhere satisfactory.
>
> The total number of C.S.M. cases for this year is 692 with 109 Deaths.[155]

Kimali was far away near the arid shore of Lake Eyasi and Mutahangarwa, with no transport, had to cadge lifts in order to visit dispensaries.[156] The CSM epidemic continued throughout his three-and-a-half years at Shanwa, although cases and deaths steadily decreased, which he attributed 'to the fact that the people have now realised the benefit of bringing their sick ones to hospitals at once for proper treatment instead of hiding them in their homes to die miserably and spread infection'.[157] During 1944, however, it was supplemented by a smallpox epidemic, initially mild but developing during 1945 into more fatal strains which spread along the cattle trails crossing the district. Mutahangarwa organised vaccination in the Shanwa area but, hamstrung by lack of transport, had to call for assistance in outlying areas. The epidemic peaked between August and October, after which Mutahangarwa was able to go home on leave. Some 86,604 people were vaccinated in the district during 1945.[158]

Meanwhile Mutahangarwa was also running a thirty-eight-bed hospital and outpatient clinic. During 1943 it had 715 inpatients, 54 of whom died, whereas in the previous year the Indian Sub-Assistant Surgeon had treated 386 inpatients, with 19 deaths. 'Work done at this hospital during the year has doubled in all respects', Mutahangarwa reported. 'This may be attributed to the fact that the natives are gradually realising the benefit of giving Medical Education to the Africans. Several patients have come to this hospital from neighbouring districts for surgical treatment.'[159] In 1944 there was a further increase to 846 inpatients and 126 operations, including 26 hydroceles, 19 hernias, and 15 fractures, along with three amputations, a malignant tumour, and an appendectomy. During the same three years from 1942 to 1944, however, the outpatients numbered 12,843, 11,208, and 9,731, which Mutahangarwa blamed on restrictions on movement imposed to check epidemics.[160] The chief complaints treated were scabies, bilharzia, filarial infections, malaria, and venereal diseases. He paid thirty visits to dispensaries during 1944.

Mutahangarwa's most inventive activity at Shanwa was an experiment in cooperation with indigenous medicine, probably the only one attempted in East Africa between the First World War and independence. He had been at Makerere during the revival of interest in indigenous medicine there, but had not shown much enthusiasm,[161] and it is not clear whether the experiment was his idea or was devised by European officials. Pulmonary tuberculosis was spreading in Sukumaland and the Medical Department could do little about it. Some local healers, however, had great reputations for treating it with herbs. Mutahangarwa took three confirmed TB cases into his hospital. One had standard treatment, while two reputed healers were paid to treat the others with what a European Medical Officer called 'a decoction of which the principle ingredient was the root of a plant called mpogoro bongole in Kisukuma. It had other ingredients never disclosed and was fermented, and we were never able to get it analysed. It certainly had a kick in it, the patients sometimes went into convulsions after a dose.'[162] The patients were regularly subjected to X-ray and laboratory tests. Mutahangarwa was initially enthusiastic. 'So far there are two cases who were T.B. positive and after treatment sputum negative on several occasions and their general condition much improved', he reported early in 1945.[163] Two years later, however, his relative and successor at Shanwa, Raymond Kafamba, explained that 'the famous Anti tuberculosis experiment by the use of unidentified native shrubs started by A.M.O. Joseph like many other experiments, failed to achieve its objects and this year saw it rapidly dwindle into oblivion'.[164]

Despite Mutahangarwa's initial pride and optimism, his years at Shanwa were probably unhappy. He was very isolated, although a second AAMO, 'Pim' Ibreck (the son of a German settler and an African mother), was sent to work with him. He was drinking heavily. He was poor at paperwork and was pestered by unsympathetic bureaucrats in Mwanza. And his financial worries grew:

> I have been during these long and trying years endeavouring to carry on with my present meagre pay. I have worked to the best of my ability and I have realised the importance of my profession. I am now 38 years old, a man with family, and must look after the education of my children. I am afraid I cannot do this with the present scale of salary lest I incur debts which I shall be unable to defray.
>
> I request, therefore, that either of the following should be granted me:
> a. that I should be put on Staff Grade which is Shs.400/- per month;
> b. that I should be transferred to Native Administration if I can be paid better there;
> c. that I should be allowed to run my own dispensary.
>
> Hoping in each case to do service to my people in my present professional capacity please.[165]

Government gave him another twenty shillings a month. In September 1946 he was posted elsewhere and Shanwa was soon reoccupied by a Sub-Assistant Surgeon. In 1951 Mutahangarwa took the first opportunity to quit government service for private practice.

Of Mutahangarwa's Tanganyikan contemporaries, the most gifted was Francis Mwaisela. The son of a hospital worker at the northern end of Lake Nyasa, he had a brilliant career at Makerere before undergoing the normal initiation at Sewa Haji. Eager to marry his Jamaican-raised fiancée, he complained bitterly in 1943 that his salary of Shs.160 a month could barely support even a bachelor, although the budget he submitted allocated twenty-seven of those shillings to cigarettes and thirty to games and entertainments. 'The general out look at present as far as my life is concerned is very gloomy', he protested:

> I have been brought up to such a level in life that I can neither cope up with my own peoples life, nor that of a civilized man. To get married to a girl of any reasonable standard, for instance, in order that I should maintain that standard of education I enjoyed at School, is literally to commit suicide.[166]

These grievances were never satisfied, but in 1944 Mwaisela was posted to Nzega, a station much like Shanwa with a dilapidated forty-six-bed hospital built twenty years earlier by the Native Administration. He married his fiancée, and there, like so many vigorous young doctors at their first station, Mwaisela flourished. He toured dispensaries, he helped the African midwife who ran the busy maternity clinic, he handled 723 inpatients and 14,010 outpatients during 1947, treating them for syphilis and malaria, constipation and ulcers, anaemia and anthrax.[167] He was centre-half of the football team and president of the Social Welfare Centre, which he insisted on making a place of education: 'knitting socks or sweaters alone is not enough'.[168] The Swahili press published a string of letters from Nzega thanking the government for sending him. The local Arab and Indian communities, who had initially denounced his appointment, came to welcome it. European officials counted him as not only a colleague but a friend, a rare occurrence at that time.[169] In 1948 he was one of the first East Africans to study medicine in Britain, taking the Diploma in Public Health at Wolverhampton. Then he returned to Nzega, and there, in 1951, he was drowned while shooting, apparently when trying to save an Indian child.[170] His death robbed Tanganyika of a man who would surely have been among its leaders at independence. But Nzega produced, in Aloysius Nhonoli, the country's most distinguished physician of the next generation.

Most medical work was not of this pioneering type. Among Makerere's outstanding early graduates was Bartholomewo Nvule, who spent his career as a clinician, doing the routine work of district hospitals while the European Medical Officer undertook the touring and administration.[171] But whatever his medical role, the AAMO was expected and aspired to be a paragon of modernity. Mutahangarwa was 'proud to say that he has taught his children English from the beginning'.[172] Visiting a hospital in distant Moyo in 1938, Sir Philip Mitchell noted it as 'clean and apparently well run. In charge of an S.A.M.A. called Kalibala a Muganda and an excellent chap. I went without any warning into his house and found it spotless, altho' his wife was away in Kampala. They really are a remarkable product.'[173] Housing was an enduring grievance for African practitioners. Because they needed to live near their hospitals but were transferred every year or two, they depended on departmental housing. This was graded by race and the African quarters were not designed for professional men with six children: 'no indoor sanitations or water supply, badly lit because of bad windows and no ceiling. There were no house boys' quarters and they were supposed to stay in the same houses with the graduates.'[174] To be a paragon of modernity in these circumstances was hard indeed, but men like Mwaisela nevertheless led the tiny groups of educated Africans who clustered at district headquarters. 'I was always happy if there was a school nearby and I could talk to the teachers', one recalled.[175] While working at Shanwa, Mutahangarwa was virtually *ex officio* president of Maswa Victory Club, confined to government servants with at least five years of education. In Uganda the AAMO would often be president of the local Old Budonians Club or, outside Buganda itself, the Baganda Association.[176] Yet there was often tension between these elite coteries and the surrounding population, especially in Uganda where there was no *lingua franca*. In addition to his native Luganda, Eria Babumba learned Runyankole, Runyoro, Rutoro, Rukiga, and some Lusoga and Luo by the end of his medical career.[177] Communities preferred a native son as their medical officer. In 1945, for example, Massai local councillors asked for Jason Likimani's appointment to Kajiado.[178] For the practitioner, service in his own district presented problems, especially the demands of relatives, but Makerere men nevertheless preferred to work there, especially if they were Ganda for whom Mengo was the centre of civilisation. They devoted much energy to avoiding up-country postings, generally with little success. Each prodigal son from a remote station was welcomed by the Luganda press as he returned on leave to the capital for a busy round of visiting. After the Second World War, as salaries rose quite quickly, many AAMOs acquired motor cars.

By the later 1940s medical graduates had become the elite of the elite. They were still relatively junior civil servants, but they were professional men, often in their late thirties or early forties, with growing families and many social contacts. They were invited to tea at Government House, became the first African members of official boards, served on the committees of multi-racial discussion groups, become governors of their old schools, or arranged splendid funerals for their parents. They quite suddenly came into demand as lecturers on public health issues related to concern about Buganda's apparently stagnating population. Sebastiano Kyewalyanga, for example, spoke on 'the advantage of hospitals and doctors', the care of babies, and how Ganda could achieve better health, stressing regular breastfeeding, hygiene, nutrition, better housing, the advantages of modern medical aid, the need 'to abandon the local way of life and adopt the British or white man's way of life', and the danger of indigenous medicines, for 'it is true that not all herbs are bad but the production and prescriptions in right quantities are not yet grasped'.[179] This gospel of public health animated Z.M. Musoke to survey the informal settlements around Kampala and then serve as African Assistant Medical Officer of Health to the Buganda Government, where he undertook the herculean task of improving Mengo's sanitation.[180] He was succeeded in 1942 by George Sembeguya, who spent more than a decade as Mengo's Medical Officer of Health.

AAMOs in government service in Uganda were permitted private practice outside government hours and institutions. They suffered great pressure from patients who believed, in the traditional manner, that they knew what treatment they needed. 'Injection practice' was never the scandal that it became in West Africa, but many practitioners were tempted. In 1946 David Kiremerwa sent Uganda's Medical Department a cheque for Shs.500 'to compensate some of the departmental losses by me', explaining 'that I have been saved by God, and I am now, in other words, what is termed here in Uganda "Omulokole"', a member of the Revival movement. 'God has shown me my sins', he went on, 'and among them there are some which are departmental'.[181] Pressed for details, he replied:

> In my private practice on the Non-Africans, I used Government medicine and dressings plus my own drugs, injections and some dressings. On getting fees from them, I did not, in some cases, pay the revenue for the mixtures or lotions, or dressings as it should be . . .
>
> In case of the Natives I used to attend them and I used Government medicine, injections and dressings. I tried to hold clinics in a private locality . . . Whether the drug or injection was mine or of government, in some cases the doses were very small, the people, most of them, were ignorant and some poor, but I did not mind provided they paid me money. Really I was an 'injection-monger', and not a doctor for the poor and ignorant. All money I received was taken by me . . . When doing all these I thought no one would discover me and I forgot that God who sees every creature on the earth, was seeing me also. It is He who has caught and instructed me to report to you so as to give me the 'Eternal Life' in exchange. This free gift can be given to every body who believes in Jesus and becomes so simple.[182]

The Department returned the cheque and overlooked the matter. Kiremerwa remained a dedicated, humble, and deeply loved doctor for more than thirty years.

Not all made their peace. In 1951 another Omulokole, E.S. Lubulwa, was dismissed after being convicted of wilfully obstructing the police following an obscure incident in which his preaching band conflicted with a local chief. He appears never to have been employed again, except on temporary terms, and described himself thereafter as an evangelist, although he practised privately towards the end of his life.[183] The greatest tragedy among Makerere doctors was Arthur Okwemba, the impoverished young Kenyan who performed so brilliantly in the final examinations of 1941. According to the DMS, he

> went completely to the dogs from the very start. I do not think that was due to any unsympathetic treatment here . . . It was partly due I think to the fact there were no other Africans of his own 'class' for him to mix with. As a consequence he got mixed up with a bad lot of taxi drivers and so on. But I think it had started before we got him. I, or perhaps it was my successor had to discharge him in the end.[184]

Okwemba appears to have been murdered.[185] He was not the only practitioner to die suddenly. J.M. Siryegana, a young houseman, treated a plague victim at Mulago in 1936 and died two days later.[186] Medicine was a dangerous career. Kiremerwa survived blackwater fever, pneumonia, typhoid, peptic ulcer, hypertension, prostatic enlargement, and heart disease.[187] And if Okwemba was not alone in dying suddenly, nor was he the only doctor to 'go to the dogs'. By the mid-1950s at least six Makerere doctors had resigned or been dismissed chiefly as a result of alcohol,[188] usually remaining sadly on the fringes of the profession, seeking reinstatement or practising covertly. One practitioner had been dismissed for 'misconduct in a professional sense' so grave that no details of it have come to light. Another had gone mad.[189] Several had resigned, either to rural tranquility or in frustration at their permanent subordination. 'Every white man in those days, whatever his rank or intellectual capacity, considered himself superior to any black person', recalled Samson Kisekka, who resigned in 1948.[190] By then the entire service was rent by bitterness.

Tension had grown during the 1930s and was intensified by the outbreak of war, when, in contrast to 1914, not a single African doctor appears to have joined the forces. Sir Philip Mitchell noted during mobilisation on 30 August 1939 that the Ugandan authorities 'are having a disappointing response from Africans as medical personnel, mainly over pay, family allowances and gratuities, wh[ich] I hope will soon be cleared up'.[191] According to a probably exaggerated account by Kisekka's biographer:

> At the beginning of the Second World War . . . the government authorities ordered Uganda's African physicians to join the war. Dr Kisekka led the group that insisted that if they served, they be given rank equal to the White physicians who served. 'Since South African Whites had been involved in fighting, the British Ugandan government had no alternative but to give up the idea of recruiting African Ugandan physicians.'[192]

Whatever exactly happened, the war certainly embittered relations, rather than harmonising them as in 1914–18. With many Europeans away, AAMOs carried additional responsibility without better pay or status. Inflation – the *official* price of imported cloth in Uganda trebled between 1941 and 1945[193] – provoked protests among all groups of Africans, but governments refused to raise general pay levels significantly, lest they merely fuelled inflation, or to reward doctors specifically, lest they destabilised the whole civil service.

Another wartime development was that a few AAMOs in Uganda, and even fewer in Kenya, became involved in medical research and gained more responsible positions within major hospitals. The pioneer of research at Mulago was Trowell, whose chief interest was the protein deficiency disease, kwashiorkor, commonly identified in Uganda at that time, like so much else, with congenital syphilis.[194] The problem, as Trowell was later to explain, was that in the absence of sophisticated equipment 'I can never get a problem beyond its initial stages. I can't get it very far, as it gets so technical.'[195] From 1946 he was reinforced by the pathologist, J.N.P. Davies, whose discipline was crucial to research because it alone could identify internal conditions with reasonable certainty. He contributed to the kwashiorkor work, identified in 1948 a heart condition called endomyocardial fibrosis which opened a new field of investigation, and in 1954 launched a cancer registry which was to provide the basis for Makerere's most famous research.[196] Africans entered this research environment at an early stage, initially as auxiliaries to white doctors. The first was Erifazi Mukiibi-Mwanjale, who had qualified with distinction in every subject and was appointed in 1938, at the age of twenty-four, as assistant to the surgical specialist.[197] His success led in 1940 to the creation of a parallel post in medicine for Eria Muwazi, a man of thirty from Buganda who was to be a key figure in the growth of the medical profession before independence. Trowell, an outspoken paternalist, later said of Muwazi:

> Oh, he was a straight-forward Muganda, and had been to Budo, and Makerere, and then a medical student under me.
>
> But he showed considerable application, and I was very anxious then to get Africans on to research, or at least associating with us, and our names published together, even putting his name before mine in the occasional journal; because it seemed to me that this lifts them into quite a different plane vis-à-vis their own doctors, and also the odd European.[198]

Nevertheless, Trowell gave Muwazi his chance. In 1942 he was first author, with Trowell and R.S.F. Hennessey, of the first scientific paper to bear the name of an East African, a classification of seventy-one cases of liver disease at Mulago. 'The bulk of the work', it was stated, 'fell upon the African Assistant Medical Officer who prepared the first draft of the paper'. Muwazi had admitted and treated the cases, while Trowell had studied some and Hennessey had performed autopsies.[199] Two years later Muwazi and Trowell – with Trowell clearly in charge – published a similar classification of 269 neurological cases admitted to Mulago and its mental hospital, showing that 137 suffered from neurosyphilis, a complaint supposedly rare in the tropics.[200] In 1945 Trowell and Muwazi produced a singularly confusing paper on kwashiorkor which nevertheless showed that fewer than 10 per cent of affected infants had congenital syphilis.[201] In the next year Muwazi published his first paper as sole author describing a small but careful experiment to treat relapsing fever with the new miracle drug, penicillin, which did not work.[202] The last paper in the series, published jointly with Trowell and Davies in 1947, finally demolished the congenital syphilis theory of kwashiorkor by showing that only about 1 per cent of Ganda children, but 26 per cent of pregnant women, suffered from syphilis, whereas 'the kwashiorkor syndrome . . . is almost universal in babies in Kampala'. The authors wrote:

> The clinical examinations were made by one of the writers, E.M.K. Muwazi. Being himself a Muganda he has great advantage in taking detailed histories and in

appraising the significance of the various symptoms reported by the mothers. In the opinion of the writers this cannot be undertaken by a European, however skilled he may be in an African language and certainly not by interpretation as it is necessary to appreciate African idiom and thought. The main lines of the enquiry were decided in consultation, and then the bulk of the work was undertaken by one of us (E.M.K.M.) and continued during the absence on leave of the other (H.C.T.).[203]

It must have been especially satisfying to a Ganda – and an emerging nationalist – to demonstrate that kwashiorkor should not be attributed to a disease whose prevalence was seen as a slur. By this time Muwazi also had an important teaching role at Mulago as the senior African in the hospital, in effect a registrar.[204]

Other East Africans also published at this time. Before Davies went to Mulago he encouraged two AAMOs at Mbale, Kadama and Kibaya, to publish short articles on unusual cases with which he had assisted them.[205] In Nairobi, Arthur Mbuthia worked at the Orthopaedic Centre with W.H. Kirkaldy-Willis, an innovative surgeon and former missionary who became a world authority on diseases of the spine. Kirkaldy-Willis was eager to train African surgeons and encouraged Mbuthia to perform operations, chiefly for tuberculosis of bones and joints, while Charles Karau gave the anaesthetics. In 1946 and 1954 they published two accounts of these operations describing new techniques.[206] The first medical article published solely by a Kenyan African, in 1950, was a brief account by Wellington Aruwa, also from Makerere, of a rare case which he diagnosed as congenital relapsing fever.[207]

The irony was that this entry into research took place amidst bitterness and conflict. These originated from long-standing grievances, wartime strains, and a political crisis in Buganda caused by a power struggle between two factions. One, representing the modernising, Christian establishment, was led by Martin Luther Nsibirwa (Katikiro to 1941) and his ally Serwano Kulubya, supported the young Kabaka Mutesa II who had succeeded in 1939, and was closely allied with the British Government. The other, led by Nsibirwa's successor, a man of peasant origin named Samwiri Wamala, was traditionalist and populist, hostile to missionaries and government, backed rival candidates to Mutesa, and had much support among peasants, traders, and organic intellectuals.[208] Medical men were first drawn into this conflict in 1944 when the British tried to remove Wamala on grounds of illness. The evidence is fragmentary and likely to remain so. Wamala consulted the young and brilliant Mukiibi-Mwanjale, who belonged to the Lugave (Pangolin) clan from which Wamala drew much support. Mukiibi apparently diagnosed neurosyphilis, which was what killed Wamala four years later. After some months a formal medical board considered Wamala's case. The members were Trowell, Arthur Williams, and Sebastiano Kyewalyanga. They heard Mukiibi's evidence, but Wamala refused the lumbar puncture needed to prove neurosyphilis, so, at the cautious Kyewalyanga's insistence, they declared only 'that there is a *serious* mental disorder and that the presence of neuro-syphilis cannot be excluded', so that Wamala was incapable of performing his duties.[209] Two months later he was obliged to take sick leave and then to resign. Mukiibi was now in great danger and wrote insisting that he had diagnosed not neurosyphilis but 'a mild anxiety state which led to some malnutrition' owing to overwork. According to another account, Mukiibi protested at the use of his clinical notes without his permission.[210] If he had previously been in danger from Wamala's supporters, he was now in danger from the government. It illustrated the risks which many East African doctors were to face during the next fifty years.

On 15 January 1945 strikes paralysed Kampala. At one level they were prompted by wage grievances arising from wartime inflation. At another they were used by Wamala's supporters to secure Kulubya's dismissal, lest he become Katikiro.[211] Most subordinate staff in Mulago's male wards walked out, demanding a 150 per cent wage increase and refusing to attend even emergency cases. Next day strikers entered the wards with sticks to force those working to leave, but were themselves chased away by European police officers and nurses.[212] At one point Mukiibi 'stood and appealed to the strikers not to drive away those who were caring for their own people – we had several badly injured rioters on that ward'.[213] Similar intimidation took place at several other hospitals. At Entebbe the long-serving Dionysius Bamundaga helped to persuade workers not to strike. 'Rioting and strikes have never occurred among hospital staffs', he reported telling them, '. . . leave rioting to other gatherings – if they get benefit therefrom, you will also get it automatically'.[214] The official enquiry blamed the riots on 'political agitators', but the collapse of order badly frightened the government and especially the Governor, Sir John Hall, who saw communists in every corner. Alarm intensified later in 1945 when Nsibirwa, who had been reinstated as Katikiro, was assassinated on the steps of Namirembe Cathedral.[215] Hall reorganised his Intelligence Department (under a former Game Warden) and launched a purge.[216] One of its targets was Mulago. The first victim was Mukiibi. The Senior Pathologist, who loathed AAMOs, reported hearing Mukiibi and a friend say of a man shot during the strike 'that this was wanton murder by the police, that deceased had no weapon'.[217] Shortly afterwards Mukiibi sought an interview with Hall at which, as the DMS recorded, 'it appeared that he was not unsympathetic with the leaders of the trouble'. Hall told him bluntly to stay out of politics.[218] Shortly afterwards Mukiibi, the best African surgeon at Mulago, was posted to Moyo on Uganda's furthest northern border, where he could not practise surgery, was kept under surveillance, suffered a mental breakdown, retired, and never recovered.[219] Attention then focused on Sam Mukasa, who was Wamala's son-in-law. The Medical Department resisted pressure to move him out of Buganda,[220] but it had no such compunction when Intelligence turned on Kagai Samba, who had charge of urogenital surgery at Mulago and had become a spokesman for civil service grievances. Mulago's Medical Superintendent described him as 'definitely politically inclined' and Intelligence identified his house as the meeting-place for leaders of the African staff who opposed government's plans to restructure the African civil service and were thought to be planning a strike in January 1947. On Christmas Day 1946 Hall ordered Samba's immediate posting to Kitgum, also on the northern border. He resigned instead.[221]

The investigation into Samba's activities had implicated many other Makerere practitioners. One informer claimed that 'Meetings are being held daily in the house of Dr Samba; usually at 1 p.m. AAMO Muwazi and Mukasa S. appear to be the leaders with Sambe [sic] . . . The objects of the meetings are to secure more pay.'[222] Another, more imaginative, reported meetings in a hospital clinic during the lunch hour and at night, together with suspicious visits by up-country doctors, the whole implicating Samba, Nfamba, Lulume, Ndugwa, Katumba, and Bamundaga.[223] Hall told the DMS to tell Mulago's African staff

> that Govt. is fully aware of what has been happening at Mulago recently and of the names of those who have attended these surreptitious meetings . . . He might speak on profesional standards and the supreme obligation of A.M.Os. and other medical staff to their patients, and say that . . . he has heard that some of them have been discussing a course of action which would be opposed to all medical ethics and would not only imperil their own careers but reflect the greatest discredit on all ranks of the African Medical Service in Uganda.[224]

The DMS did so, there was no strike (if indeed one was ever planned), the new and more generous terms of service were accepted, and nothing further resulted, although Intelligence kept watch on African medical staff until at least 1949.[225]

These events of 1945 and 1946 further soured the relationship between Makerere-trained practitioners and the colonial state and drew several AAMOs closer to Buganda's radicals, whose target was shifting from the Kabaka's Government to the British. But the events also showed African practitioners their vulnerability to the colonial state and the violence of African populism. This last point was vividly reinforced in 1949 when new disturbances struck Buganda. This time there were no hospital strikes, but suspicion nevertheless focused on Mulago. Muwazi, specifically, was reported to have paid suspicious visits to the prison ward where wounded demonstrators were admitted. But this was overborne by the fact that he was himself a victim of the riots:

> Information reached him [Muwazi] on the afternoon of the 26th April that his house had been destroyed by a rioting mob whereupon he became very emotional and demanded that the police should be asked to confirm the report and rescue his wife and family. I reported the incident to the Police who informed me of the occurrence of many similar cases and regretted it was impossible for them to afford protection to individuals in distress. Muwazi was under the impression he was a marked man and the rioters had every intention of 'getting' him. The next morning (27th) he with his wife and family, who had meanwhile rejoined him at Mulago, were packed in an ambulance and driven by Mr Hoyle to the Police Station, where I am told he demanded his rights as a private citizen for police protection, which of course, under the circumstances, were rejected . . . Even allowing for the condition of stress under which he was labouring, I do not think this sort of behaviour was entirely excusable.
>
> The above information is given in detail in case at some future date the integrity of this officer is questioned, as I have no doubt it will be.[226]

If indeed Muwazi was a marked man for the rioters, as he certainly was for the British, this was because his work in the children's ward and female outpatient clinic at Mulago created great fear among unsophisticated Ganda. 'A.M.O. Muwazi as said to kill children by taking blood', a Medical Officer reported. '. . . He is also said to facilitate the deliberate hysteriectomising of African women.'[227] Such rumours had existed throughout East Africa since modern medicine began.[228] They were probably spread deliberately by Buganda's populist leaders[229] and they surfaced in the heat of the riots. Europeans were said to have brought typhoid fever and sleeping sickness in bottles still to be found on islands in Lake Victoria, which was why Africans were forbidden to return to them. There were said to be separate drugs for Europeans and Africans. Post-mortems provided material for harmful drugs. Europeans drank the blood samples they took.[230] These rumours focused especially on George Sembeguya, the Assistant Medical Officer of Health in Mengo, whose sanitary duties had made him many enemies. He was said to spread typhoid by taking blood samples and giving TAB inoculations. He was severely beaten, his house was burned, and he and his family had to be rescued by the police.[231]

Nothing could have illustrated more vividly the ambivalent relationship between aspiring professionals and the state. It was both their enemy, blocking their aspirations, and their protector against the latent hostility of the unsophisticated. The ambiguity was to remain until independence, and beyond.

5 The pursuit of professional status

At the Makerere Medical School, technical training had fused with the most advanced education available in East Africa, attracting gifted students and giving status to their occupation. But in 1949 the status was not yet equal to that of European Medical Officers. It was not yet a professional status. The drive for professional standing took place during the 1950s and coincided with the growth of nationalism. Indeed, as Murray Last has written, 'The process of professionalisation became part of decolonisation.'[1] The doctors' career goals profited from wider nationalist pressure on colonial regimes. And through their role – in Uganda, their vanguard role – in public life and politics, doctors in turn contributed to the liberation of their countrymen.

Recognition

The spearhead of the doctors' drive for professional status was the Makerere Medical Graduates Association (MMGA). Its papers have not come to light and its origins are uncertain. The earliest surviving statements claimed that it was formed in April 1935 by 'some new energetic and enthusiastic young gentlemen' who included Eria Muwazi,[2] but the Medical School's historian described its formation as a response either to the de la Warr report of 1937 or to wartime grievances.[3] The sources disagree as to whether it was originally called the Medical Assistants' Association or the African Medical Association. By one account the association lapsed when Muwazi was posted away from Mulago, but revived in 1939. It certainly existed in 1943 as the Uganda African Medical Association,[4] and probably changed its name to the Makerere Medical Graduates Association between June 1949 and May 1950 in order to include non-Ugandans and, presumably, to stress the claim to be graduates.[5] Muwazi presided over it for much of the 1940s from his tutorial position at Mulago. In 1950 it claimed over sixty members among the seventy-nine Makerere practitioners in East Africa.[6]

The MMGA's first success was to press the authorities to implement in

1944 the long-promised conversion of Makerere's medical certificate into a diploma. In 1945 it probably inspired letters which reached the Ugandan press, the Fabian Colonial Bureau in London, and eventually the Colonial Office protesting that Makerere practitioners were not registered or allowed independent private practice.[7] In 1946 the Association memorialised the visiting Parliamentary Secretary for the Colonies, although with little evident effect.[8]

By 1949 the Association's members had four main concerns: the regularisation of their status, the right to private practice, their pay and conditions, and recognition of their qualifications by the General Medical Council. With regard to status, although many in practice served as doctors, they were still known as African Assistant Medical Officers and, although Africans commonly called them doctors, many Europeans refused to do so. Alexander Odonga remembered bitterly how, in the mid-1940s, 'A young English Nursing Sister who had just commenced work at Mulago Hospital called one of the graduates "doctor"; the specialist who was there almost shouted to the sister saying "He is A.M.O., not a doctor."'[9] Makerere's medical diploma did not entitle its holders to be registered as medical practitioners even in their own countries, a situation which the Colonial Secretary's Medical Adviser believed to be unique in the British Empire. Instead, AAMOs were licensed to practise medicine while in government service.[10]

From the late 1930s, licensed AAMOs in Uganda, like European Medical Officers and Indian Sub-Assistant Surgeons in government service, were allowed, as a privilege, to practise privately and to charge fees outside government hours and institutions.[11] Most probably took advantage of this, as Kiremerwa's confession suggests, and some probably made enough from it to show that full-time private practice might be economically viable, as the many Indian private practitioners demonstrated. Governments, however, were anxious to retain AAMOs to staff public institutions, especially in remote districts, and they also believed that many AAMOs could not be trusted to practise ethically outside government control.[12] Legislation therefore permitted Africans to practise privately outside government service only after they had retired, only if their service had been meritorious, and only if the Medical Board specifically licensed them as a privilege rather than a right. An AAMO who resigned before the retiring age – thereby forfeiting his pension rights – was not licensed for private practice, as Pim Ibreck discovered when he attempted it in 1946.[13] At that time no African was in independent private practice, but the issue was becoming urgent, not only because some AAMOs wished to resign but because others were nearing retirement and wanted to practise thereafter by right rather than European favour. The issue was raised in the House of Commons in 1946 and the Colonial Office pressed the East African governments to reconsider it, but all were opposed to change.[14] The Colonial Office returned to the issue in 1948, suggesting that, as in Nigeria, AAMOs should be able to enter private practice after five years' government service. This produced violent opposition from all the governments except Uganda, expressed most contemptuously by Kenya's Chief Native Commissioner:

> If the Makerere 'Diploma' was in fact equivalent to any registerable medical degree in England, no-one could have the slightest objection to Makerere 'diplomates' engaging in private practice. The diploma, of course, is not equivalent to any registered practitioner's qualification at home – particularly as the holder of it has had no ethical training, no tradition of service, no central body to control him, and would not be allowed in private practice anywhere where there were such traditions. But even so, it is proposed to pretend that the diploma is the same, and allow 'diplomates' to make a profit from the inarticulate African, and I have no doubt that the real good they would do would be far offset by all sorts of charlatanism.[15]

In Uganda, however, African practitioners were relatively numerous, had some political leverage, and were expected before long to exceed the numbers needed in government service. By lobbying members of the Legislative Council, the Uganda African Medical Association secured a new Uganda Medical Practitioners and Dentists Ordinance in 1949 which gave an AAMO the right to leave government service after ten years and then to be licensed for private practice provided the Medical Board considered him 'likely to be a responsible and skilful medical practitioner'.[16]

The third main issue for the MMGA was pay and conditions. The long-standing resentment which had inspired thoughts of strike action was to some extent mollified by pay increases late in 1946. David Kiremerwa, for example, saw his salary rise from £156 to £315 a year.[17] Anger intensified again in 1948, however, when the East African Salaries Commission – an exceptionally reactionary body – refused to relate the AAMOs' earnings to those of European Medical Officers, on the grounds that AAMOs were unqualified, and instead gave them a starting salary exactly half that of a European nursing sister. These terms deterred medical recruitment.[18]

The MMGA's fourth and guiding concern during the 1940s, however, was to secure GMC recognition of their qualifications. As the Asquith Commission observed, this 'has its roots more deeply in the opportunity for demonstrating intellectual equality than in the privileges of practice which registration confers',[19] although recognition also bore on all the Association's other aspirations. Many African practitioners thought, mistakenly, that Needham had predicted that GMC recognition could be secured in 1946. When Makerere requested a formal GMC visitation in 1949, the visitor chosen was Sir Henry Tidy, who had experience of medical schools in Egypt, Khartoum, and South Africa. For Makerere that was no advantage, for Tidy doubted the capacity of Africans to replace European doctors even in Sudan, where all students completing the medical course successfully were Muslim northerners.[20] His visitation of Makerere was cursory and devastating.[21] He drew attention to Needham's warning that Makerere would not find it easy to secure recognition and added that since that visit the Medical School had stagnated, largely because school standards and entrance levels were low. He thought that Mulago's staff/patient ratio was too low for a teaching hospital. He met representatives of the East African medical departments and recorded their negative view of Makerere's graduates:

> They gave willing testimony to the assistance received from Assistant Medical Officers acting under European supervision. But they were unanimously of opinion that the education traditions and ethical standards do not justify registration and the right of all Diplomates to practise without European supervision. Confidence can be reposed in a proportion after due observation and the right to practise can be granted in such instances by the present system of licences. It was the opinion that local registration when it is regarded as justifiable, should be a stage before recognition by the GMC.

Tidy gave Trowell the impression of thinking it an impertinence for Makerere even to have sought recognition.[22] Certainly, in later correspondence, Tidy claimed that since Makerere's diploma did not guarantee registration in Uganda, the GMC could not even consider granting registration in Britain, so that his visit had been a waste of time.[23] More important, Tidy reported that Makerere's diploma could *never* secure registration, because most of Mulago's patients suffered from typhoid fever, hookworm, kwashiorkor, pellagra, and other tropical diseases unsuitable to train a doctor to practise in Britain, which was all the GMC could grant. Eric Holmes thought this had some truth, but others said it was nonsense – 'Almost all the diseases of temperate climates occur in the tropics, and in addition specifically tropical disease'[24] – and it was a curious argument for an organisation which had recognised Indian qualifications for sixty years. Tidy, nevertheless, drew a damning conclusion:

> If the [General Medical] Council acts on this basis, recognition will be impracticable not only at the present time but also in the foreseeable future. I would emphasize that such a bar is independent of the standard of teaching, of the standard of learning, of the intelligence of the students and of nationality.
>
> If such be the decision of the Council, I would urge Makerere College to put aside the question of recognition. It has been a disturbing factor for many years. The belief that recognition lay, so to speak, just round the corner has been due to misapprehension in many quarters.[25]

He suggested instead that the Medical School should enter its best candidates for London degrees.

Tidy's report dismayed not only Makerere but the Colonial Office and even the GMC, whose imperial concerns caused it to evade the issue of recognising doctors trained on tropical material and focus instead on the fact that Makerere's diploma did not guarantee local registration.[26] MMGA members were equally angry that Tidy had not met them. They sent the GMC a memorandum to be considered with Tidy's report and asked that two MMGA members then in Britain, Muwazi and Ivan Kadama, should present their case. The two appear to have received their appointments too late to attend.[27] Whether the memorandum was considered is unclear, but it could scarcely have affected the decision, for it was written without full knowledge of Tidy's findings.[28] However, the Association had clearly been told his view that local registration was an essential precondition, so that the memorandum protested that 'a Makerere Graduate is denied his professional Right i.e. Local recognition of the Diploma with subsequent registration and practice', which 'would be a stepping stone to recognition by the General Medical Council'.[29] When the Colonial Secretary visited Mulago in 1951 the Association raised the issues again.[30]

The Colonial Secretary did not meet the MMGA in 1951 and it was perhaps at this point of frustration that the Association seriously considered suing Makerere for giving a false diploma which the government did not recognise, but could not find a lawyer to take up what was certainly a hopeless case. They did succeed in having the prefix 'African' dropped from their title as Assistant Medical Officers.[31] Behind the scenes, the Colonial Office was pressing the doctors' case on the East African governments, but negotiations had reached an impasse. 'To help the [GMC] President to bury the Tidy report', the GMC had to be persuaded to send another visitation, but it refused unless the East African governments first recognised the Makerere diploma for local registration.[32] The governments refused to do this until the GMC had assessed the diploma as worthy of local registration. Their grounds were that many Makerere practitioners had proved unsatisfactory. Of seventy-two licensed to practise in Uganda, so Governor Hall wrote in March 1951, two were dead, seven had been discharged, seven had resigned in circumstances under which only two could be thought registrable, and almost half of the fifty-six still in government service 'have at one time or another been adversely reported on in respect of their professional conduct'.[33] 'The grounds for adverse reporting are: reported for alcoholism 13; general irresponsibility 11; malpraxis (including illegal charging, seduction, false certification, professional negligence) 10; other defects (low standard of work, absence without leave, laziness, personality troubles, etc.) 20.'[34] As the argument grew more heated, so did the accusations: 'for example, opening up a patient's abdomen and then bringing in the relatives and demanding a sum of money before closing him up again.'[35] Eventually the GMC undertook to send a new visitation provided that the East African governments would state in advance that they would welcome a recommendation for local registration if it were made. Uganda agreed, while Kenya and Tanganyika replied that they would register such diploma-holders in a separate section of the medical register.[36]

The GMC visitation of 1951 was conducted by three experienced medical teachers who produced a thoroughly sensible report.[37] They were impressed by the Medical School and recommended that its diploma should entitle holders to local registration, with correspondingly better pay, higher status, and opportunities for promotion and postgraduate study. They emphatically denied that Mulago's clinical material was inadequate to train a doctor for GMC recognition: 'We are of the opinion that an intelligent student efficiently taught in Uganda would be at least as well qualified to practise medicine in the United Kingdom as a student trained in the United Kingdom would be qualified to practise in Uganda.' Yet they identified specific weaknesses: inadequate staffing, a lack of African staff of registrar grade, insufficient teaching of paediatrics, obstetrics and gynaecology, inadequate use of modern drugs, and a need to improve general 'therapeutic and diagnostic standards'. When these were remedied, 'in a few years' time', they believed inspection with a view to full GMC recognition would be possible.

Uganda now had a dynamic new governor, Sir Andrew Cohen, who demanded the report's urgent implementation, 'otherwise I am afraid that we are in for trouble'.[38] The Medical School drew up a list of improvements to meet GMC requirements, including a new Mulago Hospital – which they believed the visitation had taken for granted – with much autonomy from departmental control. The Medical Department vetoed autonomy, but the other plans went ahead, as did implementation of the rest of the report.[39] Local recognition of the Makerere diploma – renamed a Licentiateship in Medicine and Surgery – proved difficult to embody in law and was not enacted until 1953. The legislation provided that those who passed the Makerere Licentiateship after 1 December 1951 and served two years' internship should be registered as medical practitioners in East Africa. Such doctors were to undertake to serve government for five years after internship, although legal obstacles prevented this from being implemented. (At the insistence of European doctors, Kenya empowered its Medical Board to refuse to register a Licentiate who did not satisfy it.) Those who had secured Makerere medical qualifications before 1951 could qualify for registration either by appearing before a board of assessors for interview or oral examination and scrutiny of their career record, by passing a special examination, or by passing the current final examination at Makerere. All those registered would become Medical Officers (East Africa).[40] MMGA members resented this title, which underlined that their qualifications were only locally recognised. The Association also tried to stop its members taking the special examination, urging that it be replaced by a period of postgraduate training abroad, but the lure of registration and consequent higher pay was too strong, so that by May 1956 seventeen had secured registration by examination and eleven by interview.[41] Those refused included some older practitioners like Bamundaga, several with bad records, and those who had ceased regular practice. A number did not apply or, like Mutahangarwa, failed to attend the interview.[42]

Acceptance of the GMC's recommendations, however, meant delaying for another 'few years' an internationally recognised qualification. This was especially bitter because in 1954 the first Makerere students in other fields took London degrees under special relationship. The Medical School, publicly described as the College's leader in 1937, felt itself outpaced. Applications to read medicine declined sharply in the early 1950s, although they recovered thereafter.[43] The problem was that the GMC recognised an institution and *all* its graduates, so that it withheld recognition, in principle, until the weakest graduate was considered fit to practise in Britain. The pace was that of the slowest. This had long-term advantages in East Africa, ensuring that all its doctors had the same respected qualification, but it held back the abler students who could have taken university degrees and postgraduate qualifications. They were naturally bitter. Repeated complaints culminated in 1956 when Barnaba Kununka, an MMGA leader, moved in the Uganda Legislative Council that Makerere be requested to institute medical degrees:

> Surely, when you get two students coming up to Makerere for their courses, one taking medicine and one taking Arts, the one taking medicine receives a diploma after seven years of hard training plus two of internship, which makes nine years, to qualify for L.M.S., and yet it takes his contemporary four years to get a degree in Arts. Surely nine years for a diploma is absurd.[44]

'His friend puts on his gown', Muwazi added, 'and the medical graduate has nothing to put on'.[45] After a debate marked by mutual incomprehension, with government speakers unable to understand why this mattered so much to Kununka, and his supporters unable to grasp the long-term arguments against them, the matter had to be settled by Cohen's casting vote against the motion.[46]

Although the Medical School had few students during the 1940s and early 1950s, they were more diverse than before, breaking the long Ganda domination. Of 141 students who secured medical qualifications between 1952 and 1962, only 66 were Ugandans, together with 43 Kenyans, 27

Tanganyikans, 4 Zanzibaris, and 1 Nyasalander. The first significant number of Asian students entered Makerere in 1952; by 1959–60 they were 69 in a student body of 881.[47] In 1953 the Medical School admitted its first woman, Josephine Namboze, the daughter of a Catholic teacher at the great Nsambya mission station; she was to graduate in 1959 as East Africa's first African woman doctor.[48] Clinical study still predominated, for despite a growing concern with preventive and community work – in 1959 a health centre was opened at Kasangati, outside Kampala, to introduce students to rural medicine – nevertheless clinical research was so exciting and clinical medicine was so absorbing to learn that the school concentrated on them.[49] Clinical medicine, surgery, and anatomy attracted the ablest students, notably Wilbert Chagula, a Tanganyikan who taught anatomy briefly before leaving for study in Britain.

Study abroad – the goal of most ambitious students in the 1950s – had in fact begun twenty years earlier, when Benjamin Kaggwa, a son of the Mukwenda (a leading Ganda chief), had gone to the United States to study at Lincoln, Columbia, and New York University where he secured the MD degree, but the Uganda Government refused to recognise his American qualifications and he returned to Uganda only late in his life.[50] By contrast, Albert Kaggwa, who was no relation of Benjamin but the youngest son of Sir Apolo Kaggwa, went to Britain in 1927 at the age of eight, qualified in London, practised in the East End, married a British wife, served with the British army in Burma, and returned to Uganda in 1951 as a District Medical Officer.[51] By 1945 both the Makerere authorities and the Uganda Medical Department favoured some AAMOs undertaking further study in Britain.[52] The Medical School approached several British institutions during 1946, but most were full of ex-soldiers and Makerere's practitioners did not have the recognised qualification generally needed for admission to postgraduate courses. However, a new and ambitious medical school at Wolverhampton agreed to accept one or two students, believing that they needed practical training 'as opposed to a lot of high-faluting theoretical stuff of M.R.C.P. standard'.[53] When this was put to the Directors of Medical Services in 1947, reaction reigned, Austin and Sneath thought AAMOs incapable of profiting from such courses, and it was decided that 'no general system of post-graduate training for AAMOs should at this stage be introduced'.[54] The first Makerere practitioner to undertake study abroad was therefore L.W. Lwanga, who had gone blind while working in Karamoja and went to Britain in 1948 to take a Diploma in Physiotherapy in order to begin a new career.[55] The Wolverhampton offer was taken up later in 1948 by two Tanganyikans, Francis Mwaisela and Charles Mtawali, who both took the Diploma in Public Health. They were followed in 1949 by Muwazi, whose paediatric work at Makerere led him to study for the

Diploma in Child Health, and Ivan Kadama, who took the DPH at the London School of Hygiene and Tropical Medicine, while George Sembeguya studied at both institutions in 1950–1. Jason Likimani, the first Kenyan, was a houseman at a hospital near London in 1951–2 and studied midwifery and gynaecology at Guy's.[56] By 1956, according to Uganda's DMS, 'Practically every MO(EA) and AMO in the department is applying for one of these scholarships.'[57] And ambitions were growing. In 1952 William Ouko resigned from the Kenya Medical Service and left for Britain with funds raised among his Luo friends, returning five years later as a Licentiate of the Royal College of Physicians and Surgeons of Edinburgh.[58] Sebastian Kyalwazi, Mulago's most distinguished African surgeon, had gone one better in 1956 by securing a Buganda Government grant to spend two years in Britain studying for Fellowship of the Royal College of Surgeons of Edinburgh, the basic qualification for a specialist, involving an examination with a failure rate often approaching 80 per cent which expatriates believed was beyond Makerere doctors. Kyalwazi qualified as FRCS in 1961, the same year as John Kibukamusoke became East Africa's first Member of the Royal College of Physicians of Edinburgh.[59]

This exodus, together with local registration, had an important impact on private practice. Following the legislation of 1949, Uganda licensed its first two private African practitioners, Solomon Matovu and G.K. Makoro, in 1950. They were followed in 1951 by Sebastiano Kyewalyanga and William Sewanyana, a Ugandan who had gained a medical degree at the University of the Witwatersrand and worked for a year at Mengo Hospital before setting up practice in Kampala as Uganda's first registered African doctor, only to die a year later of poliomyelitis.[60] In Tanganyika, Joseph Mutahangarwa retired from a decade of troubled government service in 1951 and established a practice on the Uganda border conveniently remote from both authorities.[61] Muwazi entered private practice soon after returning from Britain in 1952. A year later a major exodus from Uganda Government service took place, involving Samson Kisekka, Barnaba Kununka, Ivan Majugo, and Norman Kanyarutoke. By 1955 there were nine African private practitioners in Uganda, alongside four Europeans and seventy-nine Asians.[62]

This exodus and the declining entry to the Medical School led the Uganda Government to cast around for remedies. Promoting a few doctors to Senior Assistant Medical Officers had no effect. At an interview with the MMGA in 1953, Cohen promised that any African doctor capable of performing the duties of a Medical Officer would be promoted to that grade, even without a fully registrable qualification, only for the DMS to add that he had never found an African who was so capable, just as he had never met one fit to study medicine or surgery in Britain. Cohen could only end the meeting by pointing out that a new salaries commission had been appointed.[63] This did temporarily stop the rot. Following the GMC report of 1952, the pay of registered Medical Officers (East Africa) had risen to £430–£720 a year. The new commission abolished salary discrimination by race or gender, but retained inducement allowances for expatriates. This transformed the financial position of African doctors. In 1951, for example, David Kiremerwa had earned £390; in 1953, £542; in 1954, £894; and in 1955, £1,321.[64] The effects were immediate. Whereas eleven African doctors resigned from the Uganda medical service between 1950 and 1953, none resigned in 1954, and only a trickle in 1955 and 1956, the most important being George Sembeguya. In 1957, however, resignations rose again, notably Eria Babumba.[65] The lure of private practice also spread to Kenya, where the first African private practitioner, Samson Mwathi, opened a surgery in 1957 in Nairobi, where five other Africans soon followed him, among them Munyua Waiyaki, who had qualified in South Africa and Britain, and Njoroge Mungai, trained in South Africa and America. Jason Likimani also entered private practice at this time.[66] The only Tanganyikan addition to the list was W.B.K. Mwanjisi, a Makerere graduate who left government service in 1954 to practise in his home area at Tukuyu.[67]

The growing influence of Makerere-trained doctors in Uganda was made clear by an inquiry into the country's medical services carried out in 1955 by a committee, chaired by Professor A.C. Frazer of Birmingham University, appointed in response to widespread complaints that the medical service was deteriorating owing to lack of staff. The committee's nine members included an African private practitioner, Ivan Majugo, whose influence is clear in the report, and several other members sympathetic to Makerere doctors, many of whom gave evidence. In effect, the committee accepted the doctors' case. It reported that between 1949 and 1955–6 the proportion of the Uganda Government's annual expenditure devoted to health had fallen from nearly 11 to 7.3 per cent. The chief consequence was an acute shortage of staff, and especially of Makerere-trained doctors, whose numbers in government service had fallen between 1950 and 1955 from fifty-five to forty-five. The committee blamed this on 'poor conditions of service, poor prospects and lack of security on leaving government service'. Noting that during the next five years Makerere would at best produce only sixteen Ugandan doctors, the committee recommended that the Medical School's intake should rise by 1960 to at least twenty Ugandans and between forty and fifty other East Africans each year; if it could not take twenty, the balance should be trained abroad. Although the committee thought that African Medical Officers were now adequately paid, it recommended that they should be placed on the same salary scale as Europeans in order to demonstrate their equality. The committee suggested that a Medical Officer should normally remain at one station for at least five years. It criticised doctors' housing as sometimes 'quite deplorable, poorly sited, too small, badly built and maintained'. After hearing the MMGA allege that qualified practitioners leaving government service had been denied private practice for inadequate reasons, the committee rejected 'the principle whereby people who have already passed a recognised examination, after a prescribed period of study, and worked in Government Service for many years as licensed practitioners, should be subjected to a further investigation of professional competence on leaving Government service, before they are allowed to continue the practice of their profession'. The committee also recommended that Africans should pay small fees at government institutions.[68] With regard to the sub-professional medical assistants who did much of the routine work in hospitals and larger dispensaries, the committee listened to their grievances and then consulted the MMGA:

> The Chairman asked what the attitude of the Makerere Graduates Association was to the medical assistant, and whether they would object to an increase in production and perhaps a slightly different training, concentrating more upon training them as doctors rather than nurses. He pointed out that there was a danger that this might undermine the status of the Makerere Graduates. The Makerere Graduates expressed the view that there would be no objection to this provided such medical assistants were regarded as technicians and supervised. They stressed that a great deal of supervision was required. It was agreed that it was essential that this should not lead the Government to forget to produce doctors and to concentrate upon medical assistants. They would not like them to get a license to practise when they retire.[69]

The committee wholeheartedly accepted this view. 'The medical assistant', it wrote, '. . . should on no account be allowed to become a sub-standard doctor. Technical training must not be allowed to deteriorate into a back door to a profession.'[70]

African doctors were understandably delighted by the Frazer Report, even Muwazi welcoming it.[71] Government refused to abandon its power to deny private practice to an unregistered practitioner, cautioned that finance must determine how quickly the recommendations could be implemented, and eventually decided not to introduce fees,[72] but otherwise the report charted Uganda's medical course until the 1960s. Yet one thing Frazer could not do was to grant GMC recognition. After what Makerere's Principal called 'a period of almost ceremonial wooing deemed necessary by so august a body',[73] the GMC President himself inspected the Medical School in March 1957. The report is not available, but in May he told his General Council:

> We found that the deficiencies pointed out by the former Visitors in staff, teaching facilities and accommodation, as well as the lack of status of the qualification in the Territories and the lack of status of the Diplomates, had nearly all been remedied. We were impressed by the spirit and atmosphere of the School as a whole, and we

reported to the Executive Committee that the qualification granted by the College was worthy of recognition for the purposes of provisional and full registration in the United Kingdom.[74]

While the medical students organised a Recognition Ball and their teachers found the news 'not so exciting as it ought to be',[75] legal implementation of the decision proved immensely complicated. Eventually it was decided that all holders of the LMS, including all those of earlier vintage who had acquired it by special examination, should gain registration and become Medical Officers without further qualification. The most senior of them had left Makerere in 1934. Recognition, however, only briefly boosted entry to the Medical School, for doctors still received no degree. This anomaly was finally removed when MB, ChB degrees were awarded in 1964 and holders of the LMS, some now well into their fifties, received the qualification for which they had struggled.[76]

Up-country medicine

While the pursuit of professional status during the 1950s centred on the Medical School and major hospitals, African practitioners were at work in the most remote areas of East Africa. They were less concentrated in Uganda than before, a contrast exaggerated by the chance survival of their reports, which are easily available in Kenya but not elsewhere. Medical practice, too, had changed since the 1930s. Patients were more numerous, almost overwhelmingly so in some districts. Their complaints were changing, with less attention to yaws and epidemic diseases like smallpox and sleeping sickness. The remedies available were significantly better, thanks to antibiotics and other powerful drugs. African practitioners, too, were better trained than before, with more responsibility, ambition, interest in specialisation, concern with preventive medicine, and capacity for research. Yet while much had changed, more remained the same. Most African doctors outside capital cities were subordinate to European District Medical Officers or headed one-man stations carefully chosen to avoid conflict with Asian physicians or European nurses; only late in the 1950s did any gain greater responsibility. Most African doctors, also, still saw themselves as pioneers of enlightenment, although with some of the ambivalence towards indigenous culture which some had expressed as medical students. And all were alert to political awakening and racial conflict.

To see an up-country doctor in action, it is best to focus on Jason Likimani. The first Kenyan to qualify at Makerere, in 1939, he spent the next ten years working mainly as a surgeon at hospitals in Nairobi and Fort Hall (Murang'a). Partially Maasai, speaking the language, and requested by the Maasai Local Native Council, he finally took over the small hospital at Narok in March 1950. His house, designed for a European bachelor, had to be enlarged to accommodate his family, while the hospital itself was rudimentary: 'One room was used as a Dispensary, Laboratory, Dressing Room and Out-patient department. This was most unsatisfactory and often resulted in chaos during peak periods.' About twenty new outpatients and ten repeat visits attended each day. Their main complaints were respiratory conditions, digestive problems (including worms), wounds, eye conditions, and venereal diseases – the complaints of a largely pastoral people, as were many of the more serious cases admitted, such as anthrax and hydatid cyst. At the end of 1950 Likimani could report that admissions had risen by 40 per cent over the previous year and operations by 123 per cent. In addition, he had seven dispensaries to supervise, some of them 150 kilometres away in the depths of Maasailand, and had to rely on the District Commissioner's transport. 'Safaris were made from the middle of September', he reported, 'and camps were made for an average of 3 days in Engare Nairoua, Kilgoris, the Loita hills and Lemek. These safaris were very popular with the Masai.' While visiting dispensaries he taught the dressers to use sulphonamide and penicillin for pneumonia and venereal diseases. Preventive work scarcely existed, owing to 'lack of staff, the large sparsely populated district and the habits of the majority of its inhabitants'. The spread of venereal diseases especially alarmed him. 'There is little hope of reducing promiscuity amongst the Masai which is the cause of the prevalence of venereal disease', he wrote. 'It is gratifying, however, to note that they are becoming increasingly conscious of the need for early treatment, particularly syphilis.'[77]

Likimani could do nothing further about venereal disease before he left Narok in July 1951 for a long-coveted study period in Britain. When he returned late in 1952 he took charge of the more important hospital at Kajiado, the centre of British administration in Maasailand, and spent the next six years there. He settled back into a routine of hospital work punctuated – less frequently as time passed – by tours of the dispensaries in his own unreliable car or any better transport available. If he was lucky, the chiefs would have assembled their sick, mostly demanding injections, and there would usually be emergency cases awaiting him, although many of these were brought to the hospital, often in terrible condition. 'One case of obstructed labour of several days duration was treated, subsequently developing a vesico-vaginal fistula', he noted. 'A motor truck took about two days to and from a practically inaccessible village where she was lying critically ill.'[78] He once treated at least eight people mauled by lions. He also tried, with little success, to clean up Kajiado's dreadful township and, with rather more success, to provide employment for his family. By 1957, however, Likimani's reports had lost all excitement.[79] They say nothing of his frustration, but he had been in Kajiado too long and felt that he was being denied the advancement to which his position as Kenya's first qualified African doctor entitled him. In May 1958 he resigned and shortly afterwards entered private practice in Nairobi.

For younger men, a remote first station could be an exhilarating place – 'this love of mine', as Emmanuel Lumu described his first posting on the Sudanese border.[80] However well trained, no young doctor could be prepared for all the emergencies he would meet:

I remember over a decade ago when I found myself in a district hospital. On my very first day of duty I was required to do three caesarian sections and one strangulated hernia. In those good old days government hospitals . . . did not have a maternity unit of any kind and therefore apart from what I had learnt as a student, I had not had the opportunity to revise let alone improve on it and here I was confronted by three caesarian sections![81]

Nor could an eager young doctor escape frustration with rural conservatism. Eighteen months after Likimani left Kajiado he was succeeded by a Kikuyu moderniser, Michael Migue:

1960 will probably go down as the year in which some inclination to change was detectable in this district. This change was seen in thoughts and in attitude the masai were showing. It was a year the masai showed some enthusiasm to change for the better. It was a year one Masai decided to change from his old masai type of house (hat) to that of a mud house (square with three rooms) and corrugated iron sheets and later the same year decided to change to a house built with bricks . . .

We have got to get the idea of good housing across to the masai by constantly educating them, but education is nothing more than seeing and copying more or less.

. . . while protecting the Masai we should not be blinded by that and forget that here at Kajiado we are building Kenya of the future we are not just building a district but part of a Country. The development have got to be planned to keep in pace with the other districts . . . The attitude of just letting the masai continue in their old role is absolutely futile. The Masai may think that it is the best way to live but the others will say it is not. The old Masai way of life will just drive them to extinction. A change to the modern way of life must come and come soon.[82]

Doctors who spent their first ten or twenty years moving from station to station never ceased to be surprised by the diversity of their countrymen. Posted away from the progressive Christian peasantry of western Kenya to coastal Kilifi district, Tadayo Evelia was astonished that 'it is still believed that it is wrong to harness cattle on a plough':

The occupiers of the land are the 'Midzikenda' . . . They have definite tribal traditions, beliefs and practices. They observe omens, believe in promotive medicine, their big witchdoctor Mr 'Kabwere' is supposed to have specialised in protective and promotive medicines. Children come into hospital with all sorts of charms tied round their necks, waists, shoulders, thighs, legs and arms as signs of protection for various diseases, and evil spirits. Expensive as they are to get them worn for each sacrifice may mean a loss of a goat, a chicken, etc. for the sacrifice to ward off the misfortune, cool dangerous spirits, invoke superhuman help, all mysticism.[83]

Most doctors came from dominant ethnic groups with almost unconscious prejudices. Deogratias Byaruhanga's DPH thesis on leprosy in the Toro kingdom, for example, divided its population into 'the ruling and educated Batoro' and 'the primitive Bamba and Bakonjo', the latter having most of the leprosy because 'for many years it was a well known fact that these tribes carefully avoided washing'.[84] Eria Babumba published in 1954 an article on African patients, 'with the idea that it may be helpful to the non-African medical practitioner new to the tropics', in which he discussed superstition, ignorance of disease, and fear of witchcraft, gods, and evil spirits by people 'just emerging from primitivity'.[85] Yet his contemporary William Ouko from western Kenya, with several British postgraduate qualifications, wrote a more subtle analysis of African medical thinking, stressing the demand for rapid curative results but arguing that the modern doctor must *use* this demand 'by first curing their complaints and . . . then afterwards effecting preventive measures'. Rather than pressing pregnant women to eat high-protein foods which were taboo, the health educator should encourage them to eat more of the protein foods they already ate. (Less practically, perhaps, he should not make people abandon round houses for square ones, but encourage them to build oval houses and find that the furniture would not fit.) Ouko was a keen advocate of health surveys, an enthusiast for preventive medicine, and among the first to urge the training of indigenous midwives and their incorporation into the medical system.[86]

The earliest work of this kind was undertaken by Charles Mtawali on his return to Tanganyika from Wolverhampton in 1949. He was posted to Bukoba District, where government had initiated a scheme to rescue the Haya people from what was thought to be impending extinction through female infertility due to prostitution and venereal disease, much like the crisis diagnosed in Buganda forty years earlier.[87] Probably this crisis too was greatly exaggerated,[88] but during 1949–50 an administrative officer established an experimental network of committees and injection clinics to treat syphilis. Mtawali was sent to strengthen the campaign. He found that the Haya and the administration both saw the remedy as VD clinics giving penicillin injections against syphilis, whereas Mtawali and the Medical Department did not, for the main disease was gonorrhoea and injections gave no protection against reinfection, merely fostering 'a most peculiar attitude to V.D. The disease is so common that the attitude is that it is as inevitable as a cold in the head and rather more common.' Mtawali accepted that there was a crisis, but, as a Christian and a doctor, he saw it as chiefly social and moral. 'The problem is a purely sociological one and not medical', he wrote, 'and it is extremely difficult for anybody to put this fact across to them'. Its root, he believed, lay in the fact that the prosperous coffee and banana economy of the Haya had benefited chiefly senior men. The remedy lay in 'a complete change in the structure and customs of the tribe, first through the emancipation of the women and then perhaps by introducing a change in the economic pattern so that the young men share the work with the women and marry early'. As it was, women either 'tend to live with the old men for their keep but to get their satisfaction elsewhere', or 'they emigrate [as prostitutes] in order to lead a free independent life, thus escaping from the peculiar custom in their District of doing everything for their husbands as if they were slaves'. Reliance on VD injections was misguided. 'The general impression . . . of those closely associated with it is that apart from rousing considerable public interest in the problem, it has, so far, not produced any appreciable results.' Because it was what people wanted, the scheme would probably have to continue, and he suggested mass treatment in one chiefdom to demonstrate whether it made any difference, although expecting that it would not: 'The medical view . . . is that V.D. can only be eradicated by the people themselves changing their sexual habits and any funds available should be invested in the long-term policy of providing better education etc., and not in purely curative campaigns.' The whole situation, he concluded, 'shows the practical difficulties mass education and community development are up against in some parts of Africa'.[89]

Mtawali's analysis illustrates both the intellectual confidence which the ablest East African doctors of the 1950s displayed and their alertness to current thought. Bernard Omondi, a Kenyan, had the same qualities. In the late 1950s he returned from London with a Diploma in Child Welfare to take charge of the district hospital at Kerugoya below the southern foot of Mount Kenya, an exceedingly busy hospital with over 100,000 outpatients a year where his staff included two European sisters and a European hospital superintendent.[90] The four main causes of death in the hospital were broncho-pneumonia, gastro-enteritis, pulmonary tuberculosis, and kwashiorkor. Omondi decided that they formed a syndrome, with malnutrition at its root: 'Kwashiorkor is the most accessible bus in which TB, Broncho-pneumonia, Gastro enteritis, Whooping Cough, Helminthiasis and others ride in reign.' His conviction rested partly on a geographical study of tuberculosis patients suggesting an association with kwashiorkor. He conducted a village survey showing that the survival of newborn children was adversely affected by 'early marriage before 14 years (females) and 21 years (males); advanced maternal age over 25 years; parity and large size of family; male sex; low birth weight; ignorance and low standard of living'. And, like Mtawali, he was convinced that the 'chronic malnutrition which has been increasing over the years' was due chiefly to socio-economic change:

> Whatever the actual or predesposing causes of Kwashiokor the far too common picture of the underdeveloped child with gross wasting, pallor, oedema, ulceration of skin, and pale straight fine hair was rare in the old days. The desire to get employment and earn more money, to build good houses and to educate ones children are detrimental to child life in the present stage of economic struggle particularly in the low-income class of people who value money more than food. In addition to this clamour for 'saving' the Emergency, land consolidation, communal labour, and all that these imply have added greatly to the cause of Kwashiokor as the infant is often left to the care of a child only two to four years older, or a grand mother, for almost every day of the week. The lack of maternal love and care causes psychological and physical trauma which makes the child a social and physical misfit in the community for the rest of his life. This state of affairs can be prevented by an orderly systematic approach.

His system sought to ensure that all births were notified and then inspected by a health visitor, followed by examination at dispensaries and child welfare clinics and the admission of severe cases into hospital. He tried to launch a malnutrition centre, checked an epidemic by immunising 60,000 children against polio – only the second such operation in Africa – organised a mobile team to counter another epidemic of measles, undertook a survey of handicapped people, and called in the provincial physician to diagnose a mysterious disease (trichinosis) never previously described south of the Sahara. Curiosity and intellectual energy ran through everything he wrote.

Tuberculosis was the priority disease of the 1950s, especially in Kenya and Tanganyika, much as yaws had been in the 1920s and for the same reason: drugs had become available to treat it. James Ang'awa, a colourful and abrasive character, made himself Kenya's African specialist on the disease, taking over the Port Reitz tuberculosis hospital with some 140 staff for a time in 1960.[91] For most up-country doctors, however, the prevalent diseases were still those of the past. In the remote West Nile District of Uganda, Yusufu Semambo and a European medical officer devised a method of treating the huge local ulcers by applying penicillin, cutting the ulcer out, grafting skin from the opposite thigh, adding vaseline, and bandaging it for up to three weeks until the graft had taken. They could do up to twenty a day.[92] Yet alongside these more exciting duties – to which might be added the local epidemics of polio or meningitis or measles – up-country doctors had many routine and distasteful tasks. Young African doctors seem always to have been made responsible for the VD clinic. They treated the leprosy patients, visited the gaol, witnessed the flogging of prisoners, conducted post-mortems, spent much time waiting to give evidence in court, and filled up the countless forms. The Frazer Committee found much resentment among them. 'There are four doctors in the district', the committee noted at Soroti, 'one European, one Asian and the two African. The European and the Asian do district work but the Africans complained that they are tied to the hospital all the time. They wished to have a wider scope of work.'[93] Racial barriers were always present. Kenya's doctors were barred from operating at the European Hospital and even in Uganda the anglicised Albert Kaggwa and his British wife were denied membership of the Mbale Club.[94] Studying the writings of these gifted and progressive men, one is struck, on the one hand, by how optimistic they were at this time of their ability to improve their societies and, on the other, by how rigid the structures of colonial society remained to the very end of European rule.

Private practice

The first Africans entered private practice in Uganda in 1950. During the next half-century it became the main activity for most East African doctors, but it produced little documentation and is difficult to study. Before independence, moreover, it was on a small scale.

The first African private practitioners generally had personal reasons for quitting government service. Majugo apparently resigned on an issue of principle, but Muwazi was angry that his Diploma in Child Health did not win him promotion to full Medical Officer status.[95] Kyewalyanga left because he was denied postgraduate training in Britain and 'could not support his family on his salary'; he forfeited his pension rights and was denied a gratuity.[96] Sembeguya, similarly, needed more money for his children's education and resented discrimination in favour of a younger expatriate, while Babumba had expected reward for a course in eye surgery which he had taken (but failed) in Britain.[97]

Private practice also offered attractions. One was the freedom of self-employment. A.K. Kibaya was to feel 'like a diver . . . who has surfaced after a long swim under water'.[98] Several travelled extensively abroad, as Samson Mwathi did in America in 1958, visiting many major cities, studying family planning and the chest diseases which were his speciality, receiving honorary fellowship of the American College of Chest Physicians, and returning via Lisbon, Ghana, Nigeria, and the Belgian Congo.[99] Almost all private doctors established solo practices, usually no more than a two-roomed clinic. The few partnerships usually dissolved quite quickly. Moreover, private practice offered relief from the endless transfers, loneliness, and poor housing of government service, promising instead the chance to settle among one's own: Kyewalyanga in Masaka, Majugo in Hoima. There the doctor could create the healing homestead, now translated into a nursing home or clinic:

His Nursing Home is well situated on top of a lovely hill where the breezes from the neighbouring lake create a healthy atmosphere. The buildings are modern and spotlessly clean. He has an operating theatre equipped with a large piece of enaesthetic [sic] apparatus and a diathermy among other things. He has six beds for inpatients, a laboratory and an outpatient clinic. He has a staff of three medical assistants, two nurses and a midwife. During his absence, there is a qualified assistant to carry out the job.[100]

In this idyll the private doctor, like his indigenous predecessor, could practise the holistic medicine, treating the patient and not merely the disease, impossible amidst the anonymity and workload of large hospitals:

To Bintabara's again in evening . . . Usual story of frequent postings . . . keen now he is settled to become a real family doctor, knowing his patients' social conditions and seeing members of the same family over a period in a way he c[oul]d not do in Government service.[101]

Such a practice might bring the social prestige which a Makerere student described in 1958 as his career ambition:

(Immediately): Medical Officer. (Later): I aim to be a middle aged man with a good wife and children, with my own surgery somewhat at home. I also aim to being a Councillor in Town Council or Native Council or Legislative Council.[102]

Several achieved it. Kyewalyanga, with a successful nursing home and ten children, became Mayor of Masaka, Legislative Councillor, Member of the Order of the British Empire, and Papal Knight. Mwathi became a leading figure in Nairobi society. In Uganda doctors were to be prominent in local and national politics for half a century.

Moreover, by the 1950s private practice offered real possibility of material success. Uganda's DMS estimated in 1951 that a mercenary practitioner might make between £1,000 and £2,000 a year by 'injection practice', or twice the government salary. Kyewalyanga refused £800 a year and a registrarship at Mulago to stay in government service.[103] The opportunity to prosper came from the wealth, especially in Uganda, derived from the cash-crop boom of the late 1940s and early 1950s, with its associated rapid urbanisation. Muwazi, so often a pace-setter, opened his surgery in Katwe, the African freehold township just outside Kampala's southern boundary which was Buganda's largest African trading centre, the location of its vernacular press, and home to the 'new middle class' of informal entrepreneurs and junior civil servants whose fees could make a doctor happy.[104] Eriazali Kafero, Samson Kisekka, and Barnaba Kununka chose another strategic position to the north of Kampala for their Kunonya Nursing Home, the first in Kampala owned by Africans, which the Nabagereka (Queen) of Buganda opened in 1954. It had one large ward, three private wards, an operating theatre, dispensary, store, and waiting room. Not far away, in the Kawempe township of northern Kampala, Sembeguya built the Nakasi Nursing Home, with twenty-two beds in 1964.[105] The pioneer, however, was Kyewalyanga's Nursing Home at Kako, near Masaka, begun in the early 1950s:

> Went to Kako. Met Dr Kiwalyanga [sic], who runs his own private dispensary . . . Noticed piles of journals, as in better Engl[ish] doctor's; buildings in a bit of a mess because of white ant invasion. Builders failed to put down proper damp course, termites have penetrated. It means practically pulling down and rebuilding, all at Dr K's own expense. He has an ass[istan]t another ex Makerere former doctor, not now licensed . . . also 2 assistants, man and woman, in training as dispensers, nurses, etc. V[ery] intelligent about social medicine, health education. Feels Government hospitals need supplementing by private practice. Is speaking to clinical meeting at Makerere next week. Visitors' book contained large no of distinguished visitors.[106]

At the opening ceremony in 1956, performed by the Kabaka, Kyewalyanga said, 'If we Africans tackle successfully new ventures of our own creation, we shall have opened up one of the ways leading rapidly to self-government.'[107] Nearby, on the Mbarara road, was Babumba's Muteesa II Nursing Home, built in 1961. Five years later it was valued at Shs.84,500 and consisted of a maternity block, dispensary block, office, operating theatre, quarters, kitchen, and latrines, mostly built in local brick with steel window frames, concrete floors, corrugated-iron roofs, water-catchment tanks, and electricity. Run mainly by a resident medical assistant, it had 42 inpatients and 1,528 outpatients during 1962.[108]

At that time there were some twenty-three African private practitioners in Uganda,[109] but only perhaps five or six in Kenya and three in Tanganyika. The pattern in Nairobi was similar to Kampala's. Mwathi settled in the African township of Bahati and opened a practice with such success that two other doctors followed him within the next three years, forming 'a little "Harley Street"' there. 'Doctors in private practice, hordes of patients, huge incomes, always working', it was noted at the time.[110] Kenya's first African-owned nursing home was the Sunshine Nursing Home in Kitale, which William Ouko bought from expatriates in 1960. The first in the Nairobi area was established shortly afterwards by Njoroge Mungai at Thika.[111]

Private practices were residential clinics or nursing homes where the patient sought out the doctor, rather than domiciliary visits by the doctor to his patients. The chief reasons, as Sembeguya pointed out, were 'the widely distributed nature of the population', the difficulty of transport, and 'the almost complete absence of domestic telephones'. The doctor's time was more valuable than that of his patient, who needed to know where the doctor could be found. This had been true of successful indigenous practitioners, it was the experience of midwives and mission doctors, and it was a principle which idealistic later health planners neglected at their peril. Sembeguya reckoned that 60 per cent of his patients came from more than 15 kilometres away. He described the same number (and commonly the same people) as 'working class', with only 8 per cent as 'well-to-do'. Nearly half had been ill for at least two weeks before consulting him.[112] Patient power remained strong, with patients visiting one doctor after another to demand a preferred treatment:

> One such patient came up with his eye absolutely full of pus. Enucleation was the only thing in the face of the impending danger of sympathetic ophthalmia in the other eye which might result in complete blindness. All this was explained to the patient but he would sooner have a needle thrust into the eye to drain it. His alternative was obviously rejected upon which he turned his back on this very incompetent doctor.[113]

Sembeguya complained that the private doctor's chief problem was his family: 'Patients, relatives and friends attended in large numbers and some even became squatters on the premises. Very rarely would they accept advice to go to the main hospitals but would insist on getting their treatment from the general practitioner himself!'[114]

Private practitioners with social ambitions needed assistants to act in their absence. The obvious candidates were those Makerere-trained doctors who had been denied licences to practise independently. Kyewalyanga, Sembeguya, and the proprietors of the Kunonya Nursing Home employed a sequence of them by accepting responsibility for their actions, thereby assisting colleagues in distress as well as serving their own interests.[115] Less scrupulous doctors 'covered' unlicensed practitioners who performed medical procedures on their premises or in their names. Another breach of ethics was to advertise. The Luganda press left its readers in no doubt where to find Muwazi's surgery. From 1959, it appears, an MMGA subcommittee on general practice 'dealt with the problems of alleged professional misconduct in a friendly and professional manner'.[116]

The pioneers underestimated the difficulty of making money from private practice, especially from nursing homes with high overhead costs. In 1966 Sembeguya claimed that his average annual loss during the previous ten years had been Shs.8,000, partly because the poor could not be turned away:

> There is also that human sympathy, that one finds it difficult to refuse credit where life is at stake . . . This is why Medical Institutions never make profit like business establishments . . . I treat more Bahima and Jaluo [scil. poor people] together than Baganda.[117]

Since he was seeking a government subsidy, his complaints need not be taken literally, but they were echoed by Kyewalyanga and other practitioners. One remedy was to diversify. Sembeguya claimed to survive only through his farm in Bugerere, while Samson Kisekka's share in the Kunonya Nursing Home jostled interests in a bus company, transport cooperative, fishing company, farming association, dairy cooperative, and insurance company.[118] But when the cash-crop boom ended in the late 1950s all nursing homes in Uganda met financial difficulties, worsened by Asian competition.[119] In 1962 Kafero transferred his share in the Kunonya Nursing Home to Kisekka and re-entered government employment, as did several private practitioners, while others worked part time for the Buganda Government. Kunonya eventually closed as the partners decided 'to help the Government solve its problem of acute shortage of Doctors'.[120]

At independence, African private practice was still in its infancy and its financial viability remained uncertain. In the future it would profoundly alter the medical profession. For the moment, however, its chief contribution was to provide a platform from which doctors could enter politics.

Doctors in politics

Discontented doctors did not resign from government service to enter nationalist politics as a means of protest. Some medical assistants did so, for they had deeper grievances and some used politics as an escape from a dead-end job. Doctors certainly could not avoid politics, as their experiences during the Mau Mau rebellion will show, but those who became deeply engaged did so by first entering private practice and then being drawn into politics by ambition, the natural constituencies provided by their practices, and a sense of public service. Thus doctors were not prominent in Tanganyikan politics – although medical assistants were – because there were few African doctors and still fewer private practitioners. The same was true in Kenya, where only two doctors became important in nationalist politics, both only shortly before independence. Zanzibar's doctors were more active politically, but nearly all were Arabs. In Uganda, however, the path from Medical Officer via private practitioner to politician was well trodden, not only because private practitioners were relatively numerous, but because Uganda had no mass party and recruited its politicians mainly from local notables. Moreover, in Buganda, where the pattern was most clear, the modern elite faced an agonising choice between Buganda patriotism and Uganda nationalism which drew many responsible men into public life and destroyed several medical careers.

East Africa's first semi-political organisation with a territorial structure was the African Association in Tanganyika, which civil servants could join. Its president in the early 1950s was a doctor serving his internship at Sewa

Haji, Vedast Kyaruzi, who led a circle of politically minded young Africans.[121] But Kyaruzi was posted up-country, civil servants were ordered to quit the association in 1953, and the Tanganyika African National Union which succeeded it in 1954 involved few doctors. One, Michael Lugazia, held a high position at TANU headquarters in the late 1950s, apparently after conflict with the medical authorities. Another, the private practitioner W.B.K. Mwanjisi, was TANU's first chairman in Rungwe District. By contrast, former paramedical staff were important in TANU, with Austin Shaba, a medical assistant who became Junior Minister for Health, only the most prominent.[122]

In Kenya, scarcely any prominent African could escape the ramifications of Mau Mau. No qualified African doctor is known to have participated actively, although Likimani's widow claimed that he had aided the detainees he treated,[123] and certainly his reports were remarkably silent about the political events around him. Omondi also found himself tending detainees. Mwathi was made responsible for organising the Home Guard at the King George VI Hospital in Nairobi and Mbuthia was recruited to its Psychological Warfare Committee 'to get the African's point of view'. One Kikuyu doctor formed the nucleus of a team to screen medical staff in Nairobi.[124] Paramedical staff were involved on a larger scale. Those detained included thirty-one from Kerugoya Hospital, ten Laboratory Assistants and sixteen Kikuyu medical staff at the Medical Research Laboratory, and even so trusted an assistant as the anaesthetist Charles Karau.[125] On the other side, at least two medical workers were killed by Mau Mau bands[126] and the real number must have been higher, for they were vulnerable and often associated with Protestant missions firmly opposed to the rebellion.

None of Kenya's Makerere-trained doctors appears to have been politically active in post-Mau Mau nationalism, although paramedics were again much involved, the former sanitary inspector Tom Mboya being only the most prominent. The politically active doctors were the two private practitioners trained outside East Africa, Njoroge Mungai and Munyua Waiyaki. Both were southern Kikuyu from the political heartland close to Nairobi. Both had fortunate family connections: Mungai was Jomo Kenyatta's nephew, while Waiyaki came from a chiefly family prominent in early dealings with the British. Both were educated at Alliance High School and Fort Hare University in South Africa. Both missed the Mau Mau emergency, which compromised so many political careers. Mungai went on to Stanford, Waiyaki to Britain. Returning to Kenya in 1958–9, they found political leadership in non-Kikuyu hands and collaborated in penetrating it. Mungai established a clinic and maternity home in Thika, a mobile clinic in Embu, and a (partly charitable) dispensary in the Dagoretti township on the outskirts of Nairobi where he had been born. Highly educated, urbane, and as yet uninvolved in Kikuyu factionalism, he moved quickly into a leadership position, acting as secretary to the first Kenya African National Union (KANU) conference in May 1960. He also became personal physician, and thereby emissary, to the imprisoned Kenyatta. In May 1963 he used his local connections in Dagoretti and his reputation as the champion of its poor to win the West Nairobi seat.[127] Waiyaki's path was similar but rougher. He set up practice in another Nairobi township, Bahati, and gained KANU's Nairobi chairmanship, but he was a more radical figure, 'a Socialist nationalist who believes in a Welfare State'. In February 1961 he made the mistake of challenging Tom Mboya for the parliamentary seat in Nairobi East and lost by 2,668 votes to 31,407. With Mungai's support, however, he rebuilt his career and won a new Nairobi seat in May 1963. They were the only doctors in Kenya's independence parliament. Mungai became Minister of Health and Housing. Waiyaki became his Parliamentary Secretary.[128]

Although paramedics were important in Uganda's local politics,[129] it was doctors who took the national stage. The first was Majugo, who joined the Uganda National Congress – Uganda's first nationalist party, formed in 1952 – as soon as he resigned from government service a year later and remained one of its leaders in Bunyoro for the rest of the decade.[130] More active was Muwazi, whose Katwe practice was close to UNC headquarters. He had left government service with a bitter personal grievance, had strong anti-colonial sentiments, and was on the make, talented, ambitious, perhaps rather shallow and unscrupulous. He first appeared in politics in 1955 as both treasurer of the committee organising the Kabaka's welcome from exile and Secretary-General of the UNC, whose office was for a time in his surgery.[131] The combination of Buganda and Uganda politics was unexceptional at this time when the Kabaka's exile was a nationalist issue. It was natural, too, that Buganda chose five UNC leaders to fill the Legislative Council seats allocated to it under the 1955 Agreement with the British. Muwazi was one and Barnaba Kununka another.[132] They entered the Council in September 1955, along with Kyewalyanga, who was nominated by the Governor.

Muwazi deliberately injected venom into the Council's bland debates. 'Though my knowledge of trade is scanty (applause)', he said in his maiden speech, only Africans should receive trading plots until they equalled other races in commerce.[133] Two days later all three doctors opposed the continuation of the Central Legislative Assembly, feared in Buganda as a step towards East African federation.[134] In January 1956 Muwazi moved that by 1957 all Legislative Council members should be elected directly. 'The right to vote is given, even in notoriously conservative countries like

Great Britain, to all citizens', he claimed, and when Cohen as chairman asked him to repeat the statement, he obliged.[135] With the support of Kununka, who was said to debate 'with a smooth eloquence which reflected his professional training',[136] Muwazi sustained his attack throughout 1956, helping to induce Cohen to announce direct elections on a common roll for 1961.[137] The doctors pressed for rapid implementation of the Frazer Report – even the normally silent Kyewalyanga spoke strongly on the subject[138] – and secured improvements to the medical system, including the abolition of racial segregation in government hospitals.[139] But above all they pressed the issue of Africanisation, which their experience had made central to their nationalism.[140]

Yet the doctors' position in Ugandan politics was changing. In July 1957 the UNC split over ideological and organisational issues. Kununka remained its secretary, but Muwazi helped to form the United Congress Party. In order to outbid the UNC for support among those in Buganda who opposed the kingdom's integration into a unitary Uganda, Muwazi resigned from the Legislative Council in November 1957. A year later, when Buganda refused to participate in Legislative Council elections, Muwazi instead won a seat on Buganda's Lukiiko. Once an extreme nationalist, he now became an extreme federalist.[141] He also joined two other newly elected doctors, Emmanuel Lumu and Samson Kisekka. Of the three, Lumu was the most formidable politician. One of the first doctors to leave government service in 1950, he had acquired business interests and adopted an extreme federalist or even separatist position designed to outflank the incumbent Buganda government. When the Lukiiko voted in favour of Buganda's secession from Uganda in September 1960, Lumu and Muwazi joined the committee to draft plans for independence.[142] This, however, the British would not countenance, and instead, at constitutional talks in September 1961, Milton Obote, leader of the Uganda People's Congress (the UNC's successor), proposed an alliance with Ganda leaders on the basis of a semi-federal status for Buganda. Lumu and Muwazi jumped at this and were prominent in organising a Ganda party, Kabaka Yekka, to control the kingdom's politics.[143] Muwazi became Buganda's Minister of Health and Works. Lumu – whom many younger men wished to see Katikiro of Buganda – refused a Buganda ministry and was instead elected in April 1962 to represent the kingdom in the new National Assembly. Within a week he was Uganda's Minister of Health in Obote's first government.[144]

This intensive politicking, with its important regional as well as national implications, had drawn other Ugandan doctors into politics, to such an extent that a correspondent complained in the press 'at the behaviour of our African professional men, who after our painful sacrifice to bring them up as such, give up their professional jobs in preference to politics'.[145] Kununka remained loyal to the UNC and fought (and lost) every election until independence.[146] When a constitutional conference in May 1962 discussed the status of kingdoms other than Buganda, Toro's negotiating committee included Dr D.B. Byaruhanga and Bunyoro's chief spokesman was Dr Ivan Majugo, who had led a modernising party in the kingdom since the mid-1950s and was prominent in its unsuccessful campaign for the return of the 'Lost Counties' transferred to Buganda by the British. He was narrowly defeated in the April 1962 election to the National Assembly,[147] but three other doctors joined Lumu there. Paul Kiggundu, who had studied medicine in India and Britain, occupied a specially elected seat, as did George Sembeguya, who was both a liberal nationalist and a moderate Ganda patriot.[148] The third new doctor-legislator, elected by the Lukiiko, was Eria Babumba, a private practitioner of complex background – his Ganda father had been personal aide to the Chief Minister of Ankole – who had become a Kabaka Yekka firebrand and was to have a turbulent political career.[149]

At independence, therefore, doctors held all the ministerial positions controlling health in Kenya and Uganda, although not in Tanganyika where medical men were less numerous and influential. The difference was to shape national policies for a generation.

6 The transfer of power

In their struggle for status under colonial rule, East Africa's doctors had achieved a degree of professional solidarity and organisation, more effectively in Uganda than elsewhere. At independence they strengthened this by taking over the institutions of colonial medicine – the ministries, international representation, disciplinary bodies, and professional associations – although again unevenly, for Tanganyika's less numerous African doctors did not gain the power their counterparts enjoyed in Uganda and Kenya. Yet black doctors were not content merely to sit in white men's chairs. They were nationalists and modernisers and they were eager to improve their countrymen's health, especially by increasing the supply of doctors, whose inadequacy was their chief criticism of their colonial predecessors. This meant creating new medical schools in Nairobi and Dar es Salaam, with major implications for Makerere and East African cooperation. In medical policy the doctors were at first chiefly concerned to ensure continuity, but they had to respond to pressures on the medical system which had emerged during the colonial period and were to become overwhelming after independence: pressures of demand, population growth, cost, and changing patterns of disease and therapy. This chapter describes the establishment of African control over modern medicine in East Africa and surveys the situation Africans inherited.

Africanisation of the ministries

Tanganyika gained independence in 1961, Uganda in 1962, Kenya and Zanzibar in 1963, but the sequence said more about their degrees of political unity than their preparedness for self-government. Of their medical systems, Uganda's showed much the highest measure of African control. Cohen had initiated Africanisation in 1952 by appointing a standing committee, including Dr S.M. Magezi, to oversee training and promotion.[1] In the Legislative Council, Muwazi and Kununka began to exert pressure for Africanisation in 1956. A year later Cohen's successor began the training of African doctors for higher administrative and specialist posts. Several became district medical officers and in 1960 the first, Peter Muganwa, was posted to gain administrative experience at headquarters.[2] In 1961 the government began to promote Africans over expatriates and appoint Africans to understudy senior administrators.[3] Ivan Kadama, the senior African doctor still in government service, became Chief Medical Officer in 1962 and combined the post with that of Permanent Secretary in 1963, thereby excluding lay interference until he retired in 1970. Although no innovator, he was a competent administrator much feared by his subordinates.[4] By April 1964 the ministry could report that 'all the key administrative posts have been Ugandanised . . . With regard to the other cadres of staff, out of a total establishment of 21 specialists 8 are Ugandans; 9 matrons, 4 are Ugandans; 102 nursing sisters, 24 are Ugandans; 9 tutors, 1 is a Ugandan; 141 Medical Officers, 51 are Ugandans.'[5]

By comparison, at independence Tanganyika had only twelve registered African doctors and five interns in government service.[6] Its educational system was backward and its government showed little serious concern with Africanisation throughout the 1950s. When the first TANU ministers took office in 1959, Nyerere was so aware of the lack of qualified Africans and the danger of administrative breakdown that he envisaged a long dependence on expatriate manpower. It was only when Kawawa replaced him as Prime Minister during 1962 that Africanisation of senior posts was pressed vigorously.[7] Charles Mtawali, who had made his reputation by his work in Bukoba, became Permanent (renamed Principal) Secretary in the Ministry of Health from 1962 to 1968, while the Chief Medical Officer from 1964 was Benjamin Akim, a cool-minded Makerere graduate of 1947.[8] Like Kadama, they were able and progressive administrators but jealous of anything touching their profession, which separated them sharply from independent Tanganyika's first Minister of Health, Derek Bryceson, a British settler who had abandoned the white community for TANU and favoured radical positions.

Kenya's transfer of control was less smooth. Although the first Lancaster House Conference of January 1960 provided for an elected African majority in the Legislative Council, the Medical Department continued until March 1961 to think of Africanisation purely as the few posts in the existing service which might become available to Africans each year.[9] Ordered then to train Africans for senior appointments, it generally sent them abroad, so that they were not available for employment. At independence in December 1963 Kenya had forty-nine African doctors in government service,[10] but staffing arrangements remained in turmoil for several years. There were problems, too, at the centre, where Jason Likimani, who was the senior African doctor but had resigned in 1958, was brought back into the ministry in 1962 and appointed DMS in 1964. His appointment offended some African doctors who had remained in government service and was seen as a KANU appointment, for Likimani had strong political support which was to keep him in office until 1978, much to the disadvantage of the medical system.[11] His deputy, Arthur Mbuthia, had made a name as a surgeon in the 1940s. Makerere graduates took over the other senior posts in the ministry, where it could be said in 1965 that 'the question of Africanization is finished'.[12] The weakness in its upper levels was compensated initially by Njoroge Mungai's ability as Minister, but in December 1964 he was promoted to Defence.

Independence also implied African responsibility on the international stage, which was especially important in medicine, a truly international concern where the WHO was exceptionally influential. Given East Africa's scarcity of high-level manpower, some doctors were completely lost to international duties. Vedast Kyaruzi became Tanganyika's representative at the United Nations before holding a series of other international posts. Solomon Asea became Uganda's ambassador in the United States and Britain.[13] Several younger men like Stephen Lwanga and Eleuther Tarimo took WHO posts, while a number of distinguished senior doctors, including Aloysius Nhonoli, Kihumbu Thairu, and Thomas Ogada, moved to international appointments after mid-career. Many worked in WHO projects in East Africa, which had begun in the 1950s with malaria eradication in Zanzibar and the Kigezi District of Uganda, peaked in the mass vaccination campaigns of 1967–8 which eradicated smallpox, and would continue into attempts to control AIDS.[14] Other doctors became specialists in tailoring plans to the distinctive interests of foreign donors, whether Chinese pride in indigenous medicine, Russian eagerness to display soviet technology, Scandinavian earnestness about primary health care, or the World Bank's obsession with cost-sharing. International contacts enabled a fortunate minority of doctors to maintain their elite status, but international bodies mainly advocated policies other than the hospital-based urban medicine associated with professional elitism. Moreover, international participation helped East Africans to preserve modern medicine as the skilled and literate sector of health provision. 'The most pleasant reward' of medical research, Raphael Owor, Dean of the Makerere Medical School, was to tell his students, 'is a passport to the whole world; a passport which leads one to colleagues in all corners of the world regardless of political boundaries, religions or languages'.[15]

Africanisation of the professional bodies

Although medical professionalisation among East Africans emerged as part of decolonisation, colonial doctors had created professional institutions which served both those in government service and private practitioners. The two main institutions were the Medical Practitioners and Dentists Boards, which regulated the profession in each territory, and the local branches of the British Medical Association (BMA), which acted as professional trade unions. At independence African doctors took control of these and other professional bodies, thereby strengthening their own solidarity and proclaiming their desire to follow British professional models.

The number of private practitioners in colonial East Africa is obscure because medical registers did not record whether those registered were still in practice or even in the territory. One well-informed guess was that in 1961 Kenya had some 300 private practitioners, or nearly three times as many as its government medical officers. Of the private practitioners, probably at least two-thirds were Asians, although the statistics were so unreliable that another well-informed source put the number of Asian practitioners in the colony in 1962 at 459. Half the private practitioners were probably in Nairobi.[16] Numbers were smaller elsewhere. In Tanganyika in 1961, 182 of the 403 registered doctors were said to be private practitioners, although one wonders how many actually practised; over 80 per cent were Asians.[17] In 1955 Uganda had 79 Asian, 9 African, and 4 European private practitioners, as against 124 government doctors in post, but during the late 1950s there was an influx of private Asian doctors.[18] The numbers had risen steeply during the later colonial period, for in 1926 Nairobi had only six European private practitioners and as late as 1947 only twenty-five of all races were on the register in Tanganyika, thirteen of them in Dar es Salaam.[19] The fact that non-African medicine in Kenya was effectively privatised before independence gave a special character to health provision there, much as Uganda's lead in the training of African doctors made it distinctive.

The colonial institutions controlling these practitioners were the Medical Practitioners and Dentists Boards set up in Kenya and Uganda shortly before the First World War and in Tanganyika in 1920. They were small, nominated bodies of doctors and dentists chaired by the DMS, although Kenya introduced an elected element in 1946. The boards had great power to accept or refuse practitioners for registration, without which practice of modern medicine was illegal, and to discipline them by warning, suspension, or removal from the register. Until the 1950s the Kenya board spent much time trying to control practitioners of Indian medicine, whom modern Indian doctors resented as competitors. Thereafter it heard more charges of unprofessional conduct, mainly against Asian and African doctors, for offences like advertising their practices, 'covering', drunkenness, and contravention of the law governing drugs and poisons.[20] The first African member, Samson Mwathi, joined the board in 1959. It passed into African control at independence and was described in 1966 as almost a

'Makerere Medical Council', but was not reconstituted as a more independent body until 1979.[21]

Little is known of Tanganyika's medical board, but Uganda's was active during the 1950s, mainly against Makerere graduates accused of offences involving drugs and poisons. Four were removed from the register during 1954, another eight appeared before the board during the next three years, and during the late 1950s and early 1960s there was a steady stream of deregistrations and applications for reinstatement, many of which were refused.[22] It is not surprising, therefore, that whereas in the late 1950s the board had only a token African member, by October 1962, under Kadama's chairmanship, it was in African hands.[23] The Makerere doctors tried to use it to benefit their colleagues and, as they saw it, the country, given the acute shortage of doctors. Kadama secured a legal amendment to permit the licensing for specified duties of doctors who had been struck off the register, so that their skills would not be wasted. All cases were then investigated. Only the elderly Dionysius Bamundaga was then licensed, but a pattern of short-term contract service was established and used to employ many senior doctors long after the official retiring age.[24] In 1965, at Sembeguya's suggestion, the Ministry also sought to compensate fifteen African doctors who had quit the service during the colonial period without receiving pensions or gratuities, 'because of the rather oppressive terms of service then obtaining'. Lumu backed this enthusiastically, but Obote vetoed it.[25] The board itself was reconstituted in 1968 with an unofficial majority nominated by Makerere, the Uganda Medical Association, and the Uganda Dental Association, but with ministry representation and under the Chief Medical Officer's chairmanship. Eight of the nine initial members were Makerere-trained Africans: Kadama, Muganwa, Kununka, Gesa, Kibukamusoke, Kyalwazi, Lutwama, and Martin Aliker (a dentist). Their duties included assessing the qualifications of applicants for registration by comparison with the Makerere medical degree rather than GMC recognition.[26] They were less active in disciplining the profession during the 1960s than a decade earlier, but investigation of suspected drug offences continued. One suspect was the elderly Joseph Mutahangarwa, now living on the Ugandan side of the Tanganyika border:

> I asked for his records but he informed me that the records for 1962 had been stolen from his house. I examined the records for the first part of 1963, and while the date and name of patient was entered with the diagnosis there was no record of treatment, in any case I noted that he had only a few patients every day. On questioning he stated that he did not know, he had not been told, and had not kept a record of drugs supplied to his patients. He confirmed that he had a small practise, a very small practise! I then showed to him 57 orders [for drugs] sined [sic] by a Dr Mutahangarwa, he looked at each signed order and stated that the signature on all

the orders was not his. He added that some b—g— was forging his signature and stealing his note paper and must be found.[27]

The second set of institutions to pass into African control at independence was the reconstituted branches of the BMA. This organisation, founded in 1832, was the powerful trade union of British doctors, setting their minimum fees, meeting their collective needs, and representing them in politics and government. Doctors in almost all British colonies formed branches.[28] Nothing showed better that government doctors in colonial East Africa were far from mere bureaucrats than their membership of the BMA and their use of it to further their service interests. More accurately, the BMA was so powerful that colonial governments could not prevent their doctors from belonging to it.

It was Uganda's DMS who suggested in December 1911 the formation of a BMA branch for Uganda and Kenya. The Uganda section first met in September 1913 with seventeen members, mainly in government service, under Albert Cook's chairmanship. Almost its first action was to set minimum fees. The Kenya section did not take off, nor did joint action, and in 1920 the association was launched again as two separate branches, followed by Zanzibar in 1921 and Tanganyika in 1923.[29] Between 1918 and 1921 the BMA secured major salary improvements for East African doctors by threatening otherwise to stop advising 'members of the profession to accept appointments in the East African Service'.[30] For a period in 1925 it advised doctors to boycott the colonial service entirely until the Colonial Office agreed that government doctors in East Africa might continue to practise privately outside working hours, a concession not granted to other professionals.[31] When the Labour Government threatened this privilege in 1946, medical officers in East Africa again negotiated successfully with their own governments through the BMA; at one point Kenya's DMS sent a copy of his correspondence with the Nairobi authorities to the BMA in London, where the secretary congratulated him on 'an excellent presentation of the case'.[32] The association's final intervention in this bizarre situation was to protect its members' interests during rapid Africanisation.[33]

Even without help from London, BMA branches could be effective, especially in Kenya, where the branch had 100 members in 1927 and 330 in 1960.[34] Its minute book for 1930–50[35] shows it resisting advertising by doctors, practice by unqualified persons, and the registration of those without British qualifications, trying to enforce minimum fees, proposing a postwar health scheme for the European community, concerning itself with hospital conditions and public health, publishing the *East African Medical Journal*, paying the passage to Britain for a sick member, pressing the interests of members in government service, and insisting on being consulted on medical legislation. The other branches were less active but could be mobilised when interests were threatened. The Kenya branch did not admit registered Indian doctors to membership until 1934, when they had already formed or were forming an Indian Medical and Dental Association. After much subsequent tension, the BMA branch elected its first Indian president in 1957. Probably the chief reason for admitting Indians was to stop them charging lower fees.[36] The same consideration may have persuaded some members to welcome Makerere-trained practitioners, starting with Likimani in 1940, but only James Ang'awa was active.[37] The Tanganyika branch elected its first Indian president in 1952,[38] but there is no evidence of active African members. The Uganda branch was more encouraging to Indians and Africans, but Indian doctors maintained a separate Uganda Medical Society and only about 20 per cent of Makerere-trained practitioners joined the BMA.[39]

As independence approached, the Uganda branch was the first to come under African control. Complex negotiations led it to change its name to the Uganda Medical Association in 1961 and elect Africans to its main offices, Sembeguya becoming president. The UMA affiliated to the BMA, which had material advantages but meant that only doctors registrable in Britain could be full members. In1965 only some 250 of the 600 doctors in Uganda belonged and attendance at meetings was poor. The link with the BMA was therefore broken in 1969, but with little effect on membership.[40]

In Kenya the transition was more abrasive. In August 1960 Njoroge Mungai called a meeting of African doctors and was elected president of a Kenya Medical Association distinct from the BMA. Negotiations with the Asian Medical and Dental Association and the BMA branch lasted until 1963, when the new Medical Association of Kenya came into being as a self-governing unit 'incorporated within' the BMA, a closer association than affiliation. Leadership passed mainly to Africans in 1964, when Samson Mwathi became the first African president.[41] The organisation was renamed the Kenya Medical Association in 1968 and broke its remaining links with the BMA in 1973, but not until its revival in 1981, which will be discussed later, did the KMA have much impact on the profession.[42] Much the same was true in Tanganyika, where there was a hiatus at independence until a Medical Association of Tanzania replaced the BMA branch in 1964, but despite formal African leadership there was little African involvement until 1975.[43]

It was symptomatic of the position of African doctors at independence that they could take over these bodies, give them a national colouring, provide them with leaders, protect them from state control, and preserve them for future use, but not put them to much immediate work. By contrast, the Law Society of Kenya had compulsory membership and extensive statutory powers of self-regulation but scarcely any African lawyers, so that it did not elect its first African president until 1970 and in the meantime the state reclaimed much control of the profession.[44] Even the specialist medical associations fell under African control more quickly than the Law Society. John Kibukamusoke became the first African president of the Association of Physicians of East Africa in 1965 and Sebastian Kyalwazi took the same position in the Association of Surgeons two years later.[45] Moreover, it was the medical profession, through the BMA's Kenya branch, that began in 1961 to organise an Association of Professional Societies of Kenya, an initiative later absorbed into the Commonwealth-funded Professional Centres established in the three East African capitals to strengthen professional solidarity and provide support for individual professional associations.[46]

Professional training and professional power

Alongside their personal grievances. African doctors' chief criticism of colonial medical policy was that it had confined medical training to so few Africans.[47] This they were determined to remedy, and they succeeded. Within twenty years of independence, East Africa was producing not 20 but 200 doctors a year, from three medical schools rather than one. Along with the eradication of smallpox, it was the main medical achievement of the period, and it provided Kenya and Tanzania with the bases of medical professions. But it presented its own dilemmas. One was to undermine existing plans for university education in East Africa. A second was how to preserve standards of training while rapidly expanding its scale. A third was how to order the relationship between the growing number of doctors and other medical workers.

Dissatisfaction with Makerere's output of doctors was widespread at independence. In 1960 the Medical School admitted only thirty-one first-year students. The Uganda Government reckoned that the School would produce only sixty-three Ugandan doctors during the next seven years. Tanganyika expected only sixty over ten years.[48] Even the Kenya Government, whose European medical authorities thought in 1960 that between six and twelve new Makerere doctors a year 'will be adequate to meet the needs of Kenya in the future', realised by 1962 that a rapid increase was essential.[49] Under government pressure, Makerere planned in 1960 to increase its medical intake to sixty a year over five years, but without earmarking sufficient resources to do so.[50]

One much-discussed solution might have been to move part of medical training away from Makerere. Medical administrators in Kenya had long envisaged a future medical school,[51] which became a more serious prospect in 1950 when the new King George VI Hospital for Africans opened in Nairobi with magnificent operating theatres, originally designed for all three races, and with able and ambitious European surgeons who suggested that either the clinical training of Makerere's medical undergraduates might move to Nairobi or that postgraduate training might start there. Some postgraduate surgery did begin in 1957, but the idea of undergraduate work had to be dropped as prohibitively expensive. It revived in 1961 when a British specialist recommended that Nairobi should start a medical school immediately to meet the need for doctors in the 1970s, warning that if the British did not start one the Americans would.[52] There were, however, two obstacles. One was expense, especially while Makerere still had unused capacity. The other was that a Nairobi Medical School would destabilise the planned East African university.[53]

Since 1945 Africans in Tanganyika and Kenya had demanded that colleges like Makerere should open in their territories.[54] In 1954 Asian initiative opened a technical college in Nairobi. A year later Tanganyika's governor hoped to see a university there.[55] Eventually the Lockwood Committee of 1958 recommended that the Nairobi technical college should become a university college analogous to Makerere, that a similar college should open in Tanganyika by about 1965–6, that all should teach basic arts and science courses, that professional training in each field (such as medicine) should concentrate at one or other college, and that the three colleges should form a federal university. A second medical school was ruled out for many years to come.[56]

However, the Lockwood scheme did not survive independence. First, Tanganyika's politicians decided to start their college in 1961 and persuaded Wilbert Chagula, earmarked to be Makerere's first African Professor of Anatomy, to become first its Registrar and then its Principal. The new college raised funding problems. In 1962 the Nicol Report recommended that money should be channelled away from Makerere until the other two colleges had reached parity. The new Uganda Government refused and a compromise was patched up to enable the federal University of East Africa to come into being in June 1963.[57] But that was also the month when Njoroge Mungai became Kenya's Minister of Health and reversed policy almost overnight. Without consulting the university, he sought WHO assistance to open an undergraduate medical school at Nairobi during 1966.[58] This put the pressure on Uganda, many of whose leaders already saw the federal university as retarding Makerere's development. They proposed to expand Makerere's medical intake to ninety a year as a charge on general university funds. Kenya and Tanganyika refused to contribute and Kenya suggested the additional students should do their clinical training in Nairobi. A number did so during 1965–6,[59] but by then Mungai's energy had located the funds and expatriate staff for his medical school and Kenyatta had announced that it would open in 1967.[60] This, as Roger Southall wrote, 'sounded the death knell of the University [of East Africa] as an institution of planning'.[61] It dissolved in 1970.

That left not only Makerere and Nairobi with medical schools, but also Dar es Salaam. With only twelve serving African doctors at independence, Tanganyika's need was the most urgent, but its secondary education was also the most backward, so that it had little hope of meeting its need from Makerere, which from 1959 admitted only students with higher certificate (six years of secondary schooling). In 1961 the Tanganyika Government decided to supplement Makerere by opening a medical school at the former Medical Training Centre in Dar es Salaam. It would admit students with school certificate (four years of secondary education) and give them a four-year training in rural medicine. Tanganyika benefited most from the federal university and was anxious not to threaten it, so it proposed that these rural practitioners should receive diplomas rather than degrees and should be licensed as Assistant Medical Officers. The course opened in July 1963.[62]

With its echoes of the second-class status suffered by Makerere-trained physicians before 1957, this scheme aroused much medical opposition. An Ugandan representative called it 'a retrogressive step'.[63] 'It would be very unwise', Sembeguya told the Uganda Medical Association,

> to depart from the standard of training that has been set up and which is equivalent to the highest medical training offered in the world and that is of Great Britain. It has taken well over 100 years for Britain to build up her medical curriculum which, in the course of her rule here, she has passed to us. It is my firm belief that the profession should continue to remain independent of political influences . . . What is desperately needed is not a vast number of semi-doctors with a consequent lowering of standards, but a nucleus of highly trained professionals such as emerge from Makerere now.[64]

Hilary Ojiambo, the most articulate of Kenya's younger physicians, 'did not believe in the production of pseudo-doctors'. 'Our aim', he argued, 'should be to produce an individual whose professional qualifications will not be a perpetual embarrassment to him'.[65] In Tanganyika, understandably, opposition was more muted, but it was still strong. In August 1962 Swedi Mwankemwa, Regional Medical Officer in Morogoro, told a visitor that 'Makerere doctors [are] worried about prestige. The public will regard the AMO and the R[ural] M[edical] P[ractitioner] as doctors.'[66]

These objections would scarcely have deterred Tanganyika's politicians. What destroyed the scheme was student opposition, demonstrating the same entrepreneurial pursuit of knowledge and status that had inspired indigenous apprentices and carried the first medical students through Makerere. The course opened with only sixteen of the planned twenty-five students. After three months only ten were left 'and most of these were trying to arrange avenues of escape'. Students demanded degree training, teachers were scarce, accommodation was poor, grants were inadequate, and the final qualification to be awarded was undecided. In 1966, with forty-eight students in four classes but still no agreement on the final qualification, the students struck and thirty-one were rusticated. But by now secondary school output was increasing and the federal university was doomed. In 1968 the Medical School was integrated into the University College, Dar es Salaam. Of the sixteen initial students, four eventually graduated.[67]

A second Tanganyikan scheme had been more successful. Medical assistants, normally with school certificate, three years of medical training, and often much practical experience, had become the core of colonial medical systems. For African doctors, however, they were a problem and a threat. Tension between the two was notorious: one East African novel recast the Romeo and Juliet story as a romance between the son of a former medical assistant (grown rich as representative of a drug firm) and the daughter of a doctor (grown poor on a civil service salary).[68] In independent Tanganyika, however, the politicians were in control and their concerns were, first, to increase the number of African doctors and, second, to check the outflow of ill-paid medical assistants into the enormous opportunities available in politics, government, and business, which reduced their number from some 300 in January 1961 to 198 in March 1962. Moreover, medical assistants were thought to be inadequately trained and applications for such training were falling off as schools increasingly taught beyond school certificate.[69] Tanganyika therefore abolished the training of medical assistants in government institutions and sought to upgrade most of those in service to licensed Assistant Medical Officers who would form the core of the medical service. Upgrading began in 1961 with a six-month course, eventually extended to eighteen months. Although the university and some doctors opposed the scheme and some AMOs complained of their second-class, unregistered status, upgrading checked the outflow of medical assistants and rewarded many competent clinical workers.[70] The scheme lapsed when the Medical School opened but was reactivated at intervals into the 1990s when pressure from medical assistants mounted, for by the mid-1960s it was realised that medical assistants were still needed and their training resumed in 1968.[71]

The problem of medical assistants existed also in Kenya and Uganda, but their solutions differed because doctors were more powerful. In Kenya, hospital assistants (as they were called) were the core of the medical service at independence, but their training was abandoned in the early 1960s with the intention that nurses should assume their nursing functions while the better hospital assistants were upgraded to clinical assistants and given charge of rural medical units until qualified doctors could replace them. By 1966 it was obvious that the supply of doctors would not increase quickly enough and the government began instead to train medical assistants, but it fiercely resisted pressure from the assistants and their numerous parliamentary representatives for upgrading to break through the 'parchment curtain' separating them from doctors.[72] 'Hospital assistants are not assistant doctors and we are going to place those two categories completely separate', Mungai insisted.[73] In Uganda the doctors were even more fully in control, there was no scarcity of sub-professional staff, and the treatment of medical assistants was brutal. 'Already the Uganda Medical Assistants consider they should be called Assistant Medical Officers', the Ministry of Health noted in 1962. If that happened, 'a sub-standard type of medical practitioner will have been produced. Uganda has already done this once and there is no valid reason for repeating the experiment.'[74] Although training of the cadre continued, their demands for better pay and status were rejected with disdain:

> Medical assistants have lower salary entry points as compared with state registered nurses, laboratory technicians and health inspectors because the medical assistants' course, the syllabus of which is controlled by me and may be altered from time to time to suit my ministry's needs without consulting anybody, is not at all recognised by any other commonwealth country.[75]

When Mulago's nurses struck in April 1963 rather than wear identification numbers, one Makerere-trained doctor saw even that as a medical assistants' plot:

> This section of the Ministry of Health, constitutes a thorn in the whole Ministry. They are convinced that they are half or three-quarters Doctors. And they are full of discontent and resentment because they are not regarded as Doctors. Last year they submitted a memorandum to the Ministry of Health demanding to be given the status of Assistant Medical Officers. Such overtures are an insult to the medical profession . . . the Government should henceforth keep an open and observant eye on this personnel. We are aware that our sister nation Tanganyika is presently training this type of medical men, but we in Uganda should from now set our eyes to seeing an end to their generation.[76]

As a final insult, Uganda removed stethoscopes from the training of medical assistants in 1972 on the grounds that they needed to concentrate instead on public health.[77] Professionalism in a status-conscious honour society could be harsh indeed.

Looking to the future

The Africans who took control of East Africa's medical systems at independence inherited not only structures and institutions but constraints. The underlying fact was poverty. In 1962–3 Kenya's total public expenditure on health was about £4,300,000, which amounted to 2 per cent of Gross Domestic Product or Shs.11–12 per Kenyan per year. Yet this expenditure had risen significantly during the late 1950s, so that a World Bank study of the economy in 1962 warned against any substantial further increase.[78] A similar mission to Uganda demanded 'vigorous action' to restrain demands for medical expansion.[79] The current orthodoxy was that the first priority in government expenditure must be productive economic activity, to provide the revenue for other development, and that the second priority was education to provide manpower. In Tanganyika the share of recurrent government expenditure devoted to education had risen between 1948 and 1958 from 6 to 17 per cent, largely frustrating the medical development plan for 1956–61. That trend continued after independence. Tanganyika's plan for 1961–4 devoted so few resources to health that a parliamentarian asked whether the slogan was 'Freedom and Sickness'.[80]

While public expenditure on health stagnated, demand rose dramatically. Population was growing at between 2 and 3 per cent per year, its impact multiplied by the fact that childbearing and infancy created peak demands for medical care. An enormous reservoir of illness had not hitherto been treated, estimated by a Kenyan survey in the early 1980s as between 60 and 90 per cent of all cases needing medical attention. People were increasingly alert to the benefits of modern medicine. And modern medicine itself was increasingly beneficial, especially its new antibiotic and antimalarial drugs.[81] Between 1954 and 1959, paediatric outpatients at Mulago Hospital had multiplied sixfold. During the next five years, patients attending government hospitals and dispensaries in Tanganyika doubled.[82] There the government had attempted to check demand by introducing outpatient charges in 1957, while Kenya introduced fees for many dispensary and hospital services. This generally reduced patient numbers for a year or two, but they quickly recovered.[83] And it was very unpopular. KANU's election manifesto in 1963 promised to aim at free medical treatment, radical critics in Tanganyika demanded the same, and opposition in Uganda prevented the introduction of the fees recommended by the Frazer Committee.[84]

Given this constraint, medical changes at independence, apart from the Africanisation of senior posts, were largely cosmetic. One easy victory was to replace racial distinctions in hospitals by class distinctions, but there were few other changes of policy. Kenya and Uganda had medical systems widely considered models for poor countries.[85] Tanganyika's was more rudimentary but on similar principles. The broad lines of policy had enjoyed general agreement for two decades and the question of priorities was muted so long as the little money available was committed to inherited projects. 'Kenya must copy the British model of medical services and nothing less', Njoroge Mungai insisted, and Lumu – but not Bryceson – echoed him.[86] Colonial doctors had recognised since the 1930s that medical systems which had originated to treat Europeans put too much emphasis on urban hospitals at the expense of rural and preventive medicine, but they also recognised that people valued curative institutions and disliked sanitary measures. Experience with African politicians reinforced the message: there were no votes in pit latrines. Policy, therefore, was to pursue two balanced, or perhaps contradictory, priorities.[87] One was to develop a high-quality teaching hospital in the capital and, if possible, smaller provincial and district hospitals. The other was to create a network of health centres, the fashionable panacea of the time. 'Health centres', a Kenyan doctor explained, 'are not Hospitals, but are schools for better living', places where curative and preventive medicine blended.[88] They served specified populations – the target in Kenya was one for every 20,000 people – and provided a few hospital beds and outpatient services but also undertook outreach activities: maternity care, district visiting, family planning, sanitation, health education, and eventually, as a zealot put it, 'the whole field of human endeavour, agricultural, animal husbandry, welfare, citizenship, etc.'[89] The staff was an entirely African team headed by a medical, hospital, or clinical assistant, with a midwife, a health inspector or assistant, possibly a laboratory assistant, a nurse, and a dresser to undertake the basic hospital duties and free the others to work among the community, for, as a slogan put it, one did not work *in* a health centre but *from* one, possibly using a mobile clinic. Advocates claimed that health centres were the most cost-effective form of health provision. One estimate in 1963 was that the average patient cost Shs.4 at a health centre, Shs.84 at a district hospital, and Shs.374 at a national hospital.[90] In the long term, an African doctor would head each centre and coordinate the community's development. Kenya opened its first health centre in 1951 and became the movement's pioneer in the Third World. At independence it had some 140, with plans for a total of about 300.[91] Tanganyika had only twenty-two, owing to the poverty of its local authorities, but further centres were the core of its medical planning. Uganda's policy was the same on paper, but with relatively numerous and long-established dispensaries, strong popular demand for local hospitals, and vigorous local governments, concentration on curative medicine was strongly entrenched there.[92]

Yet beneath this consensus and continuity of policy, complex changes were taking place in the medical and socio-political environment within which East African doctors acted, changes which would grow in power during the first generation of independence. Perhaps four can be identified. One concerned the state and doctors' relations with it. At one level, these relations already differed from country to country. Uganda's doctors were powerful in politics and the bureaucracy and could expect a close alliance with the state. Kenya's were less powerful, especially once Mungai moved to Defence, but they shared the political leadership's modernising and elitist goals. By contrast, in Tanganyika (from 1964 united with Zanzibar as Tanzania) the state's levelling and centralising ambitions seriously threatened professional status. Yet these contrasts, although real, would soon be overshadowed by a general weakening of the state. Perhaps it was already beginning in the late colonial period as population growth outran the mobilisation of resources, the modern sector of the economy outgrew government control, and nationalism destroyed old methods of domination. Certainly it was fully under way by the 1970s as a result of over-ambition, political factionalism, and economic decline. Not only did states become incapable of paying doctors reasonable salaries or providing them with tolerable working conditions, but it robbed them of the support against alternative forms of medicine on which professional status depended. Alliance with the state was the key to successful professionalisation outside the Anglo-American context. In East Africa state weakness destroyed that alliance.

A second set of changes affected the patterns of disease against which doctors struggled. It was not so much the balance between disease categories that changed, but the significance of particular diseases within each category. For example, colonial medicine had been especially effective against epidemic disease, so that at the time of independence plague was a rarity, smallpox was on the verge of eradication, sleeping sickness was localised and remediable, and cholera had not been seen for two generations. Yet during the 1950s two new epidemic diseases emerged to replace the old. One was measles, which had existed in the past but flourished in the growing population densities of the time; the average number of cases treated each year in Tanganyika rose between 1954–7 and 1964–7 from 6,651 to 46,049.[93] The other was poliomyelitis, which was reckoned in the 1990s to cause two-thirds of Uganda's physical disability;[94] it had probably been endemic in the past, so that most people had survived mild attacks in infancy, but it became epidemic in the 1950s, perhaps partly because new strains arrived and partly because improved hygiene prevented some people from acquiring immunity.[95] Both were primarily diseases of children, as were widespread nutritional problems and many forms of anaemia; together they reinforced the emphasis on maternal and child health which came from a rapidly growing population and the general failure of colonial medicine in this field. Similarly, although colonial medicine had successfully treated many overt diseases of poverty, especially yaws, ulcers, and (during the 1950s) leprosy, less obvious conditions may have become more common, notably helminthic conditions, bilharzia – a disease with a little-known history which probably spread widely during the colonial period, affecting over half of Tanganyika's people at independence[96] – and the venereal diseases which had often replaced yaws. Again, colonial medicine had found treatments for the two great endemic environmental diseases of East Africa, malaria in the lowlands and respiratory infections in the highlands, but malaria remained as prevalent as ever in the lowlands and had spread into many highland areas,[97] while respiratory infections had been complicated by the spread of tuberculosis. Thus the communicable diseases which caused perhaps 70 per cent of the region's ill-health[98] were changing more than they were declining. In addition, as will be seen, new behavioural conditions were becoming prominent – substance abuse, road accidents, high blood pressure – and physicians were becoming aware of cancer and heart conditions which had probably long existed but had been neglected. Ill-health was less obtrusive in East Africa at independence than it had been in the days of James Ainsworth and Adrien Atiman, but it was little less widespread or diverse.

A more dramatic influence on the evolution of the medical profession was the relentless advance of chemotherapy. The precursor had been Salvarsan before the First World War, but the major breakthrough in drug production had come in the 1930s, with sulphonamides like M & B 693, and in the 1940s, when antibiotics like penicillin and antimalarials like chloroquine became available. The techniques of research and marketing used to produce and distribute these were then applied to other products, so that by the 1990s there would be relatively cheap and simple chemical cures not only for gonorrhoea, bilharzia, and helminthic complaints but for such severe diseases as leprosy, tuberculosis, river blindness, cholera, and plague. Only slightly behind this advance went the development of cheap vaccines, first against tuberculosis and then against the child-killing diseases, especially poliomyelitis in the 1950s and measles in the 1970s. By independence modern medicine was for the first time gaining the means to cure or palliate most common East African diseases. A mission doctor caught the significance of this in 1950:

> We share with the rest of the medical world the great privilege of treating patients with the newer drugs, especially the sulphonamides and penicillin. And it is indeed a privilege. No longer must we stand by as medical students of my generation were taught. Now we have tools that can cure most cases of sepsis and pneumonia. The Africans are quick to appreciate these advances.[99]

Indeed they were. The expansion of attendances at modern medical units during the 1950s was in large measure their response.

Yet chemotherapeutic advances had three less obvious consequences. One was to make the availability of drugs the central point of public criticism of medical systems. The second was to breed immense frustration among doctors if they could not procure drugs which they knew could benefit their patients. The third was that patients needing modern drugs did not necessarily need doctors. As Trowell told the Frazer Committee in 1955, between 30 and 60 per cent of those attending Mulago Hospital could have treated themselves with drugs bought at a pharmacy.[100] Increasingly they did so, although they used a local store or itinerant pedlar. 'Aspirin and related drugs are extremely popular', it was observed of the coastal Digo people in 1959,

> and any new drug of this type, if given a little advertisement, is quickly utilized. Also eye wash, epsom salts, remedies for rheumatism, for constipation and for diarrhoea, are very popular. A number of these are prepared in India or in East Africa by Indian firms. Quinine tablets are used for all manner of *Homa* [fever] complaints . . . Black Market drugs, such as penicillin and antibiotics are also dispensed.[101]

Alternatively, those seeking modern medicine might turn to a 'needle man', as he was called in the Bunyole area of Uganda:[102] the retired tribal dresser or totally untrained practitioner with a syringe and some stolen phials of penicillin. This was where the growth of chemotherapy interacted with the weakening of the state, for it was colonial governments that had enforced the provisions in the Medical Practitioners and Dentists Ordinances and the Pharmaceuticals and Poisons Ordinances prohibiting anyone but a qualified doctor from administering modern medicines and anyone but a qualified pharmacist from selling them. By the 1950s the repression of needle men and drug sellers was increasingly difficult, as can be seen from amendments to the law raising the penalties and specifically outlawing injections, the spate of prosecutions reported in the press, and the parallel increase in professional sanctions against errant doctors.[103] As post-colonial states weakened, enforcement sometimes collapsed entirely. Faced with rivalry from self-medication with powerful and easily available drugs, medical professionalism could survive only with the support and protection of a strong state, even in Britain and America. In East Africa those states ceased to exist.

Attractive as modern drugs might be, there were other reasons for the enthusiasm for self-medication, for it also extended to indigenous medicine, where herbalists gained over other practitioners, moved increasingly from the countryside into towns, and began to standardise herbal remedies and sell them as much as possible like modern pharmaceuticals. As Susan Reynolds Whyte has suggested,[104] the attraction of self-medication in all its forms was its simplicity, convenience, and privacy when compared with ritual remedies which were increasingly difficult to organise amid religious diversity and spatial mobility, much as East African townsmen preferred to blame their misfortunes on sorcery because that was the cause easiest to counter in an urban environment.[105] Behind the triumph of self-medication lay not only the power of pharmaceutical companies but a larger process of social change.

The implications of chemotherapy for the African medical profession were very complex and need study throughout the continent. On the one hand the proliferation of drugs might deluge the modern doctor with patients. On the other it might deluge him with rivals. Some of his activities were deskilled, as could be seen in the tendency within and outside hospitals for nurses and paramedics to take over functions hitherto reserved for doctors,[106] so that chemotherapy became in one aspect a means by which paramedics struck back at doctors with their own weapons. Elsewhere in the world this deskilling was compensated by the growing skill required in other medical functions, but that probably happened less in East Africa because those functions often needed expensive equipment. Nevertheless, chemotherapy did offer East African doctors new opportunities, for it enabled them to treat complaints which had hitherto required hospital facilities. The removal of many tuberculosis cases from chronic wards to outpatient treatment illustrated the process. This benefited the private practitioner rather than the government medical officer.

At this point changes in the state, in diseases, and in therapies came together with changes taking place within the medical profession itself. No longer did it have unique status as the only true profession open to Africans; now there were African lawyers and engineers and architects to claim equal status and earn larger salaries as state finances collapsed. No longer did all the best students read medicine. No longer were doctors the admired apex of African ambition. Increasingly, indeed, they were the targets of bitter public criticism as medical facilities deteriorated. Moreover, the increasing number of African doctors weakened the profession's exclusivity and solidarity. Differences of generation, wealth, and outlook divided it, especially between private practitioners and public employees. Not only chemotherapy encouraged private practice; so did urbanisation and the formation of an elite African clientele.

There is no simple way of summarising all these changes affecting East Africa's doctors as they entered their independent future. The status of the medical profession was certainly to decline. The Anglo-American model of professionalism which doctors had been taught to admire was to be gravely, perhaps fatally, weakened. Elements of what might become a different professional pattern would emerge. And in each country doctors were to pass through a generation of anguish and struggle.

7 Uganda: doctors and a disintegrating state

At independence, Uganda's modern African doctors, although few, outnumbered those in all the other East African countries. They took control of the medical system and generally retained it throughout the 1960s, with necessary political compromises. Their professional base at the Makerere Medical School won an international reputation at that time for research and teaching. There were signs that an increasingly authoritarian state might threaten professional status, but what in fact undermined it was the near-disintegration of the state in the 1970s and 1980s during General Amin's military tyranny and the prolonged succession struggle that followed. Those years created terrible dilemmas for doctors, destroyed much of their professional standing, and forced them to compete in the marketplace with rival suppliers of modern drugs. When, in the late 1980s, a new regime tried to rebuild the state, the medical profession was not among its priorities. The doctors, too, were divided, some eager to restore the glories of the 1960s, others groping for new forms of professionalism.

The Obote years, 1962–71

Independence brought Uganda's Makerere-trained doctors to power. Lumu was Minister of Health, Muwazi his counterpart in Buganda, Kadama Permanent Secretary and Chief Medical Officer, Kibaya the Medical Superintendent of Mulago. By the end of the decade, Lumu was in detention, Kibaya either detained or recently released, Muwazi in disgrace, and Kadama in retirement. Yet beneath this political turbulence there had been an underlying continuity of medical policy, threatened only by political pressures.

Lumu and Muwazi were both high-profile politicians deeply engaged in the disputed relationship between Buganda and Uganda. Policy therefore lay with Kadama and the medical bureaucrats, whose priority was to keep the medical service working amidst the scarcity and kaleidoscopic changes of staff until Makerere's expanded output of doctors became available in the late 1960s. The figures are contradictory, but at independence Uganda probably had about 450 practising doctors, of whom 90 were Ugandans; in 1969 there were 647, including 194 Ugandans.[1] They had contained a smallpox outbreak in 1965, launched Africa's first national immunisation campaign against polio, reorganised the public health of Kampala, and generally maintained services, all despite severe financial constraints.[2] As Lumu explained in his first budget speech, medical expenditure was pegged until it had fallen to the 8.5 per cent of public revenue recommended by the World Bank. 'We shall not be building new hospitals', he warned. Real expenditure dropped by nearly 10 per cent between 1959 and 1963–4.[3]

Yet this stringency conflicted with an immense pressure of demand. Attendances at government medical institutions doubled between 1958 and 1963, then doubled again by 1969. The new Mulago was swamped by Kampala residents with minor complaints.[4] More effectively, the constituencies and their parliamentary representatives clamoured for local hospitals, partly perhaps because the chief cost to patients at government facilities was getting there – travel amounted to 75 per cent of outpatients' costs at one hospital studied in 1964 – and partly, as Colin Leys suggested, because people felt they could endure the complaints treated at dispensaries or health centres but wanted rapid access to a hospital in life-threatening conditions like obstructed childbirth.[5] The Member for Pakwach, in distant West Nile, told Lumu to go and *find* the money for a hospital there.[6] Such pressure was effective because Obote believed that Uganda's survival depended on the coherence of the ruling UPC, which was a loose conglomeration of local notables threatened in almost every constituency by the opposition, and that what voters wanted were government services. Moreover, not only did people want hospitals, but hospitals were all that the central government could give them in the field of health, for the constitution left all other medical institutions to local authorities.[7]

These considerations lay behind the decision in 1964 to abandon World Bank policy, ignore medical opinion, and build twenty-two (later twenty-three) hundred-bed rural hospitals outside district centres. They were allocated evenly among the country's four regions, but local competition within each region was intense.[8] Although GDP was growing at nearly 6 per cent per year, the hospital scheme imposed severe financial strains, helping to raise current health expenditure by 90 per cent between 1963–4 and 1968–9 and forcing the Cabinet to order drastic cuts in 1966, especially at Mulago, 'in order to avoid financial chaos'.[9] It also strained manpower resources to staff the new hospitals, a consideration which led elements in the Ministry to oppose a scheme prepared in 1968 to increase the number of new hospitals to thirty-five. 'The cry by every Ugandan . . . is . . . more hospitals, more dispensaries, more aid posts, more medicine and so on', the Minister complained in 1970. 'I am afraid that we cannot keep up with the demands of the country.' The third development plan drafted for 1971–6 reduced the share of expenditure devoted to health and increased the emphasis on training and rural facilities.[10]

Doctors flourished financially during the 1960s. An intern's real earnings doubled between 1963 and 1972, with similar increases for senior consultants.[11] Politically, however, harsh competition swept away the professional men prominent in the 1950s. Of the four doctors in leading political positions at independence, the first casualty was Muwazi. As Buganda's Minister of Health and Works, he was at the heart of the major conflict between 1962 and 1964 concerning the Lost Counties. In an attempt to win the referendum which was to decide their future, the Buganda Government planned to settle some 5,000 Ganda war veterans at Ndaiga. Muwazi, christened 'Katikiro of Ndaiga', was made responsible, but the central government declared the veterans ineligible to vote and in November 1964 the counties chose by a large majority to leave Buganda and rejoin Bunyoro. The Buganda Government resigned and another doctor, Kisekka, took over Muwazi's ministry. Muwazi abandoned politics, presumably for the private practice which was the doctors' enviable refuge. He appears to have died in the mid-1970s in exile after practising at the Machakos Provincial Hospital in Kenya.[12]

Ironically, the government victory that destroyed Muwazi also in the long term ended Lumu's political career. He had left Kabaka Yekka for the UPC in June 1963 as the only way to save Buganda and its throne.[13] As other Ganda leaders followed him, the UPC leadership began to split between southerners and northerners. In February 1966 a parliamentary motion demanding an inquiry into the conduct of Obote's military ally, Colonel Idi Amin, split the two UPC factions. Lumu warned parliament that Amin must be suspended lest he launch a military takeover.[14] Eighteen days later Obote had Lumu and four other southern ministers arrested at a Cabinet meeting. They spent the next five years in detention.[15]

Obote now suspended the constitution, declared himself president, took the Kabaka's palace, and abolished the Buganda kingdom. This made it a third doctor's turn to face the ruthlessness of politics. George Sembeguya, private practitioner and part-time lecturer in medical ethics, was a specially elected parliamentarian, a Buganda patriot, and a liberal nationalist. When Obote ordered parliamentarians to approve his new constitution without debate, Sembeguya was one who voted against and refused the oath. Two months later he faced the hostile House:

> I know that it is extremely dangerous to stand up and criticise the Government but one has to do it . . . Mr Speaker, when the new Constitution was introduced, we Backbenchers did not smell it, maybe some did, I never knew anything about it, and therefore, Mr Speaker, I could not swear to the Constitution without having read it,

I therefore decided not to swear and went home and studied the Constitution and decided to swear to it to make the best of it and that is why, Mr Speaker, I am here to air my views, because I thought it was cowardly to run away.

Amid interruptions, he went on:

I said, Mr Speaker, that Uganda had been a very peaceful country, we have always sat at the round tables and settled our difficulties amicably without the use of arms. The use of arms at the Lubiri [Palace] was, to my mind, beyond our expectations . . . If I did not have the interest of the country at heart I would not take the courage to speak. But because I want stability to return to this country, I want everybody to live in peace without any form of fear or suspicions, I stand up to tell those who are in authority that these changes were too rapid; they were major changes, they have not been done in consultation with people who are concerned, not with me as a Member of Parliament who should know about this, and then I am just a rubber stamp.[16]

As a UPC member in Buganda, Sembeguya's life was threatened and his nursing home boycotted. 'I am a refugee in my own country', he wrote.[17] At the same time his criticism of the state of emergency in Buganda led him to be assaulted by uniformed men, expelled from the UPC, and detained after there had been an assassination attempt against Obote.[18] Other Ganda doctors also suffered, including Kibaya, who was detained in 1967.[19] It was characteristic that Sembeguya should have used the hiatus in his practice to return to the Medical School to prepare for the FRCS examinations, feeling that he 'must have more qualifications'.[20]

Only one doctor-politician profited from this turbulence. Once a Kabaka Yekka zealot, Eria Babumba was quick to join the UPC in 1963, although it led to the boycott of his nursing home near Masaka. He endorsed Obote's new constitution in 1966 and became Minister of State for Foreign Affairs.[21] When Sembeguya made his parliamentary justification, it was Babumba who interrupted him: 'This was a revolutionary Constitution . . . and it was necessary.'[22] Babumba was now a fervent unitarist and socialist. As Minister of Marketing and Cooperatives in 1968 he introduced legislation establishing government control of coffee marketing, provoking the coffee-growing Sembeguya to protest that 'Dr Babumba and his colleague will be remembered in history of the coffee industry as the men who wrecked it.' Later analysts have agreed.[23]

Babumba's movement to Jacobin authoritarianism was typical of the UPC regime between 1966 and 1971 as it struggled against Uganda's centrifugal forces. Late in 1969 the government decided to restructure the legal profession under a Law Council rather than the previously self-regulating Law Society. When Makerere became an independent university in 1970, its new statutes gave the government control even over senior academic appointments.[24] The medical profession was not yet attacked in this way.

Obote was a critic of private medical practice. He had refused to subsidise private nursing homes. In 1968 he barred university medical staff from practising for profit. A year later he urged young doctors 'to fight the "mercenaries" who are undermining their profession'.[25] He was probably moving towards state control of medicine on Tanzanian lines. In the event, however, the threat to Uganda's medical profession came not from a strong state but from a weak one.

Makerere at its peak

During the 1960s the Makerere Medical School became a research and teaching centre of international reputation. The new Mulago Hospital was magnificently designed. Foreign funds flowed into one of the three leading centres of research in new African nations. Indigenous staff began to take control, notably when Joseph Lutwama became Dean in 1965. Their research was probably the most important intellectual achievement by East Africans before the 1980s. Most worked in the tradition of Trowell and Davies, charting and seeking to explain East Africa's disease patterns, but their work was infused with national and racial awareness. The combination was both distinctive and distinguished. With regard to teaching, the undergraduate curriculum was made more integrated and locally relevant, with a research project and more attention to preventive medicine at the Kasangati Health Centre. External examiners' reports were laudatory. Scarcely any medical students failed their final examinations.[26]

The students had changed somewhat since the 1940s. By the late 1960s about one-third were Asians. More were women: 53, as against 360 men, in 1968–9. Ugandans regained their dominance as medical schools opened elsewhere.[27] Educational opportunity was still open, especially for men, but the hereditary element was growing. By 1970 Blasio Mukungu, one of the first medical students of 1923, had sent both a son and grandson to the Medical School.[28] Kadama, Likimani, Odonga, Babumba, Kununka, Matovu, and Latimer Musoke all had children there. Doctors' families intermarried, strengthening group consciousness. Students in the mid-1960s no longer aspired to private practice but to government service as 'a technocratic upper-middle class of organization men', above all by gaining specialist qualifications. Only 20 per cent said they belonged to a political party.[29] 'Their feet were already marching to the rhythm of 1, 2, 3, 4: one spouse, two children, three rooms in a bungalow, and four wheels of a motorcar.'[30] Ironically, within twenty years most were probably private practitioners with more political experience than they wanted, but that was because the world changed.

The Medical School's chief innovation during the 1960s was postgraduate training. It had prepared graduates for British examinations since the 1950s. By 1975 some twenty-seven had become Fellows of the Royal Colleges of Surgeons and forty-eight were Members of the Royal Colleges of Physicians.[31] The introduction of three-year MMed courses in 1967 was designed to make training more relevant, strengthen local research, and discourage specialists from emigrating. In 1970 there were twenty-five students, released grudgingly by the Medical Department.[32] Some believed that the Medical School was becoming too specialised, too technological, too expensive, and too big. 'Gone are the days when the teachers used to know their students personally', the student president warned in 1970.[33] A graduate pointed to another implication:

> In my first few weeks at an up-country hospital I was very unhappy. The authorities in charge of training had certainly not impressed upon me the conditions prevailing in up-country hospitals . . . When I was called to see a patient with delay in the second stage of labour after examination I automatically asked the staff to prepare for a vacuum extraction . . . Nobody on the station had heard of a vacuum extractor. I had to do my first foreceps delivery under the most unfavourable conditions and with no guidance . . . Surely a student should be taught to use the instruments he is likely to have available to use.[34]

Research, however, flourished. It followed many lines laid down in the 1940s and 1950s by Trowell, Davies, and their pupils, notably Muwazi. There was the same concern to identify and explain the distinctive features of East Africa's disease environment. Initially, too, there was the same interest in kwashiorkor and venereal diseases. But just as Muwazi had helped to demonstrate that kwashiorkor was not due to congenital syphilis, so the next generation of researchers set out to demonstrate that in so far as East Africa's disease patterns differed from those elsewhere, the reasons were generally economic or environmental rather than ethnic or cultural. In a muted form, this appeared in the work of Latimer Musoke, who was Muwazi's successor in paediatric medicine and eventually headed the Paediatric Department. He showed that whereas in 1950–1 gastroenteritis had been a rare reason for paediatric admission to Mulago, by 1959 it was the most common, especially among Ganda infants from Kampala's most prosperous ethnic group. Rather than seeking a cultural explanation, however, Musoke blamed 'a falling off of breast feeding in the towns' in favour of 'early supplementary feeding . . . prepared in an unhygienic way'. Similarly, when discussing the tendency to bring rural children to hospital too late, he blamed not ignorance or conservatism but poverty:

> The life of the mothers of most of our patients is very arduous. She has the responsibility of growing food for the family, assisting the husband in cultivating fields of cash crops, providing water and firewood for the family and looking after her own four to eight children. Means of transport are difficult, although getting

easier in most parts of the country. It is with these problems that the mother has to forsake her home and other children to bring her sick infant to hospital. This is reflected in the late arrival of many of the cases admitted and the high mortality soon after admission.[35]

Another environmental factor of special concern to researchers was malaria and its wider impact on disease patterns. Aaron Masawe, a Tanzanian, argued, for example, that the severity of syphilis in Ugandans, despite the disease's prevalence for about a century, might be due to the immunological consequences of malaria.[36] The most elaborate research on these lines was by John Kibukamusoke, the first East African physician to obtain a Membership and perhaps the most productive and ambitious of all Makerere doctors. His main interest was the nephrotic syndrome, a form of kidney damage, commonly with oedema (accumulation of fluid) and high levels of protein in the urine, which was between 60 and 90 times more common in the Kampala area than in temperate countries.[37] Davies had observed the condition but been unable to explain it.[38] Malaria had been suspected for centuries and demonstrated in children,[39] but Kibukamusoke demonstrated, by studying damaged kidneys, that the most common mechanism in adults was for the body's resistance to malaria to create immune deposits which damaged the kidneys. He published this in his doctoral thesis,[40] edited a collective volume setting the subject into the general field of immunology,[41] experimented with drugs to treat nephritis,[42] and sought funds to start an artificial-kidney treatment centre at Mulago.[43] At the same period his colleagues, Raphael Owor and Samuel Kajubi, were studying chronic pancreatic disease, a cause of malabsorption and malnutrition.[44]

Mulago's other and major area of research during the 1960s concerned cancer and heart complaints. This had stronger ideological implications, for these had been thought 'diseases of civilisation' from which Africans seldom suffered, so that blood pressure became a barometer of progress. But there were other reasons for concern with these diseases. They were the cutting edge of medical research throughout the world, African students often learned the techniques in Western hospitals, the complaints were expected to multiply in East Africa in the future, and, perhaps most important, Makerere's staff realised that they could make a major international contribution in this field. As usual, the opportunity went back to Davies. In 1954 he established a cancer registry to record all Ugandan cases.[45] He also analysed Cook's magnificent case records at Mengo Hospital from 1897. These showed that cancer had been almost as common at Mengo in 1897–1906, representing 0.73 per cent of admissions, as in 1947–56, when 0.89 per cent of those admitted had cancer. Cancer was as common among Ugandans aged under forty-five to fifty as it was in Western countries; the differences were that older Ugandans were less susceptible and other diseases were so prevalent as to make cancer appear less significant. The types of cancer in Uganda in the 1950s were similar to those fifty years earlier but were strikingly different from those in the West, 'with the infrequency of lung and gastro-intestinal cancers in Uganda and the lesser frequency of breast cancer and the great frequency of primary liver cancers, Kaposi's sarcoma, and penile and ovarian cancers'.[46] There were also considerable differences within Uganda between ethnic groups and regions. The researchers suggested chiefly environmental reasons for these, which had great potential significance for all cancer studies.[47] Moreover, the work had interested a government surgeon, Denis Burkitt, who noticed that a common cancer of the jaw in children was not only extraordinarily malignant – the tumour could potentially double its size in twenty-four hours[48] – but was often associated with tumours elsewhere in the body, and these could also appear without symptoms in the jaw.[49] He thus described a form of cancer – it became known (to Davies's irritation[50]) as Burkitt's lymphoma – which could manifest in several parts of the body. This suggested that it might be caused by a virus, which was known to happen in animals but not in human beings. In 1964 external researchers identified the Epstein–Barr virus as probably the main causative agent. Subsequent research associated several other human cancers with latent viruses.[51]

These findings were of major international importance. In 1967 the United States National Institute of Health financed a lymphoma treatment centre at Mulago which later became the Uganda Cancer Institute. The senior investigator was Uganda's leading surgeon, Sebastian Kyalwazi, who conducted research on Kaposi's sarcoma (another multicentric tumour) and cancer of the liver and penis.[52] He was especially interested in the chemotherapy of cancer,[53] a major subject at Mulago because the hospital lacked radiotherapeutic equipment, multicentric tumours were susceptible only to chemotherapy, and Burkitt's lymphoma, in particular, responded to it as dramatically as yaws or syphilis had responded to penicillin.[54] 'What has not been appreciated', Kyalwazi wrote with characteristic compassion in 1974, 'is that cancer is common in Africa; that every patient who gets cancer is almost certain to die from it if not treated, and that the mode of death is very agonising in most cases'.[55] At his own death in 1992, from cancer, he had the unusual distinction, for a doctor, of a state funeral.[56] Younger men were then extending knowledge of cancer in East African conditions, notably Charles Olweny, who worked on liver cancer, Burkitt's lymphoma, and another multicentric tumour called Hodgkin's disease.[57]

Makerere also gained an international reputation for the study of heart diseases. The interest had two origins. One was Davies's definition in 1948 of a newly observed condition, endomyocardial fibrosis, which he described as 'a huge white plaque of fibrous tissue on the endocardial [i.e. internal] surface' at the apex of the left ventricle.[58] It chiefly affected the young and poor. By the 1990s, according to some accounts, it was Uganda's most common heart disease, but its aetiology, which Davies suspected to be related to malnutrition, was still disputed.[59] The other stimulus to research was that by the 1960s high blood pressure, which had been thought rare among Africans, was becoming either increasingly common or increasingly observed among them. In 1961 tropical Africa's first conference on the subject took place in Kampala and by the end of the decade a WHO Cardiovascular Research Unit was operating there. The chief Ugandan specialist, Paul D'Arbela, wrote in 1975 that the problem was no longer why high blood pressure was so rare in Uganda but why it was so common.[60] A similar demonstration that 'diseases of civilisation' were as common in East Africa as elsewhere in the world took place at the same period in the field of mental illness.[61] Medical science and racial assertion joined to give a new perspective on disease.

Doctors under military rule, 1971–9

On 25 January 1971 army units led by General Amin overthrew Obote and established a military tyranny which lasted until 1979. It devastated a state, an economy, a medical profession, and a medical school which had generally flourished during the first decade of independence. It further destabilised Uganda's precarious ethnic balance and created an environment of violence, corruption, and illegality which made professional behaviour exceptionally difficult. 'Darkness fell over Uganda', wrote the historian of the Medical School; 'civilisation, human rights, value of lives, decency, freedom of speech, justice, rule of law and order and love, all fled from darkness'.[62] Doctors are always in special danger at times of civil violence. This was their Passion.

It was not apparent in January 1971. Many Ugandans were delighted at Obote's overthrow. Amin was quick to release political prisoners, including Lumu, who returned to private practice declaring that 'God has liberated this country through his servant, Idi Amin.' Makerere students welcomed the coup 'as a truly popular revolution'.[63] Kibukamusoke, as Chairman of the National Research Council, congratulated Amin

> on ridding the country of a regime that had become increasingly unpopular, oppressive, and corrupt . . . By your action and through your courage, simplicity and honesty, and the generosity and clemency you have shown to those who plotted against you, you have set an example to all of us and opened the window of our national life to let in the fresh air of truth.[64]

One wonders whether Amin, who was neither simple nor honest, caught the patronising tone. He and his military subordinates from northern Uganda loathed the intelligentsia. But doctors were a special case, for Amin had a soldier's lively appreciation of their value, and perhaps of their danger. They had no role in his regime outside their medical work, but within that sphere he took considerable, and often alarming, interest in their welfare. Haranguing assembled doctors at Mulago became one of his favourite activities.

The most revealing response by a doctor to the military takeover was that of Justin Gesa, who had recently succeeded Kadama as Permanent Secretary and Chief Medical Officer and therefore became Minister of Health in February 1971 when Amin formed a Cabinet mainly of senior civil servants. Although the ministers were promptly recruited into the army, Gesa

> said the Government of the Second Republic of Uganda is being run by professionals and men with long administrative experiences.
>
> 'The decisions of the Government are not going to be swayed by votes, but by the people's needs, the availability of funds and personnel to run the essential services in the spirit of brotherhood, unity and equality' he said.[65]

For Gesa, an active Christian and a keen athlete in his youth, military rule was a fresh beginning, free from 'the vagaries of politics and other weaknesses of our society'. 'From now on', he insisted, 'people are going to be appointed or promoted on merit and nepotism is out'. Doctors were to concentrate on their official duty rather than private practice. And this purified health service would be a rural service, not building new hospitals for political advantage but focusing on health centres accessible to the people.[66]

Yet Gesa must have been anguished by knowledge that killing of doctors had begun. The first was George Ebine, who owned a house where an officer loyal to Obote was hiding. Ebine was taken from Mulago in the middle of an operation and most brutally killed at an army barracks.[67] Also dead by the end of 1971 was Vincent Emiru, Makerere's gifted young Professor of Ophthalmology.[68] During 1972, moreover, Gesa's cherished medical service was thrown into disorder by the expulsion of almost all Asian doctors, along with the departure of many other expatriates.[69] An even more serious crisis took place in September 1972 when Obote's supporters invaded south-western Uganda from Tanzania. Although they were repelled, the regime's paranoia and brutality now became uncontrollable, even by Amin himself. Doctors found themselves tending victims of cruelty, certifying the results of summary executions, threatened by armed men invading their hospitals, beaten by soldiers picking a quarrel, and surrounded by fear and rumour.[70] A doctor committed suicide after an unsuccessful abortion on one of Amin's former wives. A dentist was bundled into the boot of a car and never seen again.[71] Most cruelly of all, in March 1973 George Sembeguya, who had defied Obote's authoritarianism, was taken from his surgery by military policemen with a rope round his neck and was later found dead in a nearby forest.[72] Perhaps he, of all men, thought of the Uganda Martyrs.

By now many African doctors and their families were leaving the country when they could safely do so. Kibukamusoke left in March 1973 after hearing that his name was on a death list.[73] In June 1977 the Ministry drew up an 'almost comprehensive' list of fifty doctors who had fled by the end of 1976 and another fifty-seven during the first half of 1977. The latter included the Dean of the Medical School, Alexander Odonga, who moved to the University of Nairobi when, in Amin's words, 'it was reported that he was going with bad companies'. In September 1979 the Ministry stated that Uganda had only 450 doctors. At that time only 45 of the 172 posts at the Medical School were filled.[74]

Gesa managed to retire in October 1973. His eventual successor, Henry Kyemba, had a high public profile but concentrated on keeping Amin happy until himself obliged to flee in 1977, after which Amin took over personally.[75] By then everyone in the medical service was intent on surviving. Working for Amin was an extraordinary experience. He was so full of unpredictable and contradictory ideas that almost none could be implemented. 'On his jubilant tours, he promised paradise', Kyemba remembered. 'If he found that a place needed a hospital, he would promise one. "The Minister of Health is here", he would say, and turn to the poor man. "You build one."'[76] In April 1978, when scarcely any medical unit had a working vehicle, Amin told the ministry staff that 'each hospital should have at least three ambulances and the Ministry of Health as a whole should have from 50 to 100 ambulances at the headquarters serviced and ready for use in case ambulances in hospitals up-country broke down'.[77] Senior people had to respond to these whims. Some chose unctuous flattery. Exceptional men like Kyalwazi balanced deference and dignity:

> Professor Kyalwazi told the President that before he talked to them most of them had different thoughts on what the President was going to tell them. They were happy when the President came and spoke to them in a fatherly manner, hence calming their fears.
>
> As doctors, Professor Kyalwazi said, they feel challenged by the President's address and that in the name of all doctors in Uganda, he is grateful to the President for reminding them of their duties. He added that they will not let the President down.[78]

By the mid-1970s Uganda's economy was disintegrating amidst insecurity, misgovernment, international isolation, and the oil-price increases of 1973–4. Statistics have little meaning, but one estimate is that between 1973 and 1980 real per capita income declined by 6.2 per cent a year. The World Bank estimated that the Ministry of Health's real expenditure per head of population fell between 1972 and 1982 by 85 per cent. In 1973 over 70 per cent of Ugandan children were immunised against tuberculosis, seven years later fewer than 10 per cent.[79] As control measures collapsed, Amin's rule saw two small cholera epidemics, one typhus epidemic, a major expansion of sleeping sickness in the east (with 7,445 cases in 1980), and the worst measles epidemic in Uganda's history.[80] Institutional decay was most visible at Mulago. Its piped water supply broke down in 1974 for a decade. The mortuary's refrigeration system was out of action from 1975 and sewerage ceased to function at about the same period. In 1978 the DMS described the food store as 'full of rats and vermin'. A year later, George Kirya, Head of Medical Microbiology, found the floor of the main operating theatre 'covered with a pool of faecal stinking material' leaking from the wards above. At that time not one of the hospital's twelve X-ray units was functioning. Amidst these conditions, and with salaries eroded by inflation, doctors spent increasing time in private clinics and nurses concentrated on caring for their families. Yet they kept the hospital functioning.[81]

The position at the Medical School was similar. By the mid-1970s almost all expatriate researchers and several leading Ugandans had left, research funds had virtually ceased, publications had fallen by 90 per cent, the WHO had transferred its cardiovascular research centre to Accra, and the lead in East African medical research had passed to Nairobi.[82] Yet Mulago's cardiac clinic registered 3,383 patients between 1969 and 1979[83] and the Uganda Cancer Institute continued to operate at a low level. This was the period when Olweny published extensively. Staff worked in great danger, especially Joseph Lutwama who was promoted to Vice-Chancellor in 1975. So did students, who showed great courage in defending their colleagues and the university.[84] Yet teaching held up surprisingly well. External examiners' reports on undergraduate performance during the mid-1970s were almost universally favourable, cooling somewhat at the end of the decade. The MMed candidates, by contrast, were considered poor, although the course did at least continue.[85] The bitter disappointment was the withdrawal of GMC recognition in 1976, a direct result of Amin's refusal to allow a visitation but also part of a general hardening of GMC policy towards medical qualifications acquired outside Britain.[86]

Some doctors took advantage of Amin's strange blend of tyranny and anarchy, chiefly those who took over practices or other property in the scramble following the expulsion of Asians. The irrepressible Eria Babumba, for example, operated a Nursing and Maternity Home in premises formerly owned by the Ismaili community. The Uganda Muslim Supreme Council opened the country's first Islamic hospital in similar premises. Sharp-witted men took advantage of the 1975 Land Reform Decree to appropriate large tracts as private property.[87] Moreover, doctors were so scarce that many elderly men continued in government service long after the medical authorities would have wished, Amin personally reinstating several whom Gesa had retired.

Yet these were exceptions. Not only did doctors' real salaries decline under Amin, but so did their relative status, both against the new rich (*mafutamingi*) of the time and against other professions. One symbolic act was the regrading of senior consultants below High Court Judges and Permanent Secretaries. In September 1977 a Uganda Medical Association delegation met Amin to present its grievances. He began by denouncing renegade doctors enticed away by Uganda's enemies, assured the delegation that the government was buying more drugs than ever before, and told them how much he admired them. After enquiring about blood donations, he told the Permanent Secretary, 'as a matter of urgency, to have refrigerators made available to all medical hospitals in the country'. He ended by assuring them that if they had transport problems they could always call on the army. Charged to reply, Barnaba Kununka thanked Amin for giving the Association a clubhouse (the former military police officers' mess). Other delegates then set out their several grievances. D'Arbela stressed the need for equipment, drugs, and books, enabling Amin to berate the luckless Permanent Secretary again and explain that he was discussing with Russian experts the possibility of building nuclear reactors. Charles Ssali, an ear, nose, and throat specialist, expressed pleasure at the acquisition of Asian property but complained that 'the doctors were not given the opportunity to become Mafutamingis'. Kajubi stressed the doctors' need to attend international meetings, which gave Amin a second opportunity to denounce those who fled. Finally, the Medical Superintendent at Mulago unwisely complained that security officers hunted doctors there, at which the General told him to set aside an office for three or four permanent security officers. The Association did not repeat this hallucinatory experience.[88]

As real salaries declined and controls lapsed during the early 1970s, many government doctors opened parallel private clinics, which apparently had not happened on a large scale before. Often these were former Asian practices. Unqualified medical workers followed their example.[89] Complaining 'that instead of being concerned with people's lives, the Ugandan doctors are interested only in money', Amin closed all private clinics in December 1974 and ordered that they must obtain ministerial approval. During the next two years Kyemba licensed about fifty, but the order's chief effect was that more doctors left the country. During 1976 government doctors argued that they had to supplement their earnings and that medicine was more sensible than farming. Amin resisted initially but lifted the ban in 1978.[90]

Survival and the maintenance of services were the predominant concerns. The mission hospitals, although weakened by expatriate departures and loss of government grants, acquired a new importance because their standards of care often survived better than those of government institutions. Some surgeons preferred to operate in mission facilities and for the first time young doctors volunteered to serve there. The Uganda Medical Association struggled to continue up-country meetings.[91] Most important of all were the doctors who stayed to keep things going. Kununka and Majugo occupied many sensitive public positions. Kyalwazi's name was said to be on a death list and he could have worked as a surgeon anywhere in the world, but he remained instead at Mulago. 'At the present moment the Medical School is being challenged from many angles', he told medical students in 1977,

> but those who are the guardians of its good name to-day must endeavour to pass its reputation untarnished to their successors – they have to keep the flame burning till their turn comes to pass it on to those who will take over the guardianship from them. One way of fulfilling our obligation is to maintain a high standard of research in all the fields of Medicine.[92]

Two years later, when Tanzanian troops and Ugandan refugees ousted Amin and took Kampala on 10 April 1979, Mulago treated casualties from both sides.[93]

The interregnum, 1979–86

The loose coalition of military factions and exiled professional men who now took power as the Uganda National Liberation Front quickly fragmented into a series of unstable governments, in which many doctors served, until Obote's UPC regained power in the election of December 1980. By then the Ministry of Health had been held by four incumbents, including Arnold Bisase, a London trained dentist, and Peter Sebuwufu, a Cambridge-trained anatomist.[94] Early in 1985 Obote's Cabinet contained four doctors, notably John Kirunda, the Minister of the Interior, a Makerere-trained gynaecologist who had worked in exile in Zambia. A few experienced politicians who had survived Amin's rule also gained office, especially Barnaba Kununka who held several ministries during 1979–80.[95] Moreover, Amin's overthrow brought into politics younger doctors associated with Yoweri Museveni, then a military faction leader. They included Ruhakana-Rugunda, an articulate Third World radical and former president of the Makerere Students' Guild, who served for a time as Deputy Minister of Health, and Crispus Kiyonga, a gynaecologist who in 1980 won Museveni's party its only parliamentary seat. Samson Kisekka, who had remained in Uganda and joined Museveni's side because its 'courage, compassion, and sincerity' meshed with the hope that it might protect Buganda against Obote, lost heavily in that election. Several other senior doctors stood successfully as favourite sons, notably Yusufu Semambo in Luwero Central and Eriab Muzira (Amin's last DMS) in Jinja East. Even Kyalwazi joined a delegation demanding greater democracy.[96] Uganda's urgent need for peace and recovery helped to preserve the tradition of public service among doctors when their counterparts in Kenya and Tanzania had largely abandoned politics.

Yet peace and recovery were far away. Amin's departing troops looted Mulago in 1979. The Ministry of Health headquarters was looted by its own workers.[97] Even when the Uganda National Liberation Front was established in Kampala, armed robbery and murder remained common. Of fifty-five doctors who died in Uganda between 1964 and 1986, at least fifteen died by violence.[98] Three of these and a dentist were killed in Kampala in July and August 1979, and at least three others wounded, by gangs suspected of targeting doctors in order to discredit the new regime. One gang told a witness, 'We are members of the movement and we are on a mission; we have killed the person we wanted.'[99] When a dentist, Jack Barlow, was killed after leading a protest delegation, Mulago's doctors struck for six days, together with other hospital workers, as a display of 'mourning' and a demand for protection. At Barlow's funeral, Olweny, as Chairman of the Uganda Medical Association, added to the prayers the words, 'May Jack Barlow's spirit NOT rest in peace until there is peace in this country.'[100] The strikers were accused of opposing the UNLF regime,[101] although perhaps they expressed more the anger of those who had worked throughout Amin's tyranny and resented the exiles lording it incompetently over them. Killing of doctors in Kampala did largely cease, but insecurity continued throughout the country during the next seven years. Although a number of doctors returned to Uganda when Amin was overthrown, the exodus soon resumed, especially by young men who saw no future in Uganda. Of fifty-three medical students who graduated at Makerere early in 1983, twenty-four had left Uganda by August. More senior exiles included Kisekka, who was warned that he was a wanted man, Olweny, who eventually settled in Canada, and Bwogi Kanyerezi, who later claimed to have fled to escape revenge for failing UPC youthwingers in their Makerere examinations.[102]

In April 1979 the incoming UNLF regime appointed a Sub-Committee for Rehabilitation of Medical Services. Merely restoring the curative system of the 1960s, however, conflicted with intervening changes in international thinking, especially the Primary Health Care policy espoused by the WHO at its Alma Ata meeting in 1978. One section of the Ministry of Health, led by Ruhakana-Rugunda and the able epidemiologist Samuel Okware, advocated this approach. But the UNLF politicians, with elections to fight, reverted to Obote's formula in October 1979 and announced plans for twenty new hospitals. A vigorous policy dispute ended with rehabilitation and PHC as the two chief priorities.[103] The Ministry's targets under Obote's Recovery Programme for 1982–4 were to raise and spend $5 million on rehabilitating Mulago, $5 million on restoring other hospitals, $10 million on PHC, and $5 million on the purchase of drugs.[104]

In reality, however, the state did not have these resources. Economic collapse continued into 1981, when there was some recovery until 1984 before civil war and international depression bred further economic crisis. In 1985 GDP per capita was still some 43 per cent lower than in 1970.[105] Both rehabilitation and PHC therefore depended on foreign aid, and although individual organisations responded, world health aid stagnated amid depression and the total provided to Uganda was small. By 1985 only half the capital cost of rehabilitation had been funded, all but $1 million by foreign donors.[106]

The need for rehabilitation was great. Five hospitals had been destroyed during Amin's defeat. The Ministry spent nearly $1 million simply to find out what needed to be done. Priority was given to restoring basic services like water, plumbing, and sewerage. UNICEF provided funds for elementary refurbishment of some hundred health centres. The greatest difficulty was drug supply, for in 1979 there were virtually none in the country, foreign donors refused to finance purchases, the Uganda Government would not provide foreign exchange, the Ministry's lack of transport obliged district staff to collect such drugs as were available, and it was estimated in 1985 that over 40 per cent were lost by spoilage or theft. Many doctors tried to keep all available drugs under their personal control.[107] Staff at all levels often spent most of their time on other means of survival, for by 1986 the total range of salaries in the medical service extended only from $2 to $12 a month. At these levels the number of employees had little importance, so that a survey in 1982 suggested that although the Ministry had 6,359 established posts it employed 14,410 people, 'employment' providing access to government housing (where available), other fringe benefits, and opportunities for corruption.[108]

These problems were most obvious at Mulago, whose restoration was a matter of national pride not only for Uganda but for Britain, which made an emergency grant of £2 million. There was some success. By 1983 six operating theatres and four X-ray units were working. But the crucial water supply was not – water was fetched in buckets or delivered by a tanker regularly diverted to the homes of military commanders – and nor were sewerage, electricity, and other services dependent on the general rehabilitation of Kampala and Uganda.[109] Between 1974 and 1988–9 Mulago's postoperative infection rate for clean wounds rose from 4.3 to 14.0 per cent, against the 2.0 per cent generally considered the acceptable maximum. The increase was partly due to resistance to antibiotics, although perhaps also to failure to administer them, for in 1985 J.G.M. Jagwe, the Medical Superintendent who struggled for five years to keep the hospital going, estimated that half its antibiotics were stolen, most commonly by not giving them to patients.[110] Nurses and doctors, of course, received much of the blame, although they bitterly resented working in such conditions and watching their patients suffer and die.

The second element in the recovery programme was primary health care. Some, especially in the World Bank, held that it should have been deferred until rehabilitation was well advanced, but the idealists who controlled donor funds saw Uganda's crisis as an opportunity for a radical break with the curative medicine of the past. Some Ugandans agreed, others wanted the funds.[111] The Ministry established a PHC section in 1980 and drafted a PHC plan in 1982, while NGOs began to encourage communities to select local representatives for training as community-based health workers to teach hygiene, administer first aid, and eventually, under local pressure, distribute the drugs which were what people chiefly wanted.[112] By the mid-1980s NGOs provided about half of Uganda's health services, to the anger of some officials and politicians.[113] NGOs and international organisations were especially important to the most urgent priority, to reactivate the immunisation programme. This had been launched in 1978 but had collapsed during the war, just when Uganda suffered a severe epidemic of measles, whose share in hospital deaths rose between 1970 and 1981 from 5 to 26 per cent. UNICEF funds revived immunisation in 1981, but reported coverage rates among infants in 1985 were still only 13 per cent for poliomyelitis, 17 per cent for measles, and 37 per cent for tuberculosis. The programme then collapsed again amidst violence and a second, less severe measles epidemic.[114]

The continuing disintegration of the state further demoralised the medical profession. The Medical School had shown great resilience under Amin but now suffered severely. Rather than expanding its annual intake from 100 to 150, as planned, it reduced the intake to 80 in 1982. Between 1981 and 1984 only half the students sitting final examinations passed. Reasons included deteriorating schooling, admission of unsuitable students, lack of staff and resources, the teachers' need for a second source of income, the breakdown of Mulago's facilities, general insecurity, and political conflicts dividing the student body. The MMed programme was also gravely damaged and the only research unit still working effectively was the Cancer Institute.[115] Doctors' earnings were devastated by inflation and they complained bitterly that 'Their rightful position in the post-independence Uganda has increasingly become bleak as showers of blame rain on them as if it was all their fault.'[116] Increasingly they took refuge in parallel private clinics, of which the Ministry seems to have been almost completely ignorant. Thirty private clinics in Kampala alone were said to have closed during a drug famine in 1979. A newspaper reported more than ten in Mbale in 1980.[117] 'There was no control against private practice', Jagwe declared in 1980:

> Clinics in the city were to a great extent attracting doctors and nurses away from working with the hospitals. Many applied for leave for the purpose of entering these clinics. Junior officers posted upcountry dodged their postings and are doing private practice. All this havoc caused a number of clinical laboratories to mushroom in town some of which are run by technicians. These were charging exhorbitant prices for instance a pregnancy test was charged Shs.1,000, yet it is suspected that the medicine they charge for is stolen.
>
> The Ministry ought to find a solution to such problems.

'The problem has been discussed for a number of years', Okware commented wearily at a later meeting. 'The law takes care of everything, only it is to be enforced.'[118] Yet, as the Medical Council found when it tried, the law was in fact unenforceable, for if government doctors' private clinics were closed, they would leave the service and possibly the country.[119] Nor was anything effective done about the illegal sale of pharmaceuticals which became 'rampant' in the early 1980s, apart from the occasional raid, for the new Pharmacy Board's mandate to protect the public against such abuses was a large task for its one inspector of drugs.[120] Self-medication with theoretically illegal drugs was emerging as the real surrogate for a collapsing medical system.

The medical profession in Museveni's Uganda

When Yoweri Museveni's National Resistance Army took Kampala in January 1986 it intended to recreate a strong state and economy. The question, as it affected the medical profession, was whether that meant restoring the medical order of the 1960s, as senior doctors broadly wanted; whether, even if desirable, that was any longer possible; and if not, what alternative medical order could possibly emerge from the medical stratagems which Ugandans had learned to practise and the medical strategies with which the outside world bombarded them. In this contestation, which was completely unresolved a decade after the NRA's victory, professionalism played an ambiguous role, exercising limited control over behaviour but remaining powerful as an ideal. The ambiguity at the notion's core can seldom have been displayed so vividly.

Even under National Resistance Movement rule, medicine was practised against a background of violence. Twelve Ministry of Health vehicles were hijacked during 1987. Two years later northern rebels seized the senior African doctor at Lacor Hospital. In 1993 they held a doctor from Ministry headquarters for a month to tend their troops. In 1995 the Minister of Health himself was kidnapped by dissidents operating only a few kilometres from Kampala.[121] And just as doctors lived in danger, so they remained active in politics. The first NRM Cabinet contained a record of six medical men.[122] The most prominent was the seventy-three-year-old Samson Kisekka, the movement's chief external coordinator in exile and now Prime Minister and then Vice-President until replaced in 1994 by a Makerere-trained surgeon, Specioza Kazibwe. Ruhakana-Rugunda was the NRM's first Minister of Health. His successors included James Makumbi, a neurosurgeon, and Crispus Kiyonga, formerly Minister of Finance and of Internal Affairs. The NRA's two senior doctors during its guerrilla campaign, Ronald Batta and Kiiza Besigwe, also sat in its first Cabinet. As in the past, however, Cabinet ministers were only the horn of the rhinoceros, for doctors were prominent throughout the regime, often as chairmen of local resistance committees – Babumba inevitably held that office in Masaka[123] – and contesting many constituent assembly seats in 1993. Moreover, not all doctors were with the NRM. At least two served with the northern rebels of Alice Lakwena and Joseph Kony.[124]

Given the movement's composition, it naturally turned to doctors to formulate its medical policy. In 1987 it appointed a thirteen-member Health Policy Review Commission dominated by senior Makerere doctors, notably Owor, the Dean of the Medical School (as chairman), his predecessor Odonga, Gesa, Josephine Namboze, and three other medical men. Working quickly and with no attempt to cost their proposals, they outlined how to restore the medical system to the standards of the 1960s. This included increasing the share of public recurrent expenditure devoted to health from 4 to 20 per cent, rehabilitating institutions, implementing laws against unqualified private practice and drug selling, restoring professional dominance, adding primary health care, and reintroducing fees. It was a wildly unrealistic programme which nevertheless embodied what most senior doctors wanted. The government accepted it as the basis of national health policy, which retained the two priorities of the early 1980s: institutional rehabilitation and primary health care.[125] Of the $203 million expenditure projected in the 1988 rehabilitation plan, $28 million was to restore Mulago, $40 million for other hospitals, $23 million for other existing facilities, and $111 million for primary health care (55 per cent of it for immunisation and an essential drugs programme). Donors were appalled by the cost and critical of attempts to do everything at once.[126]

From the government angle, however, the programme was a shopping list for donors, because the government had no intention of providing the funds. Not only was per capita GDP only three-fifths of that in 1970, but the share of GDP taken by government had declined equally sharply. Even in 1996, tax revenue in Uganda took only 11 per cent of GDP, against 15 per cent in Tanzania and 25 per cent in Kenya.[127] Fifteen years of state disintegration had privatised the economy on a massive scale, often illegally, so that Museveni's government had to abandon radical, state-directed recovery in favour of a structural adjustment and privatisation strategy which worked partly because potentially resistant structures had become so weak. This strategy raised GDP at an average of 5.6 per cent per year between 1986 and 1994,[128] but the health sector benefited little because government decided not to spend its scarce resources on health, giving priority to security and the productive economy and probably calculating that health could attract donor funds. One indication, infuriating to doctors, was that veterinary drugs had a higher foreign exchange priority than human drugs. Figures were quoted loosely, but in 1995 about 80 per cent of the Ministry of Health's budget was donor-financed.[129]

Rehabilitation was the first priority. Destruction during the war had probably been less than during Amin's overthrow, but accumulated deterioration made the late 1980s the nadir of the health services. The Owor Commission 'were appalled by the gross state of disrepair' in the hospitals they visited. Many lacked water, electricity, sewerage, equipment, transport, and drugs.[130] 'It is common knowledge', the Ministry confessed in 1993, 'that in Government hospitals little, if any, of their food budget is used to feed their in-patients. In some hospitals food is served to the hospital staff; in others the money finds its way into private pockets.'[131] Corruption was rife, although much at the lower levels consisted of ways in which staff rewarded themselves for services for which they were not paid. 'While my wife was in agony of labour pains', a husband complained,

> the Doctor asked for 3000/- prior admission and I paid of course expecting help. The porter rolled my patient to the Labour Room where there was no midwife at all. The midwife was at home and the doctor who called her came to me saying the midwife wanted 2000/- plus a piece of soap then she can help the patient.
>
> I raised the cash for the midwife but failed to get money for soap.
>
> After all this my wife delivered unattended to but after sometime died in her labour room most likely due to bleeding.[132]

Such accusations of negligence and callous indifference against doctors and nurses were repeated endlessly throughout East Africa during the late twentieth century, perhaps most frequently in Uganda. Many must have been true. The general view was certainly that medical workers were especially demoralised and perhaps especially tempted, because their patients were so vulnerable. At the same time, however, patients' urgent needs may have given special significance to levels of inefficiency and corruption which were normal in most public services. High expectations of altruism derived from missionary precedents compounded the disillusionment, as did the tendency to view nurses as servants. Large hospitals like Mulago were also easy targets for muckraking journalists. One indication that medical staff were no more corrupted than others was that so many continued to work with little or no pay.[133] Another was that selfless workers were easy to find among the pain and squalor of dilapidated hospitals, especially among staff with a strong religious faith. The circumstances of their work polarised their responses, breeding both callousness and compassion:

> Mulago might have some of the most insensitive nurses and doctors in the profession. But it also has the best. When women who have given birth by Caesarean section develop infections, the hospital often doesn't have the medicines to treat the infections should they become very complicated. The best medicine which some nurses give the women is the spirit to fight.
>
> They will come and place their nose close to the wound and sniff it. Then they will turn and say, 'See, if the wound was so bad, I wouldn't put my nose near it. You will be fine.' No medicine can beat that . . .
>
> This 'miracle' [of birth] in our hospitals is possible only because of the hundreds of very decent doctors and nurses who work hard and faithfully in some of the worst conditions you will find anywhere. They are the unsung heroes of a dead health system.[134]

As this account suggests, Mulago in 1996 still suffered severe problems, especially drug shortages and difficulty in holding expenditure – in 1990–1 over 2 per cent of the entire national budget – within limits,[135] for during the previous decade the hospital had gained much autonomy from the Ministry.[136] Yet major improvements had been made with foreign aid from many directions, starting with the restoration of running water in 1987, progressing especially during the period around 1990 when David Kihumuro-Apuuli (with hospital management training) was Medical Superintendent, and continuing apparently without end into the late 1990s.[137] In 1996 Museveni claimed in his election manifesto that eleven of Uganda's fifty-five government hospitals (including Mulago) had been fully rehabilitated and twenty-one partially so.[138]

One major problem was to persuade doctors to work in remote districts. Of approximately 700 doctors in 1990, 309 were working at Mulago. A year later centrally located Jinja District had 228 more medical staff than establishment patterns permitted and Kisoro District (in the extreme south-west) had 111 fewer, only 21 of its 132 posts being filled.[139] Many doctors simply refused to move when posted to remote areas, for dismissal was no credible threat when government had so few doctors and paid them so little. One reason for refusing distant postings was simply violence, especially in the north. Arua Hospital, threatened by the self-styled West Nile Liberation Army, had only two of its thirty allocated doctors in November 1994.[140] But there were other reasons. 'Dumping, as assignment to the rural areas is referred to in the service, means professional deterioration to many', one observer recorded, 'and for those with children of school going age, it also means lack of competitive educational opportunities for their children'.[141] Moreover, no doctor could survive on his salary. In a town or centrally located district he could practise privately, if illegally, or he or his family could find other earning opportunities. That was less possible in a remote district, where the expenses, too, might be considerable:

> On assumption of duty I found a huge unfurnished house which I set about furnishing with the bare essentials such as a mattress and two hurricane lamps. The money to purchase them was donated by my family. The hospital has a generator but the government provides no money for petrol to operate it. Therefore I get money from my family living in Kampala. They also top up my salary.
>
> To treat patients without the assurance of power I got hospital users to come with their own charcoal and charcoal burners. With these they boil water to be used in treatment and they use the burners to sterilise the syringes to be used. I make regular trips to the medical stores at Entebbe and I may have to wait for three days before I am attended to. I am jokingly referred to as the 'Man from Mubende . . .'[142]

One Italian NGO recognised these financial problems by paying a $200 monthly salary supplement to Ugandan doctors working in West Nile, but, for obscure but probably self-interested reasons, the Ministry ignored repeated advice to make incentive payments to doctors in remote areas. Instead it made at least two years of up-country service a condition for postgraduate training.[143] Despite these obstacles, a few doctors did accept distant postings, especially in the rare cases where those were their homes. Nathan Eriamu took over Atutur Hospital in Teso country in the late 1980s during bitter fighting between NRA units, for a time stationed in the hospital compound, and rebel forces. He ran it as the sole doctor, with ten medical assistants, twenty-five nurses, no functioning motor vehicle, generator, refrigerator, or X-ray unit, and a water system which had broken down in 1978. Three other doctors posted to help him never arrived.[144] Lawrence Ojom, as an Acting District Medical Officer in war-ridden Acholi, had overall responsibility for three hospitals (with 750 beds), five health centres, six dispensaries, and seventeen sub-dispensaries. 'All the health units except the hospitals are in poor state and require urgent rehabilitation', he reported in 1993, while his four vehicles were 'old and often break down'. 'I appeal to the Ministry of Health', he wrote, 'to post immediately to Kitgum District any staff willing to work here'.[145] Other Ugandan doctors worked in even more critical situations, such as Damian Imana, for many years Medical Superintendent of Mutolere Hospital on the much-disturbed Rwandan border, and Faustin Eriya, the paediatrician at Nsambya, who helped to evacuate Rwandan patients after the massacre of 1994.[146]

The second plank of NRM health policy was primary health care. At the policy level Uganda subscribed to this with almost millennial fervour, for it was the fashionable programme of the time, meshed with the radical element in NRM thinking, and promised to open NGO and donor agency safes. By 1993 the programme had been introduced in all thirty-nine districts, but three years later over 80 per cent of health expenditure was still on curative services.[147] There was a strong cosmetic element about PHC, sometimes crudely applied. In 1995 the Ministry proposed to meet its target of one health centre per 20,000 people by decreeing that all 1,300 health units smaller than hospitals should be called health centres.[148] One PHC programme designed for Karamoja would have paid $28,000 of foreign money over three years to a Ministry official who planned to spend at least forty days a year there. On the other side, both NGOs and local activists dedicated great energy to creating the community organisations and village health workers who were in principle the basic units of integrated local programmes, although it soon became plain that workers wanted paid employment and communities wanted drugs.[149] In practice, reliance on external funding and top-down medical planning ensured that PHC consisted chiefly of vertical national programmes. By 1990 there were eight, and others were added in following years. Immunisation remained the simplest and most effective. Revitalised for a second time after 1986, by the mid-1990s it had achieved immunisation levels among infants of 96 per cent for tuberculosis, 85 per cent for measles, and 78 per cent for poliomyelitis.[150] The other priority programme of the 1980s, to treat infant diarrhoea with oral rehydration salts, proved harder to implement.[151]

Despite continuing problems, NRM rule saw major improvements in certain areas of the health system. One was the Medical School. Makerere was in turmoil as expanding student numbers – in 1992 it had 6,800 undergraduates in accommodation for 3,984[152] – clashed with declining government funding. Staff struck for higher pay in 1989, 1994, and 1996.[153] Students struck over a variety of material issues in 1989, 1990, and 1996.[154] Medical students were divided over participation in the earlier strikes, although they shared the material grievances and suffered from poor facilities and results: only half the finalists in 1989 passed and the marks in 1990 were so poor that an inquiry blamed failures in paediatrics on 'inadequacy in staffing textbooks and consultation, let alone of seriousness among the students'. 'We will not allow you to pass if you cannot do simple everyday things', the head of the department told his students. 'You will pass by going into the ward and not in your halls of residence or offices.'[155]

Thereafter, however, morale began to recover. Curriculum reforms in 1988–9 introduced an emphasis on primary health care, students spending nine months of their three clinical years at a health centre, which they were said to welcome. The symptoms of academic revival appeared. The *Makerere Medical Journal* was published in 1990 for the first time since 1978. Student research resumed. The student association organised ward rounds. There was growing rivalry with the Mbarara University of Science and Technology, which in 1989 admitted its first medical students to a course stressing community-based medicine.[156]

Mulago's research was also regaining vigour. Most new work was on AIDS and will be considered later. The rest was largely within established traditions. The Uganda Cancer Institute received new radiotherapy equipment from America. Uganda's first hospice for terminal cancer patients opened in 1993 and began to train physicians in their management. Uganda's Chief Surgeon, Francis Omaswa, struggled to establish a Uganda Heart Institute which by 1996 was undertaking relatively complex operations.[157] Perhaps the most interesting work from a historical viewpoint was C.L. Sezi's study of endomyocardial fibrosis, which he described as the product of over forty years of Mulago's research. Sezi's analysis of cases from 1969 to 1990 convinced him that it was specifically a disease of childhood and of childbearing age in women, especially among the poor. Common in the past among the families of Rwandan migrant labourers, by 1991 patients were chiefly impoverished Ganda who 'can hardly afford a balanced meal but fill up their stomachs with protein free cassava'. Lack of protein when especially needed for growth or childbearing, he suggested, left sufferers vulnerable to stress on the heart: 'Cell repair is not possible.' In linking heart disease to malnutrition, Sezi was bringing together two of the major strands in Makerere's medical research.[158]

Alongside the revitalisation of the Medical School, the new regime struggled to rationalise the medical service. A study in 1991 could come no closer than to estimate that the Ministry employed between 8,500 and 10,000 staff, excluding unskilled workers, divided into 57 personnel categories. The average doctor in a government hospital treated 471 patients a year, as against 2,441 in an NGO hospital. Investigations covering only half the country found over 2,000 non-existent 'ghost workers' on the Ministry's payroll, including 134 at headquarters and over half the staff of one hospital. Ironically, pay was so low that overstaffing had little effect on government expenditure, but the two together undermined morale and efficiency by destroying differentials and incentives. This thinking inspired massive civil service reform. Mulago began retrenchment in 1993, making over 1,000 employees redundant. No figures were available for the Ministry of Health, but the government aimed to reduce the entire civil service from 320,000 to 135,000.[159]

The NRM also wanted to motivate the health service. Initially it attempted politicisation at training seminars, but they were seldom mentioned after about 1990.[160] Instead the regime adopted two other strategies. One was decentralisation. The NRA and NRM had successfully constructed democratic local government through resistance councils from villages upwards and often saw them as a panacea. Uganda's medical system, in contrast to Kenya's, was already decentralised, because local authorities owned and financed all institutions below district hospitals. In 1992 a sweeping programme transferred the hospitals also to local management committees and made District Medical Officers responsible to local authorities. Although some local committees were soon in financial difficulty, others made significant improvements. By June 1995 some thirty-eight district health plans had been completed and health was the leading sector of the decentralisation programme.[161]

Decentralisation helped to motivate staff chiefly by facilitating the introduction of cost-sharing into government health units, as was already the practice in church hospitals and government schools. From the mid-1980s, international bodies, the Owor Commission, and doctors all urged the reintroduction of fees.[162] During the late 1980s a few government hospitals began to levy charges and spend the money on improvements, drugs, and staff.[163] In 1990 the Ministry proposed to make this national policy, distributing half the fees to staff in order to 'boost the morale of the health workers', but the National Resistance Council vetoed the plan, allegedly for fear of political unpopularity.[164] The World Bank maintained pressure, however, the Ministry authorised health facilities to manage their own programmes, and the practice continued to spread as a 'silent grass-root health revolution', until the Acting Director of Mulago told an angry Public Accounts Committee in December 1993 'that all hospitals had adopted it'.[165] There was local opposition, with complaints that absenteeism and extortion continued. The scheme was also difficult to implement in remote areas and often created conflict among staff over their respective shares (usually proportional to salaries) or charges of embezzlement.[166] Criticisms were roughly balanced by accounts of improved services.[167]

Yet neither rationalisation, decentralisation, nor cost-sharing substantially improved the doctors' position. In 1991 the Ministry estimated that Uganda had 811 registered practising doctors, 586 of them in government service, 80 working for the university, and 50 in private practice.[168] Each doctor served an average of 21,000 people. In 1969 there had been 647 doctors, each serving 15,000 people, the difference resulting from population growth. More doctors in 1991 were Ugandans, far more were Africans, and more were also women, although no figures were available; a Uganda Women Doctors' Association was launched in 1988. A medical officer's official salary in 1994–5 was about $90 a month,[169] an improvement on the late 1980s when the Uganda Medical Association estimated that a senior consultant earned about $16 a month. At that time the Association had memorialised Museveni, complaining of their pay, housing, access to transport, and conditions of work, the unfair public criticism to which they were subjected, the formal exclusion of government doctors from private practice, and the exploitation of the public by unqualified practitioners and drug sellers.[170] Despite minor salary improvements, government still gave doctors low priority in the mid-1990s and expected them to find most of their income extra-legally, either by private practice, cost-sharing, or corruption. In reality, many continued to leave the country. In 1991 the Ministry estimated that 660 were working abroad. Saudi Arabian recruiters were said in 1995 to offer $3,200 a month. 'We could have earned perhaps twenty times in greener pastures as much as we earn here', a Medical School professor told Museveni in 1988, 'but we preferred to serve our country'.[171] It is remarkable that so many stayed.

One reason was certainly that in addition to full-time private practitioners, many government doctors concentrated on private clinics. Official policy from 1989 was that they might not own clinics but might practise in them outside working hours, but this was widely ignored.[172] The Kampala area allegedly had well over a hundred private doctors in 1987, some full-time and others part-time. A year later there were over fifty private clinics in Jinja town alone, fewer than ten of them registered, while Masaka town had twenty-one clinics in 1992, eleven of them specifically run by doctors. The household budget survey of 1989–90 found that private expenditure on health (including modern drugs and indigenous medicines) was 14.5 per cent more than all government health expenditure including donor funds and development spending.[173] The most elaborate private institutions were small hospitals or nursing homes like the Kololo Hospital in Kampala, established in 1995 with bank loans to treat 'expatriates and some top Ugandans'. Another substantial investment was the laboratory servicing private practitioners. In 1995, for example, Dr Y. Mpairwe set up the Naguru Medical Laboratory in Kampala with a staff of seventeen medical workers.[174] On a smaller scale some private practitioners ran old-style private clinics in their home towns as bases for community leadership. Eriab Muzira, former DMS, owned such a clinic in Jinja; 'if funds were not forthcoming, the patients would be admitted and they would pay later at their own pace'.[175] But serving government doctors found it far from easy to combine hospital and private practice, as occasional reports of disasters testify. At the worst, they might be tempted to perform abortions. A study of 1,180 illegal abortions which reached Mulago between 1988 and 1993, and had therefore gone wrong, showed that 94 per cent had been performed by medical doctors, mainly on women under twenty; the price varied from \$5 to \$50, depending on the facility, the practitioner's skill, and the duration of the pregnancy.[176]

During the 1980s much private practice came to be conducted by less qualified medical staff or totally unqualified laypeople. Some of these clinics were registered in doctors' names, although a study in Bunyole did not find any doctor who actually supervised one. Whereas doctors themselves generally practised in towns and probably treated the more prosperous, many less qualified practitioners worked in the countryside.[177] In the Ibanda county of western Uganda in the early 1990s, for example, the three private clinics owned by doctors – and it is striking that such a remote place had three – were all in Ibanda town, but ten of thirteen clinics owned by other medical staff were in the countryside.[178] In the nearby Rwampara county, fifteen of twenty-two clinics were owned by 'nurses' (some perhaps with lesser medical roles), two by midwives, three by doctors, and two by untrained people. Nine had a thermometer, ten a stethoscope, eleven a delivery bed. Fifteen gave injections, twenty provided elementary drugs. Eight saw fewer than twenty patients a week. 'Most of the medical services were maternity and family planning services . . . Others mentioned include simple casualty services, services for headache, cough, malaria and abdominal pains.' Proprietors also stressed their first-aid function.[179] This was probably the normal pattern in rural Uganda and many informal urban areas. Studies in 1994 suggested that 61 per cent of those making prescriptions were not doctors and that 50 per cent of those giving injections were untrained. Given the risks of antibiotic resistance, AIDS, and other complications, this alarmed professionals, but it could also be said that instead of training neighbours as community health workers, rural communities were relying on members already trained.[180]

A greater threat to professional dominance came from the sale of drugs for self-medication. A survey in 1994 found some 850 drug retailers in Kampala,[181] mostly unlicensed and untrained:

> A typical Kampala pharmacy of the new type is owned by a former hospital dresser and the pharmacists he employs are highly-qualified relatives, most of whom completed primary school and can read the labels on medicine containers. The pharmacy, or drug store, covers several square metres and is sandwiched between two retail shops, with an overflowing dustbin in front and a busted sewer behind. Between processing drug demands, the pharmacists peel *matooke* [bananas], wash

babies, plait hair and do their laundry . . . The government does not interfere in the people's right to prescribe what they want for themselves. And in keeping with the global trend for free market economics, the people's freedom of choice of which drugs to put into their bodies is protected as long as they can afford it.[182]

At one end of the spectrum, drug stores merged into clinics and their operators performed injections and gave advice. Indeed, some clinics, even when run by doctors, were in practice drug stores. At the other end of the spectrum, no special licence was needed to sell aspirin or some anti-malarials and drugs were sold in general stores or peddled in markets, streets, and villages, either alone or together with other goods. Between these extremes were the bulk of drug shops operated by medical auxiliaries. In one group of sixty-three drug shops inspected in Kampala in 1992, forty-five were run by nurses of some kind, eight by dispensers, and seven by other paramedics.[183] But it was not true that the authorities ignored them. The Owor Commission urged the creation of a National Drugs Authority and the effective implementation of the Pharmacy and Poisons Act. Doctors pointed to the danger of creating drug resistance by undermedication, especially where poor patients bought in very small quantities, and the risks arising from expired, contaminated, or counterfeit drugs and ignorance of proper dosage.[184] The government shared these fears. In 1988, for example, it ordered all unlicensed drug dealers to wind up their businesses within a fortnight. The authorities then had no staff to enforce the order, but drug inspectors were trained for posting throughout the country and a long-mooted National Drugs Authority was established in 1993 to control the importation, manufacture, and quality of drugs. In December 1997 it was reported to have closed over 500 illegal drug shops around Kampala during the past six months.[185]

It was feared, however, that many distributors had gone undergound. To re-establish a professional monopoly of modern drugs was massively difficult, far more difficult than the task in Western countries of maintaining an established monopoly. Relatively cheap and very effective drugs were the core of modern medicine. Ordinary Africans had considerable knowledge of drugs; one study found that at least half the customers at drug shops demanded a specific drug.[186] Self-medication did not necessarily conflict with professional medicine, for patients commonly treated themselves or their children first with a purchased drug and sought professional help only if it failed. Like unlicensed clinics, this relieved the pressure of minor complaints on beleaguered health facilities. And since in Uganda health facilities frequently had no drugs, the alternatives to self-medication were often no medication or indigenous medication. The privatisation of modern drug distribution presented doctors with a particularly clear choice between trying to recreate an idealised professional monopoly or rethinking their role in new circumstances.[187] Not surprisingly, most opted for the past.

Ironically, the revived campaign against illegal distribution of modern drugs coincided with greater sympathy towards indigenous medicine, indicating perhaps that modern doctors did not see the latter as a real rival. The main interest was in the testing of indigenous herbs for possible exploitation within the modern system. Government had launched such investigations in 1962 at the Natural Chemotherapeutic Research Laboratory at Wandegeya. By 1972 it had tested over 1,000 plants, but had generally found their active principles less safe and specific than those of existing drugs. The laboratory then suffered severely under Amin and his successors, so that although it had some twenty research workers in 1986, the Minister of Health found it 'absolutely non-functional'. Ten years later it had been rehabilitated and its director, Nathan Mubiru, and his collaborators had published seventeen volumes of a catalogue of herbal remedies used in different regions, although little of practical use had emerged.[188] Similarly, a WHO meeting in Kampala in 1976 made it respectable to advocate collaboration between modern doctors and indigenous healers, but in practice this chiefly meant training traditional birth attendants in hygienic methods – by the mid-1990s several hundreds had been trained, not always effectively – and an intellectual respect, coloured by nationalism and displayed in the Makerere Medical School's inclusion of 'traditional medical practices' in the new curriculum of 1988–9.[189] The main exceptions were collaboration in the treatment of sickle cell anaemia, joint research into remedies for AIDS (discussed later), and the work of Brother Anatoli Wasswa, based in Rakai District, who sought to separate indigenous herbalism from religious or magical associations and blend it with modern medical skills provided by Makerere-trained doctors. Many Ugandans consulted indigenous healers, perhaps increasingly so as modern services decayed, but this rarely threatened the professional power of modern doctors or affected their practice.[190] As earlier in the century, the people in real competition with indigenous healers were the paramedics who ran rural clinics, perhaps especially if they were nurses whose training had demonised indigenous medicine.[191] Nationalist sentiments led the NRM to place a representative of indigenous healers on the National Drugs Authority, but a proposal to recognise herbalists was defeated.[192] The healers themselves were generally eager to learn modern techniques but probably not to be subjected to the subordination and supervision which modern doctors had in mind for them. The Owor Commission, for example, recommended that 'Traditional Healers should be encouraged to form a National Association, which should be the nucleus through which the Ministry of Health should regulate and supervise their practice.'[193] An association, Uganda n'Eddagala Lyayo, was apparently founded in the early 1980s and claimed to have over 30,000 members in 1991,[194] but, like such associations elsewhere in Africa, managerial crises and factional rivalry made it scarcely an effective channel of ministerial control.

That was also true of its modern equivalent, the Uganda Medical Association. Politicians demanded that it should discipline the profession. 'The medical command structure is like in the army', the Minister of Health insisted in 1996. 'An intern is like a recruit, who does not defy the orders of a consultant who is commander. How can these small boys defy the commander. This is wrong, it should be stopped.'[195] UMA leaders might have agreed, but had no capacity to discipline their members. Like many Ugandan institutions, the association's main achievement had been to survive. It had maintained a skeleton programme of meetings, presented professional grievances, and claimed seven up-country branches in 1992. But attempts to reactivate it or engage it in activities such as the continuing education of doctors failed for lack of funds. In 1993 an angry junior doctor described the association as 'defunct'. Its leaders, by contrast, insisted that it did not defy professional ethics by behaving like a trade union.[196]

There was an enormous gap between the doctors' inherited ideal of professionalism and their real situation. In this status-conscious society, their loss of status and income was more extreme even than that of teachers. The marks needed to enter the Makerere Medical School were by 1996 lower than those demanded by commerce, law, or pharmacy.[197] Indigenous healers called themselves doctors with only occasional squawks of protest. Worse, doctors had lost a degree of self-respect. The Uganda Medical Council complained that 'the majority of doctors in the country do not render even 25% of their expected output. They have no facilities to do the job, no transport to take officers or patients to hospital, there is no job satisfaction.'[198] This was doubly bitter when others measured doctors by a missionary ideal of altruism which no ordinary profession observed. In 1995, for example, a medical officer confessed that because he had written over fifty police reports without payment, he no longer took trouble over them. 'The judge told him to stop being money minded since his profession concerned the life of people. He told him to be committed to his job or resign if he cannot work where there is no money.'[199] Such doctors felt, with justice, that they were made scapegoats for the disintegration of state and society, as the Uganda Medical Association protested to Museveni in 1989:

> Given the deteriorating standards of medical care in this country the public is justified in crying but what is at issue now is *to whom the cry should be directed and about whom*. Government has, in our opinion, misdirected this cry, bringing disrepute to the medical profession . . .
>
> This is a national crisis and we think it should be taken in that vein. It would be

a pity for Government to use the health workers as a scape goat for sooner or later when the majority have either left the country or left Government service, there will be no more scape goats. At that stage Government will have to face the reality.[200]

The state had reneged on its side of the implicit bargain which made professionalism possible.

Moreover, in many respects the state no longer wished to support the doctors' professional aspirations. In 1996 the NRM's populist element defied the doctors' opposition and accepted the medical assistants' long-standing demand for their own professional status. Adopting a new title advocated by the WHO, the Allied Health Professionals Act created a council, parallel to those of doctors and nurses, to discipline and license paramedics for private practice. The National Resistance Council also considered representing nurses on the Medical Practitioners and Dental Practitioners Council, to parallel the doctors' representation on the Nurses and Midwives Council. The doctors' position of authority within the medical system was in question.[201]

The most turbulent element within the medical service was the interns. Between 1972 and 1987 their real monthly pay had fallen from $244 to $4.80.[202] Not only were their living conditions squalid, but they did most of the doctors' work in large government hospitals while fully qualified staff attended their private clinics:

'I have a patient . . .' I started to tell an exhausted intern. But he cut me short. 'Not again . . . we have had 5 anaemia – one passed away and the mother almost chewed us, then you can see the crowd. I have been here since 8.00 a.m. and now it is 12 hours sitting in this position.' . . .

The bulk of work is shouldered by interns. Other categories of doctors spend most of their time in private practice. With a meagre pay of 89,000/- per month, an intern at Mulago toils like a horse.

They work on 'admission' four times a week, attending to caesarean cases and others. They also do ward rounds and other duties throughout the week including Saturdays and Sundays.

'It is normal to do nine caesarean sections at night, then do ward work in the morning up to 5.00 p.m. Then rest before returning to admit the next. On weekends, we can spend 48 hours without sleep . . .' said an intern.[203]

Exploited and pivotal, interns also resented domination of the profession by conservative senior men on whose favour they depended. 'The medical profession has . . . stalled because the older generation of doctors who are in administrative or influential positions have completely ignored the well-being of younger doctors', it was complained.[204] These grievances gave rise to strikes at Mulago in 1985, Jinja in 1989, Mulago in 1990, Jinja and Lacor in 1993, and Mulago in 1994 and 1996. During the 1994 protest the fifty-eight striking interns 'said what they were doing was for the good of the coming generations and the good of the country'.[205]

As that statement suggested, a new attitude towards medical behaviour was emerging among younger doctors. Elsewhere in the world there was nothing new about doctors' strikes. Australian and German doctors struck several times before 1914.[206] After 1950 doctors' strikes became commonplace,[207] including, as will be seen, in Kenya. Yet a first strike was a traumatic decision, challenging notions of medical ethics by threatening suffering and death to patients. Uganda had seen strikes by paramedics, nurses, and interns, but, with the exception of the quasi-political strike at Mulago in 1979, its doctors did not strike until 1995, when the changes and grievances of the previous twenty-four years came together in action.

Early in 1994 several pressure groups threatened pay strikes. Government made concessions to doctors and Makerere staff, but resolved to resist further wage claims. The medical strike that followed in September 1995 had two immediate precipitants. One was the restructuring of civil service pay scales to extend differentials, in which medical workers had low priority, so that only consultants benefited significantly and a lay magistrate's salary rose to three times the Shs.151,124 ($150) a month earned by a medical officer. (Members of Parliament received over Shs.100,000 a *day* as a sitting fee.[208]) The other precipitant was the formation in 1992 of the Uganda Medical Workers Union, embracing both doctors and other medical staff in government service, an innovation made possible by changes in trade union law. The leaders were radical young doctors, notably Sam Lyomoki, the General Secretary, a twenty-five-year-old, born-again, former student leader from the Makerere Medical School.[209] Frustrated that pay increases promised in the 1995 budget had not materialised, UMWU delegates from thirty-five hospitals met on 8 September 1995 and decided to strike. The Minister of Health, James Makumbi, immediately declared that it would be illegal because the union was not properly registered, which its leaders disputed.[210] Makumbi was a respected and largely apolitical neurosurgeon active in public life since Amin's overthrow, but he belonged to the generation which bewailed the ethics of younger doctors. 'How can health workers supposed to save human lives just close hospitals like factories?' he asked.[211] The union leaders insisted equally strongly that *they* were the people 'determined to restore the dignity of medical professionals'. 'Let us stay around and work together to improve the country's health services', Lyomoki later urged cheering medical students. '. . . We must be recognised as a noble profession and remunerated as such.'[212] New trade union ideas were thus infused with older notions of honour.

The strike began on 19 September 1995, paralysing health services at Mulago and in most other parts of the country. 'Frail patients lay on their beds in agony without attention' at Mulago, the press reported, for the doctors only slowly arranged to treat emergency cases. According to the union, at least fifty-seven patients died for lack of care during the first eight days. Medical School students nevertheless described the strike as a 'Just, noble and good cause'.[213] Government refused to negotiate and local officials put much pressure on hospital staff to work, but the most remarkable aspect of the strike – in contrast to Kenyan medical strikes – was that it embraced all levels of medical workers: 'A paramedic could talk and a doctor listens.'[214]

After a week the government was quietly seeking a settlement, promising to investigate grievances and meet some of them, but it refused the leaders' demand for a written undertaking – 'They must know that government can't lose face' – and instead arrested Lyomoki and two colleagues.[215] The scale of suffering was now losing the strikers public sympathy. Upcountry workers were returning to duty. Museveni refused to meet union leaders but told representatives of professional associations, who condemned the strike, that the government could not afford large wage increases and that the strikers must return to work or face dismissal. By now Mulago was almost the only hospital on strike and the police moved to evict its interns from their accommodation. On 28 September the union leaders suspended the strike.[216] Makumbi demanded stiff disciplinary action, but other politicians insisted on reconciliation, and instead he announced that medical workers would receive a 'living wage' from July 1996.[217] By then Makumbi himself had been replaced, but the 'living wage', when it came, was mainly a consolidation of fringe benefits, except for higher-paid workers. Further strikes were threatened.[218]

The strike highlighted two points about Uganda's medical profession in the mid-1990s. One – revealed equally by strikes elsewhere in East Africa – was its powerlessness against the state when bereft of public support. The other was that professionalism nevertheless remained a remarkably powerful ideal for all parties: to Makumbi as an ideal learned in the days of Makerere's glory, to patients as a guarantee of altruistic service, and to union leaders as a hope of dignified status and reward as employees. All were contained within the ambiguity intrinsic to professionalism. The younger men, moreover, had begun to think about what medical professionalism might mean in Museveni's Uganda, where a government doctor might need to be a trade unionist and a referral authority for patients who had initially attempted self-medication with drugs which doctors could no longer monopolise. But that thinking was still at a very early stage.

8 Kenya: doctors and a capitalist transition

Unlike their counterparts in Uganda, Kenyan doctors at independence were not yet sufficiently numerous to form an influential profession. One important development there during the next thirty years was the expansion of their numbers through the new Medical School in Nairobi. Moreover, neither did the state disintegrate nor did it crush professional aspirations. Rather, state, society, and profession experienced a transition towards capitalism which was already under way in the colonial period, as the proliferation of European and Asian private practitioners had indicated. The chief themes in the history of the Kenyan medical profession after independence were therefore an expansion of medical provision, a yet more rapid increase in African practitioners, a marked differentiation between the majority of private practitioners and the discontented minority of doctors in the neglected state sector, and the difficulty of bringing the two together in united professional action.

The years of expansion, 1963–73

As in Uganda, Kenya's first decade of independence saw rapid economic growth. GDP increased at 5.9 per cent per year during the 1960s and most sections of the African population except the very poorest benefited.[1] Medical policy changed little, continuing to balance rural health centres against urban hospitals, although with a bias towards curative care. The need to expand and Africanise the health service absorbed medical energies and resources.[2]

The need came from the pressure of public demand. One reason was the world's highest rate of natural population growth, at 3.6 per cent per year between 1965 and 1980.[3] Prosperity enabled people to seek remedies for part of their enormous backlog of untreated sickness. Although many consulted indigenous healers, there was a shift towards modern medicine, noted among the Kikuyu in the 1950s and the Kamba and more remote peoples during the 1960s.[4] But the most important reason for increased demand was government policy. Whereas the late colonial government had introduced fees at medical facilities, the successful Kenya African National

Union (KANU) made free basic medical treatment a campaign promise at the 1963 election. Taunted by its opponents, KANU introduced free outpatient treatment for all and free inpatient treatment for children in July 1965, without warning or preparation for medical workers.[5] Mombasa's outpatient attendances multiplied five times before settling back to a threefold increase, while many other districts reported a doubling of outpatient numbers. Some one-man dispensaries in Central Province found themselves treating a patient every two minutes.[6] These rural units were the responsibility of county councils, some of which had to close dispensaries to reduce costs. By 1967 there were complaints that payment had been better because it had at least ensured treatment.[7] Free treatment exacerbated Kenya's shortage of doctors. Many expatriates left at or soon after independence, so that despite Makerere's new graduates and recruiting all over the world, the number of active doctors rose only from about 750 at independence to perhaps 1,100 in 1974, roughly in step with population growth.[8] In retrospect, this swamping of the health service came to be seen as a critical moment in its deterioration. At the time, however, it was the firstfruit of independence for many Kenyans and medical staff responded generously to increased workloads.[9]

Further pressure on the medical service came from the self-help (*harambee*) movement which President Kenyatta especially encouraged. Many communities tried to secure local dispensaries or health centres by building rough structures and expecting their politicians to induce the Ministry to supply staff. During 1967, for example, 96 *harambee* dispensaries were added to the previous 640. Health centres needed more staff and equipment, so that government accepted responsibility only for those built in accordance with the current five-year plan.[10] Many buildings consequently stood empty or half-completed. In 1967, for example, Kenya had 157 health centres but Eastern Province alone had over 50 *harambee* health centres in various stages of construction. Functioning health centres were generally so inundated with curative work that they neglected the preventive outreach work which was their distinctive function.[11] Demand for hospitals, too, was as insatiable as in Uganda. Ministers presenting annual health estimates to Parliament generally turned immediately to hospital building, sometimes district by district throughout the country. Members then crowded to press the case for their constituencies, regardless of cost:

> Whenever asked to do something they [Ministers] say, 'When funds are available.' This is the time when the Minister should ask for exactly what he wants. It is up to us to decide whether or not to give that amount.[12]

In reality the Treasury decided, and only the most powerful politician – notably Kenyatta himself – could secure the construction of an unplanned hospital.[13] Country members therefore denounced the huge cost of developing the Kenyatta National Hospital (KNH) in Nairobi into a teaching hospital or lobbied violently for a new hospital offered to Kenya as Russian aid and eventually built in Kisumu.[14] The regionalism which underlay Kenya's independence constitution caused great difficulty for doctors posted outside their region of birth. One Provincial Medical Officer in Western Region, a Kikuyu, reported that 'the Chairman of the Regional Public Health Committee and the PMO had very strained relationship':

> At one time the Regional Assembly even tried to interfere with the recruiting of the staff and even recruiting of trainees, and pre-trainees in the Institutions under the Region. It was found, for instance, that some of the students taken as trainees in Bungoma were either undesirable in that they did not have the necessary qualifications . . . or in that they were married . . . Very firm measures had to be taken . . . I am told that these students had been taken, under the instruction of some Regional Assembly Members, and it appears the move was sanctioned by someone in pretty high position.[15]

The Ministry commonly posted doctors outside their regions to promote a Kenyan consciousness, but in 1973 it introduced regional recruitment quotas for paramedical training in order to secure staff acceptable to backward areas.[16]

The Ministry incurred further strain in 1969 when it took over the medical responsibilities hitherto borne by county councils but made unbearable by free services. This freed doctors from an awkward dual loyalty, but it raised the Ministry's staff from 5,000 to 13,000, made it responsible for many dilapidated buildings and vehicles,[17] and added largely to its budget. Between 1968–9 and 1973–4 the Ministry's annual current expenditure, as approved by Parliament, rose from £4,566,502 to £11,900,534. It was regularly overspent by nearly 10 per cent, making the Ministry notorious as financially the least disciplined branch of government. In 1969–70 it was responsible for 48 per cent of all state overexpenditure. At the same time it seriously underspent its development budget, by a peak of 45 per cent in 1967–8.[18]

Part of the reason for this was that staff were even scarcer than money, but parliamentarians fixed the blame on the DMS, Jason Likimani. By 1969 there were public demands for his resignation.[19] Recalled from private practice to head the medical service at independence, Likimani had no administrative experience above the district and was plainly bored by departmental detail. He was seriously ill in 1971 and was described in 1976 as 'little more than a figure-head',[20] although he clung to office until 1978, when Kenyatta died. The Ministry was highly centralised, Likimani was barely on speaking terms with the Permanent Secretary,[21] and both jealously guarded their independence from 'political interference', so that successive ministers were reduced to exasperated impotence and seldom bothered to defend their officials:

> The position, Mr Speaker, is very difficult for me, in that the advice I get from my chief officer, as it is written here and in the answer I gave, does not seem to have any relation to what hon. Members have put down as facts . . .
>
> The question of movement of staff is governed by the Civil Service Regulations. Therefore, unless I am given the information, I cannot know what goes on in the Public Service Commission or inside the office of either the Director of Medical Services or the Permanent Secretary.[22]

Given these circumstances, it is no wonder that by the 1970s control of district medical work was visibly weakening. Almost every medical unit exceeded its budget and justified it by the urgency of its work: 'The figures are clear. We overspent all the votes already. The services must continue.'[23] Transport began to break down: by 1973 over 200 of the Ministry's 680 vehicles were off the road. Drug supply was a problem throughout the 1960s because many local authorities could not pay for their requirements, but in the early 1970s incomptence, corruption, and financial stringency made it such a major scandal that all fifty-five officials were removed from the Medical Stores and their head was imprisoned for five years. Major parliamentary criticism of the health services began in 1969 and escalated irregularly thereafter.[24] Studies showed that the public resented long waiting times, an alien environment, and hurried treatment. They wanted to be examined with a stethoscope or other instrument, treated with an injection or medicine, and told the nature of their complaint.[25] 'Doctors come to your room just for a few minutes in the morning and that is all for the day', one complained. But free treatment with potent modern medicines was highly valued. Amidst the many criticisms, it is important to remember that Kenya's hospital beds increased between 1962 and 1973 from 10,617 to 18,186.[26] The proportional increase in outpatient attendances was even greater, but no comprehensive figures are available. Medical expansion was a major achievement of Kenya's new African government.

For doctors, too, this was often a time of optimism. Thomas Ogada, a future DMS, was twenty-eight when he was posted in 1964 to his first independent station at Tana River near the eastern coast. He was the son of a railway driver and chief on the shores of Lake Victoria, 600 kilometres away, had schooled at Maseno and Alliance, sung in the Makerere chapel choir, and married a nurse.[27] He found his new posting in crisis. The Tana flood had failed, throwing agriculture, tax receipts, and local government into disorder. Somali bandits were raiding the east bank of the river. 'However the spirit of Harambee has been shown in the self help work which has gone in the building of dispensaries latrines and digging.' These were vital, for Ogada found the local Pokomo people relying on grossly polluted river water and practising 'unhealthy habits' of sanitation. Mindful of the preventive medicine taught at Makerere, Ogada resolved that these 'must be combated by vigorous campaign by political leaders, church and health department', enforcing new public by-laws 'with all our might'. This would require other government departments to provide the district with services as good as its medical provision. 'Anaemia and infantile diseases are diseases associated with poverty and ignorance. The medical department alone cannot fight the battle.' But there were things it could do. It could attempt to eradicate the bilharzia and malaria which caused 90 per cent of the district's sickness. 'A lot has been done in the field and laboratory about these diseases. Statistics have been collected for decades. What do we wait for?' The department could also give him use of a mobile laboratory and X-ray equipment to screen the population for tuberculosis. It could give his hospital a Landrover so that patients did not arrive 'almost moribund'. He concluded with a list of 'Resolutions for 1965':

> The medical problems of Tana River are not curative. They are public health problems. We want our ideas to reach people in their homes so that they change their environment for better.
>
> Concentrating on curative medicine and only paying lip service to public health education is in the long run very expensive . . .
>
> If we are not successful in bringing to reality the above . . . items, then either because we fail to press our views with sufficient force (which will not happen), or because our advice is rejected (which sometimes happens), then Tana River will have taken a step backwards towards the limbo from which she has only so very recently emerged.[28]

Several keen young doctors like Ogada spent these years in remote stations. 'I thank the Ministry for having posted here our Kenyan Doctor to serve his people Kenyans, and this rules out the idea of foreigners who quoted that No African Doctor can willingly like to work in this remote area', Joseph Obare wrote at the beginning of his two-year tour among the Samburu pastoralists of Maralal.[29] More, however, mustered such influence as they could command to remain in the densely populated areas of central and western Kenya where there was hope of further training and specialisation.[30] In the meantime, a government doctor in mid-career might expect to head a district hospital, treat a mass of respiratory infections, gastroenteritis, malaria, and anaemia – all especially in children – supervise chemotherapy for tuberculosis cases, handle difficult childbirths, and conduct those major operations like caesarean sections and laparotomies which did not require a specialist's skills. He might have to contain an epidemic, most probably of poliomyelitis or cholera.Above all, government doctors were responsible for maintaining services at a time of rapid transition, and this was their main achievement. Nearing the end of his career and looking back on 1975 as Provincial Medical Officer in Nyanza, Tadayo Evelia regretted the disappearance of hospital flower-beds but concluded:

(i) That we have done a great deal to improve the existing services and are pleased to report that whatever achievements we have made has been towards the rural areas.

(ii) Despite the limiting factors of insufficient funds inadequate transport, shortage of qualified staff especially Enrolled Nurses, the services were run up to a reasonable standard.[31]

The Medical School and medical research

Until 1967 Kenya lacked the medical school which has generally been the core of professional formation in the Third World. Thereafter the school at the University of Nairobi, with the Kenyatta National Hospital as its teaching institution, expanded Kenya's stock of doctors, provided them with a professional focus, and during the 1970s took over the leadership of East African medical research from Makerere while continuing to work largely within traditions established there.

At independence Kenya had about 750 doctors, of whom 49 were Africans. By 1993 there were about 3,700, a very large majority of whom were Kenyans, plus some 1,300 in training. The increase had outpaced very rapid population growth. In 1993 there was roughly one doctor for every 7,000 people, a ratio three times as good as Uganda's. About 1,200 of the 3,700 doctors were in government service.[32]

Most of this increased manpower came from the Medical School in Nairobi, which admitted its first thirty students for a five-year course in July 1967 and expanded to its planned annual intake of about a hundred in 1972, when the first students graduated. The syllabus was similar to Makerere's, with up to four months of community health in Machakos district, but there was more integration of specialities into a single teaching programme appropriate to local conditions. 'East Africa's crying need is for doctors to work among the masses who constitute the great majority of the peoples of East Africa', wrote the first African Dean, Joseph Mungai. '. . . This at once requires drastic changes in the conventional curricula that have been imported here from areas where their rigidity and conventionalism have often yielded undesirable results.'[33] An anatomist who had been a distinguished athlete, head prefect of Alliance High School, and chairman of the Makerere Christian Union, Mungai had an important influence on Nairobi's first students. Another dominant figure from Makerere was Nimrod Bwibo, who built a department largely responsible for expanding Kenya's stock of paediatricians from one in 1963 to eighty-five in 1984, many of them women.[34]

A medical school for 500 undergraduates necessitated major changes in the Kenyatta National Hospital, hitherto smaller than Mulago. The Ministry resisted attempts to make KNH a university teaching hospital, but a £5 million scheme began in 1968 to expand the hospital from 700 to 1,500 beds, increased further in 1982 to 2,000, although unit costs and managerial difficulties were widely believed to increase in any hospital larger than 700 beds.[35] Moreover, KNH, like Mulago and the Muhimbili Hospital in Dar es Salaam, served also as a local hospital in a swollen capital city for which it was politically impossible (because of up-country objections) to build a separate institution. Originally KNH had no outpatient department – the outpatients were to go to city council clinics – so that outpatients swamped the casualty department, especially after the announcement of free treatment increased outpatient attendances from 110,456 in 1965 to 457,489 in 1968. An outpatient department was then built, only to be swamped by a further increase in attendances to 980,623 in 1980, or 2,700 a day. The surgical wards, similarly, were overwhelmed by road accident victims, while inpatient admissions quadrupled between 1973 and 1983.[36] By 1980 the hospital took over 40 per cent of the Ministry's recurrent budget and employed more than half of all government doctors.[37] Its expense encouraged the Ministry to exercise direct control through a management committee chaired by the Permanent Secretary, despite numerous schemes for autonomy which faltered in the face of rivalry between doctors and hospital administrators, doctors and civil servants, and academics and consultants.[38] As financial constraints tightened after 1973, the hospital's facilities deteriorated badly. In 1976 it had not a single ambulance and half its toilets and one-third of its water taps were broken. In 1979 the operating theatres closed for a week for lack of drugs, surgical gloves, and other supplies.[39] The hospital became a favourite target for press, politicians, public, and doctors themselves:

> The recently published K[enya] I[nstitute of] A[dministration] report on the K.N.H. blues was not news to the many doctors and nurses who have trained or worked at this hospital. They know it all. They have lived through all that nightmare. There was nothing new about lack of maintenance of hospital vehicles and equipment . . . Stories of drug racketeering have been told like grandmothers tales; inefficient administration is perennial; the word 'out-of-stock' would as fittingly apply to medicines, syringes and needles as it would to sweepers, nurses and doctors. You have to memorise it if you are to remain sane at K.N.H. Administrators brag when they frustrate a doctor into resignation; sweepers become peer-heroes when they abscond from duty and get away with it. In short K.N.H. is decadent. It is a place where mediocrity is institutionalised.[40]

The Medical School and its students could not escape infection by this bitterness. The whole university was already racked by conflict between students and the government which began in 1969 and repeatedly closed the university. Medical students generally avoided these disturbances, describing themselves as 'usually meek and cool-headed to the extent of a near docility save for voracious devouration of their academic texts'.[41] Although medicine was no longer a uniquely prestigious and well-rewarded profession – in 1988 entry to the Medical School required fourteen points at A level, compared to seventeen for law and fifteen for commerce – the expansion of secondary schooling ensured that competition was still rigorous. Between 10 and 20 per cent of students failed in whole or part at the end of each year, generally passing at a supplementary examination. Medical students were therefore serious people, often with strong Christian beliefs. About 20 per cent were women in the late 1980s.[42] Students were expected to spend long hours in the wards. 'Diseases don't read textbooks', Bwibo told them: 'Remember, only those things we do are really remembered.'[43] On completing his internship, the qualified doctor was normally posted to gain experience at a district hospital, before perhaps taking charge of a small and distant unit where his responsibilities would be multifarious and his contact with medical centres negligible. 'In several years of up-country practice', two such doctors wrote, 'we have never seen even one of our referred patients returning to us from the referral hospital with advice on management'. Too long there might make him a 'Penicillin-Aspirin-Chloroquine Doctor'.[44] To escape that, the ambitious applied for one of the one hundred places in MMed postgraduate courses which the Medical School introduced in 1972.

By the late 1980s students and young doctors were deeply concerned about the quality of training at the Medical School:

> Clean well equipped theatres do not exist, laboratory investigations are taught in theory, bed side teaching is almost nil, the drugs of choice for many diseases are not available, rudeness and indiscipline are common place and absenteeism from work is tolerated . . .
>
> It seems that the general state of KNH has demoralised the teaching staff.[45]

External examiners were equally critical. But so were the teachers, who in 1990 urged President Moi to disband the Medical School until it could be provided with a satisfactory teaching hospital.[46] The government granted the hospital greater autonomy, introduced cost-sharing, and arranged for rehabilitation with World Bank funds, but it also introduced an expatriate management team whose presence and tactlessness infuriated Kenyan doctors. They insisted that the hospital did not need appointed outsiders but should be entrusted to the control of the doctors who worked there.[47] In 1995 the Medical School lost some autonomy when legislation entrusted supervision of medical education to the Medical Practitioners and Dentists Board, whose senior doctors suggested the use of private hospitals for teaching purposes.[48] Privatisation was infiltrating education as it had infiltrated other areas of Kenya's medical system.

The Board was also concerned about the medical training offered at the

Moi University Medical School near Eldoret, which had opened in 1990 under the leadership of a cardiovascular specialist, William Lore. Like the new medical school at Mbarara, Moi University had a community-orientated curriculum, much encouraged by the WHO, described as including 'socio-economic, demographic, cultural, ethnographic aspects of the community as well as teaching of health care economics, concepts of appropriate technology and improvisation and the inculcation of appropriate positive attitudes towards the community'.[49] Lore argued that this had been the Nairobi School's original intention but had never been fully implemented owing to lack of resources and 'lipservice to the philosophy, disbelief, lack of faculty staff and student motivation, lack of staff commitment, lack of full perception of societal needs based upon priorities and negative professional attitudes'.[50] There had been little consultation with the medical profession, however, some of whose members doubted whether the graduates could be registered to practise. And initially the School had to use the Eldoret District Hospital, whose inadequacy led in 1995 to student protests that it lacked even thermometers and stethoscopes.[51]

Although KNH had conducted little medical research before the Medical School opened, during the 1970s the two institutions took over from Makerere the leadership of medical research in East Africa. The *East African Medical Journal* is not an impartial source because the Kenya Medical Association controlled it, but from the 1940s to the early 1970s many of its contributions were from Makerere, whereas between 1978 and 1987 some 47 per cent of articles came from Kenya, 24 per cent from Nigeria, and only 29 per cent from other sources including Uganda and Tanzania. Between 1988 and 1993 about 44 per cent of the journal's articles were from Kenya, 7 per cent from Tanzania, and only 2 per cent from Uganda, although by then much Kenyan research came not from the Medical School but from the Kenya Medical Research Institute.[52] The reason, of course, was Makerere's decline under Amin and his successors. In the early 1980s some forty Ugandan doctors were thought to teach at the Nairobi Medical School.[53] Yet Nairobi had already been established as a medical research centre, chiefly by Kenyans who had graduated at Makerere and undertaken postgraduate work abroad. As at Makerere, they charted the local disease environment and attacked in particular the notion that there were 'diseases of civilisation' from which Kenyans seldom suffered.

One outstanding physician within this tradition was the cancer specialist Edward Kasili, who graduated from Makerere in 1968 and took up a post at the Nairobi Medical School. Cancer treatment had begun at KNH during the 1960s, using both drugs and radiotherapy, but Kasili's MD thesis on leukaemia, submitted in 1979, was the first full-scale research report. 'The main objective of the study', Kasili began, 'was to show that leukaemia was more common in Kenyan Africans than has been the belief from impressions'. He studied 456 cases at KNH and found its behaviour broadly the same as elsewhere in the world, 'although it appears to be more aggressive, probably due to the late presentation of patients'. Statistics suggested that leukaemia in adults was as common in Africa as elsewhere, although perhaps somewhat less common in children. It was also of growing prevalence and must be treated: 'The debate of whether to treat or not to treat is an age-old scandal that should be relegated to the past.'[54] Kasili pursued this work at KNH for another fifteen years. It showed him that leukaemia was in fact common in children, especially those aged between five and nine, and he opened a special ward for them.[55] 'The incidence of some childhood cancer in Africa is one of the highest recorded in the world', he wrote in 1986, adding that patients came so late that few could be saved. His studies also convinced him that cancer caused 20 per cent of all adult and 9 per cent of child deaths in Kenya, figures approaching those of developed countries.[56] Long experience of treating those in agony showed him how difficult it was to nurse terminal patients in a Kenyan home and how little the average regional hospital could help them. 'Pain relief is grossly inadequate due to the fact that effective analgesics are not available', while most doctors simply did not know what to do.[57] Kasili therefore explained how a patient should be informed of his condition – truthfully but gradually – and the treatment protocols to be followed.[58] He was also chiefly responsible, in 1989, for founding the Nairobi Hospice, the first institution in tropical Africa specialising in care of terminal cancer patients. He died there in 1994, of cancer.[59]

Kasili carried out Nairobi's outstanding work on cancer and younger doctors carried it on.[60] Replying to the arguments against expenditure in a poor country on hopeless cases, he had pointed to the prevalence of cancer and the suffering it caused. This issue was more acute for those treating diseases of the heart or kidney, where very sophisticated and expensive treatments – possibly even transplants – might be medically indicated. In 1978 a team led by Nelson Awori carried out tropical Africa's first kidney transplant, from a dead donor. Awori performed several further transplants, including the first from a live donor. 'Professor Awori has made Kenya Medically great', the eulogist declared at his funeral in 1986.[61] Occasional transplants and more regular dialysis continued thereafter, generally financed by *harambee* fund-raising. Heart surgery was altogether more difficult, as Peter Odhiambo, one of Kenya's leading heart surgeons, recognised in 1984 when arguing that renal transplants were possible in a Third World country but heart transplants were not a priority. Yet Kenya was

Africa's most active centre of cardiac research, after South Africa.[62] Its most articulate advocate was the physician Hilary Ojiambo, a dominating figure in the Medical School as Professor of Medicine. Ojiambo attacked especially the notion 'that heart diseases . . . are "diseases of civilisation", and do not warrant much attention in developing countries'. Not only were they already 10 per cent of admissions to major referral hospitals in East and Central Africa, he argued, but 'These are the diseases of tomorrow.'[63] The most important was hypertension, 'the greatest killer of the heart diseases commonly seen here', which was spreading with urbanisation and dietary change among the middle class. In 1976 the Consultative Committee on Cardiology Research in East Africa identified this as the first priority for study. By contrast, rheumatic heart disease, also very prevalent, was, Ojiambo thought, a disease of malnutrition and poverty. Thus, echoing much research during his time at Makerere, 'The incidence of heart disease in different societies appears to be governed largely by social and environmental determinants as opposed to hereditary and similar factors.'[64] Ojiambo's views on medical policy shifted, alongside prevailing African opinion, from the outspoken elitism of his early years – 'In developing countries there is a tendency to overemphasise the role of public health, in some cases to the detriment of clinical (curative) medicine' – to greater sympathy for primary health care.[65] But he remained convinced of the importance of cardiac medicine, and younger specialists carried it forward.[66] Cardiac surgery, however, had a chequered career. Transplants were not feasible, but open-heart surgery – requiring temporary replacement of the heart by a heart–lung machine – began in 1975 with equipment funded by a public appeal and was first performed by a Kenyan in 1979. Nearly 200 operations were completed before the equipment broke down in 1983, and it worked only sporadically thereafter. As Odhiambo, the pioneer, wrote sadly in 1992, 'It is as if we are always starting.'[67]

The discovery that 'diseases of civilisation' were in fact frequent among Kenyans gave a common theme to much of the Medical School's research. In addition to cancer and renal and heart complaints, it was demonstrated for peptic ulcers, gout, diabetes, and especially mental illness, whose prevalence came to be thought 'similar to, if not higher than, that found in the Western culture'.[68] There was less emphasis on the better-understood communicable diseases, which were left mainly to government institutions, especially the Kenya Medical Research Institute (KEMRI), founded in 1979.

KEMRI introduced a new element into the medical scene. Its chief architect was Kihumbu Thairu, specialist in brain function, Professor of Physiology, Dean of the Medical School, and author of *The African civilisation*, an exposition of racial ideas most common among black intellectuals in the Americas which, as a Kenyan reviewer put it, 'confirm and give the aura of academic respectability to what many Africans feel deep down in their guts'. Thairu argued that colonialism, 'one mammoth conditioning laboratory', had robbed Africans of a culture and creativity which had been responsible for much of the world's progress. It must be recovered and blended with modern technology to gain the power without which Africans would never win respect: 'We can never be a superpower unless we are proud of ourselves and of our *Utamaduni* [civilisation].'[69] Appointed chairman of a committee to establish KEMRI, Thairu persuaded the Japanese to build a modern laboratory to concentrate on common diseases like malaria and bilharzia affecting the mass of the people.[70] By 1987 KEMRI employed some thirty doctors and filled much of the *East African Medical Journal*. Projects included malaria, bilharzia, tuberculosis, respiratory diseases, diarrhoea, leprosy, and AIDS, together with indigenous medicine.[71] Thairu remained the institute's intellectual patron, but by the mid-1990s its director was the very ambitious Davy Koech:

> If we are to prevent our societies from sliding into geographical artefacts, we have to overcome the development philosophy of the later half of this century which invited us to passively accept the products of technology transfer by bringing science and technology into the core of our development process . . .
>
> For Africa to move forward, we must provide effective, competitive and appropriate solutions to our problems by utilizing and managing the available expertise for the exploitation of the vast natural wealth in this continent. By seeking to harness the vast wealth of knowledge in our midst, this journal provides one such effort. This is because if we can truly make full use of information that is available to mankind today, we can skip decades of slow development and 'leap frog' into the 21st century.[72]

This was written to introduce KEMRI's *African Journal of Health Sciences*, one of several new medical journals launched in Kenya during the 1980s and 1990s,[73] partly on the grounds that international journals were prejudiced against research papers by Africans, partly because the new journals could be financed by advertising for drug companies and other private medical interests, but also as a characteristically positive Kenyan response to medical crisis.

Doctors and the state, 1963–81

During its first generation of independence, Kenya experienced three doctors' strikes, in 1971, 1981, and 1994. They illustrated the progressive alienation of professionals from the state and the ethical dilemmas they faced in a capitalist and increasingly corrupt society. Doctors' strikes were always traumatic. The strikers' motives were mixed, blending material interests with concern for the health system. The doctors were commonly divided, between private practitioners and state employees, professional leaders and discontented juniors, conservative upholders of inherited ethics and radical advocates of new ideas. The one thing they shared, as in Uganda in 1995, was devotion to an ideal of professionalism, interpreted in the many different ways its ambiguity permitted.

The strike of 1971 – probably the first doctors' strike in tropical Africa – originated in long-standing discontent over pay exacerbated by the Ndegwa Report of 1971. This had recommended large increases for senior civil servants but disregarded the professionals' claims that their starting salaries should correspond to the length of their training and that the salaries of their higher ranks should match the earnings of senior administrators or private practitioners.[74] Following a stoppage by KNH doctors in July 1971, the Ministry of Health passed the doctors' complaints to the President's Office. It offered small increases which were rejected. Parliamentary debate on 5 October showed almost universal sympathy for the doctors, even among the health ministers, one of whom declared, 'If the [Ndegwa] Commission did not give doctors anything good, it is not the responsibility of the Ministry of Health.'[75] On 21 October representatives from hospitals all over Kenya decided to strike, maintaining only emergency services, despite government warnings of strong measures. Next day KNH was deserted, except for senior doctors on emergency call.[76] The Minister insisted that no variation from the Ndegwa Report was possible, for other professional groups 'are probably waiting round the corner to stage a strike', but the Minister of Labour commented 'that the doctors' issue has been handled in a queer manner', met the doctors' leaders, and persuaded them to suspend the strike while he chaired a commission to produce a settlement. Political and press sympathy were still overwhelmingly with the doctors.[77]

Conciliation failed, apparently because either the President's Office, the Ministry of Health, or the Cabinet vetoed concessions. Over 200 doctors at KNH therefore struck again on 5 November, this time bringing out colleagues elsewhere. The Ministry said all government doctors were on strike. There was little overt criticism from within the profession, but consultants, lecturers, and private practitioners in Nairobi helped to maintain emergency services at KNH, where Likimani joined them. Government now acted on its threats. Twenty-two striking doctors were arrested on 5 November.[78] Three days later, with the strike continuing at KNH and Machakos but other hospitals back at work, twenty-nine Nairobi doctors (including Joseph Aluoch, a future leader) were charged with striking illegally in an essential service, the prosecution adding that a charge of conspiracy was being considered. They were released on bond after undertaking to return to work, the magistrate reminding them that they 'are professional people who have sworn to serve the people'. Next day all doctors were at work,[79] having learned the danger of challenging the Kenyan state.

Yet the underlying problems worsened during the following decade as public demand multiplied while oil-price rises and international depression checked Kenya's economic growth. Between 1974–5 and 1978–9 the share of government expenditure devoted to health fell from 7 to 5 per cent.[80] Important developments did take place. Smallpox was eradicated, a cholera epidemic was controlled, mass immunisation against the six major childhood diseases began in 1974, the first experiments with community-based health care were launched, and an essential drugs list was published in 1979.[81] Yet overcrowding, deteriorating facilities, drug shortages, and corruption caused growing discontent.

The doctors' chief response was to enter private practice, either full-time or, more often, while retaining their government posts and taking advantage of the Ndegwa Report, which had encouraged civil servants to engage in private business because Kenya needed their entrepreneurial skills. In 1978 the Medical Practitioners and Dentists Board reported that 500 of Kenya's 1,364 registered doctors were private practitioners, 138 of them Kenyan citizens. What proportion of the 579 in government service (466 of them Kenyans) also owned private clinics is unknown.[82] The government's difficulty, as in Uganda, was that if it tried to stop its doctors dividing their time, many might resign. As one said in 1977, 'The salary only equals pocket money; the main income comes from private practice.'[83]

In that year the government attacked the problem with a new Medical Practitioners and Dentists Act which strengthened the Medical Board, made it less dependent on government, but also required private practitioners to obtain an annual licence in which the Board might stipulate where in Kenya the recipient might practise. Government claimed that this would not prohibit government doctors from also practising privately but would enable the Board to allocate non-Kenyan practitioners to the less crowded regions, leaving the more desirable areas to Kenyans.[84] But doctors were alarmed by the licensing provision, which proved cumbersome in operation. Open protest came in 1979, when President Moi (who had succeeded Kenyatta a year earlier) lost patience and banned government doctors from practising privately with effect from January 1980, saying, 'I do not want to lead a nation of mercenaries.'[85] Some thirty doctors promptly resigned to beat the deadline; resignations during 1979 included the Medical Superintendent of KNH and Likimani's successor as DMS, who was replaced by the forty-year-old and strong-minded Karuga Koinange. To check resignations, the Medical Board allegedly delayed licences for private practice. The major problem faced those government doctors, especially the majority of younger ones, who could not afford or did not wish to resign. They wanted compensation for loss of private practice, eventually demanding a 50 per cent salary increase.[86]

These grievances were exacerbated by a civil service pay review, the Waruhiu Report, which paid special attention to lawyers and teachers but not doctors, offering no compensation for loss of private practice. Contrary to service regulations provincial doctors' representatives met in Nairobi, drafted their own conditions of employment and forwarded them to government with the threat of a strike. Moi exploded: 'The president challenged the doctors to go on strike and said he would "deal with them", adding, that even if they quit government service, "I can do without them."' He also warned that government might refuse them private practice licences and demanded an apology, which doctors' representatives were said to have given.[87] Yet negotiations proved difficult. The Ministry proposed a new scheme of service which was accepted by doctors' negotiators but rejected by a meeting at KNH which resolved instead to strike. This was to be a more substantial action than that of 1971, but initiated more hastily and thereby forfeiting public sympathy.[88]

On 7 May 1981 over 300 of the approximately 600 doctors in public hospitals struck. 'Thousands of patients were turned away [from KNH] without treatment while chaos reigned in the wards.'[89] Stories of patient deaths and lurid press photographs circulated, although emergency services continued. The precipitate action caused confusion and division at up-country hospitals. The Ministry warned that the strike in an essential service was illegal, the Medical Board denounced it as professional misconduct, Koinange insisted that it 'cuts across all professional ethics', the *Sunday Nation* described it as 'a crime against society', and even the Convention of Trade Unions condemned it.[90] Many senior doctors were probably hostile, although medical students proclaimed their support.

Arrests began on 9 May and doctors started to trickle back to work, but on 15 May the situation was transformed by the students at the University of Nairobi, who rioted in support of the doctors' case and against the government's ban on the opposition leader Oginga Odinga, thereby introducing politics openly into the dispute. Riot police raided the student hostels. The university closed. Doctors withdrew again from KNH for fear of violence. On 21 May police began to arrest all they could find and oblige them to return to work under bond. By 3 June the situation at KNH and most other hospitals was said to be normal.[91]

The strike had four main consequences. The doctors eventually received much smaller allowances than they had sought, although government permitted specialists a degree of private practice, thereby widening the profession's divisions. Activists attempted to convert the Kenya Medical Association into a body which would make future strikes unnecessary. Experience of repression left most doctors fearful of further stoppages, so that an expatriate who later counselled strike action was told 'that we have done that before and some of us were handcuffed for it'.[92] Instead, yet more doctors withdrew into private practice.

Private practice

Strikes by government doctors were a method of asserting professional interests, but another and arguably more substantial form of professionalisation took place among private practitioners. Little is known about them – no study has been published or probably even attempted – but they were the majority of the profession. In the mid-1990s Kenya had some 4,000 registered doctors, of whom slightly over one-quarter were in government service and the others mainly in private practice.[93] A doctor had to work at a public institution for two years after registration before seeking a licence to practise privately. From the late 1980s, under its privatisation programme to please international financiers, government positively encouraged the private health sector, promising 'a system of incentives, including underwriting the cost of land for the establishment of hospitals and clinics especially in the rural areas, favourable tax rebates and the acquisition of drugs at cost'.[94] A few doctors saw this as a threat to the health of the poor, but most welcomed it. 'By offering alternative services for those who can pay', the Kenya Medical Association's journal *Medicus* argued,

> private practitioners reduce the number of people that would demand government health services . . . These government free services will remain for those who really need them, that is, those who cannot afford to pay for alternative services . . .
>
> It appears that doctors, who by nature tend to avoid confrontation with authorities, have decided to seek for themselves other means of professional and financial satisfaction. In all the previous confrontations between doctors and the authorities, it is the innocent patients and doctors who have been the losers.[95]

In reality, free treatment, by overcrowding government facilities, encouraged all who could afford it to seek private medicine,[96] while deteriorating working conditions and defeated strikes in government service drove many doctors out of the public sector or, increasingly, led them scarcely to enter it, as one wrote in 1989:

> Family doctor or GP-doctor is now the cornerstone of all medical promotive, preventive and curative services in Kenya . . . Many or a few years back GPs used to be retired civil service doctors who after a full service in Ministry of Health could now retire to a Private Clinic . . .

> Nowadays it is completely different, there are very many young Doctors who have for varied reasons opted to go for GP (General Practise). These are dynamic Doctors full of knowledge and energy.[97]

Behind the process, of course, lay the growth of a largely urban African middle class.

To practise privately still required the annual licence from the Medical Board introduced in 1977. This caused irritation and for some years it was difficult for a new doctor to obtain a licence to practise in Nairobi (except, it was said, by influence or bribery), but in 1984 the Board appears to have abandoned the restriction. The formal prohibition on government doctors practising privately remained, but after a renewed attempt to enforce it in 1983 led to resignations, it was 'tacitly waived', in words attributed to the Minister.[98] There is no evidence on the extent of the practice, but it was said in 1994 to be widespread and a directory of private clinics in Nairobi at that time included almost all well-known names in Kenyan medicine, whether based in government service or in the universities.[99] Specialists could profit from a foot in each camp, while for younger men it was probably often a means of accumulating sufficient capital, reputation, and patients to enter full-time private practice. In 1994 the Minister said government needed 'alternative methods of sharing the burden of paying Government doctors', which suggested acceptance of the Ugandan pattern of a poorly paid but largely part-time medical service.[100]

Many part-time private practitioners employed a clinical assistant or other paramedic to run the clinic in their absence.[101] An Inspector of Drugs described one in 1968:

> This place is a village and a trading centre as well. On arrival there, I observed no sign board bearing the name of [the doctor-proprietor] or other person's name. But I met a . . . clinical Assistant in charge of the said clinic. This clinic is part of a shop which has been partitioned off and made into two rooms. One is used for receiving patients and the other is a treatment room . . . I was informed that [the doctor] does visit the clinic once a week or twice a month to attend to some cases referred to him by his clinical assistant . . .
>
> Patients are received by the Clinical Assistant who eventually diagnoses the drugs to be given, and gives treatment to patients. He is assisted by a man who is neither a nurse nor a dresser . . .
>
> Registers of patients and their cards were properly kept and at least every drug used was being accounted for at the clinic by the Clinical Assistant. Fees paid by patients ranged from 5/- up to 20/-. The payment was said to be in cash . . . [The clinical assistant] said that about 10 patients do visit the clinic, but on market days, the number is more than ten. Serious cases are normally referred to Kajiado District Hospital, but [the doctor] is sometimes summoned by telephone to attend to some of the serious cases. Drugs are normally delivered to the clinic by [the doctor] himself. Most documents in the clinic bear a rubber stamp of the name of [the doctor].[102]

This was perhaps carefully on the legal side of the borderline separating it from 'associating with unqualified persons' or 'covering for unqualified persons', both offences under the Medical Board's code of conduct of 1979.[103] But the relationship between paramedic and doctor could range from employee through partner to virtual franchise holder paying the doctor for use of his name.[104] The latter two relationships were certainly illegal. The greyest area was how many clinics a doctor might open. The Medical Board directed: 'If more than one private clinic is operated, at the discretion of the Board, the second clinic should as far as possible, be within 30 kilometres of the parent clinic and they should be adequately covered and supervised.'[105] Some rule was much needed, for entrepreneurs had multiplied clinics during the 1970s, often locating them close to government medical institutions to attract patients seeking treatment but deterred by enormous queues. One doctor described himself in 1972 as having 'a travelling practice in various Rift Valley towns', while another (a Member of Parliament) was struck off the register in the mid-1970s for 'the opening and running of 35 or so clinics and the staffing of them with unqualified persons'.[106] Such disciplinary action by the Medical Board was rare, but it did seek to control the doctors' use of dangerous drugs,[107] while the police occasionally closed scores of clinics operating without medical supervision and arrested the doctors responsible.[108]

African doctors entering private practice competed with established European and, especially, Asian practitioners who were the great majority of private doctors until probably as late as the 1980s. The earliest African private practitioners in the late 1950s had opened clinics in Nairobi's African townships. In the 1960s, it appears, some settled in small country towns like Kitui or Machakos, where there was less established competition, or opened multiple clinics at trading centres. It was said in 1986 that 'an ever increasing number is going rural'. In 1983, for example, Kiambu District, just outside Nairobi, had twenty-five private clinics, ten owned by Asians and fifteen apparently by Africans, while in 1989 there were said to be fifteen private practitioners even in a district as remote as Kitale.[109] But successful private practice generally depended on urbanisation and by the 1970s African doctors were beginning to challenge Asian and European dominance of large towns, a trend perhaps illustrated by the first major parliamentary attack on Asian private practitioners in 1973 and by the licensing legislation of 1977 ostensibly designed to favour Kenyan citizens.[110] The only detailed evidence comes from a Nairobi medical directory for 1993–4, which did not claim to be exhaustive. It listed 161 private clinics (excluding church and obviously charitable clinics) in or close to the city, but their names did not permit a racial breakdown. Of the 492 individual private practitioners listed, 269 appear to have been Africans. They included 47 of the 108 who described themselves as general practitioners, 28 of the 48 surgeons, 41 of the 53 physicians, 32 of the 44 paediatricians (a tribute to Bwibo's teaching), 45 of the 77 obstetricians and gynaecologists, and 33 of the 85 dentists. Of 357 specialists and 106 general practitioners whose location in the city can be identified, 188 specialists and 52 GPs were clustered in the city centre, 70 specialists and 9 GPs in the zone including the high-status Parklands residential area, and 12 specialists and 22 GPs in a low-status zone including Mathare Valley. One is struck by the high proportion of African specialists – many with government or academic posts – and their concentration in middle-class areas, but also by the fact that general practitioners and even some specialists were at least geographically accessible to the poor.[111]

The medical directory also listed twenty private hospitals and nursing homes in Nairobi. They included the Nairobi Hospital (formerly the European Hospital, subsequently managed by the Kenya Medical Association) and the Aga Khan Hospital, both high-quality, non-profit-making survivals from the colonial period which admitted those Africans who could afford it but had many non-African patients. In 1988 the Nairobi Hospital had 194 beds, employed 14 full-time doctors, and was regularly used by over 300 private doctors for the treatment of their patients.[112] Among the more entrepreneurial private institutions was the Masaba Hospital, opened in 1989 by Dr J. Momanyi. In 1993 it claimed 200 beds, advertised in three categories: 'the private fully-contained rooms, a two-bed sharing ward and a six-bed general ward in an atmosphere of immaculate cleanliness and decor'. It claimed a laboratory, X-ray unit, ultrasound scan, HIV-testing facilities, two operating theatres, and dental and physiotherapy units. Like the Nairobi Hospital, Masaba either provided physicians and surgeons or allowed the patient's medical adviser to use its facilities, an arrangement much strengthening the position of private practitioners.[113] Smaller institutions on these lines existed in the mid-1990s in Mombasa, Eldoret, and probably elsewhere.[114] The number of private hospitals in Kenya doubled during 1993–4 alone, but during 1995 some forty-one private hospitals and nursing homes were closed and fifty doctors, proprietors, or administrators arrested, allegedly for defrauding the National Hospital Insurance Fund, a compulsory and contributory insurance scheme for higher income-earners established in 1966 which paid between 40 and 80 per cent of inpatient bills for its over one million members The only substantial fund of its kind in tropical Africa, it was 'the life-line of the private hospitals', but by the mid-1990s it operated on a financial knife-edge, allegedly in part because some hospitals claimed reimbursement for non-existent patients or kept patients in the wards longer than was warranted.[115]

Hospitals like Masaba were the exception. The normal pattern of private medicine was the solo practice, whose main obstacle elsewhere – that it was difficult to start – was perhaps obviated by moonlighting from government service. It is striking that Nairobi lawyers, with fewer opportunities for moonlighting, often formed partnerships,[116] and that there is little evidence that medical practices were bought and sold. The doctor practised almost entirely at his clinic(s). Solo practice isolated him from medical criticism and encouraged him either to treat cases which he should have referred to a specialist or to enter into unethical fee-splitting arrangements with specialists, which were said to be common. Solo practice also made him dependent on his patients' favour. But it permitted him to become a family doctor, which was said to be emerging during the 1980s, and it avoided the intricate financial disputes which partnership would probably have bred.[117] Little is known about earnings. By comparison with the consultation fee of 5/- to 20/- quoted at Kajiado in 1968, the average in the wealthier parts of Nairobi in 1975 was said to be 40/-, with additional charges for specific procedures and probably sale of medicines.[118] A study in the early 1990s found that most private practitioners in Nairobi treated over five patients a day for sexually transmitted diseases, and over three a day in Kisumu, often charging over Shs.200 for drug treatment and more for an injection; the patients were mainly low-income people seeking private and accessible treatment with available drugs. Many doctors probably gave some free treatment to the poor, although there were allegations that some contravened medical ethics by requiring prior payment. Of the twenty-five complaints received by the Medical Board during 1978, ten were for 'abuse of financial opportunities'.[119] After tentative and unsuccessful attempts by the Kenya Medical Association to standardise fees, the Medical Board issued guidelines for standard procedures like consultations, operations, and hospital visits, but there is no indication of their effectiveness.[120] The only extensive data on earnings come from questionnaire replies by 376 doctors in 1989.[121] Since 39 per cent of these doctors lived in Nairobi and slightly over half had practised for less than ten years and were under thirty-nine years old, they were probably a fairly representative sample, although how accurately they reported earnings is another matter. Some 39 per cent claimed to earn less than Shs.10,000 ($435) a month, 31 per cent earned Shs.10,000–Shs.20,000 ($435–$870), 20 per cent earned Shs.20,000–Shs.35,000 ($870–$1,522), and 11 per cent earned over Shs.35,000. The figures are hard to interpret, but one inference might be that there was a large (and probably young) category at the bottom struggling for a middle-class lifestyle, quite a substantial number of prosperous doctors at the top (probably older men, some of whom may well have had business interests), and a middling group which was the largest of the three but by no means dominant. This might suggest a hierarchy not unlike that within a large hospital like the KNH, whose influence within the profession was very great. But this is speculation.

The established private practitioner might well become a community leader. Eric Mngola was briefly Mayor of Nairobi. William Ouko was Ker (President) of the Luo Union. Samson Mwathi came within range of winning the Parklands seat in Parliament and belonged as firmly to Nairobi's elite as any man in the city.[122] James Munene had a turbulent career in Thika, where he opened his practice in 1962, became Chairman of the Town Council and much else, launched into business and farming, held a parliamentary seat from 1969 to 1973, and was finally driven from politics by the town's notoriously bitter rivalries, losing his medical licence.[123] His business interests, including the classic Kenyan beer-distribution franchise, were probably crucial, for doctors generally fared badly in Kenyan politics after independence, especially when compared with Uganda. Several stood for election during the late 1960s and 1970s, but only four newcomers (including Munene) were elected. Success in Kenyan politics probably needed money and alliances on a scale more available to businessmen than doctors. The two exceptions were the pioneers, Mungai and Waiyaki, although neither had an entirely successful career and neither seems to have been very active as a doctor. Mungai was successful as Minister of Defence and then of Foreign Affairs, but in 1974 he lost his Dagoretti seat, which obstructed his challenge to Moi's succession to the presidency in 1978 on the death of Kenyatta, with whom Mungai's intimacy was a positive disadvantage. Thereafter Mungai remained on the political fringe.[124] Waiyaki succeeded Mungai at the Foreign Ministry and his populist gifts held on longer to his even more turbulent Mathare seat – during the 1979 election one of his speeches 'was subjected to a minor distraction when someone began splashing human faeces on his audience' – but he lost it in 1983 and failed to make a political comeback when multi-partyism was restored.[125] Nevertheless, both men were still politically active in the mid-1990s.

The private doctor competed with a wide spectrum of medical workers, all catering to a rapidly growing and very young population. At the legal end of the spectrum, midwives could run maternity and nursing homes provided they had an arrangement to call a doctor in emergency, a provision which aroused suspicions of 'covering'.[126] Clinical officers, the best-trained paramedics, long demanded the right to independent private practice after retiring from public service, but met the doctors' stubborn resistance. In 1985 the doctors secured the abandonment of a bill for this purpose, *Medicus* denouncing clinical officers as a colonial anachronism, equipped only 'to follow simple signs and symptoms to make probable diagnoses, and then provide uncomplicated remedial measures', quite incapable of independent practice and not on any account to be equated with professionals. Soon afterwards, however, legislation did permit clinical officers to practise independently under a separate council and specified the diseases and conditions they might treat.[127] Further along the spectrum, many former nurses and paramedics with less training operated small illegal clinics or simply dispensed drugs and injections from their homes.[128] So did many people with no training at all, especially in outlying districts:

> A new type of health worker now taking advantage of the situation is the 'bush-doctor' a person with some formal education who has acquired needles and syringes illegally and some antibiotics and chloroquin. Such a person has no clinic and does his medical work part time. He tries to combine both traditional and western medicine in his practice often with tragic results.[129]

Many toured the countryside on bicycles. Their practice merged imperceptibly into drug-selling, which was probably as common as in Uganda but apparently aroused less alarm in Kenya's highly commercialised society. Any trader could legally sell drugs not scheduled as poisons under the Pharmacy and Poisons Act. Scheduled drugs could be sold legally only by registered retail chemists, of whom Kenya had over 1,200 in 1997,[130] and then only on a doctor's prescription, although this was widely ignored. In practice, thousands of traders sold all kinds of drugs:

> We were overwhelmed to find that at every place visited that had large mobile crowds of Kenyans, there were people selling drugs; in every case these were men. At bus stations, open-air markets, the so-called 'shanties', in the train and even on board the lake steamers, there were people selling drugs. The majority of these people either had temporary open-air stalls at which they sold clothes (mainly new cheap clothes), blankets, crockery, soap, sweets, stationery, etc., or they carried some of these articles and sold them as they moved in the crowd. With remarkable regularity, they announced in low but clear voices their drugs in order, 'M.B.,[131] suta, capsules'.
>
> The drugs were often kept in plastic bags, in jacket pockets or on the roof of the stall. There was no word of greeting to the prospective buyer; all that was asked was the type of the drug required and the quantity. We found that we could purchase as little as even a single tablet or capsule. There were several types of capsules evidenced by the different colours but the choice was left to the buyer. No word of dosage or even the type of illness that could be treated with these drugs was forthcoming, except one was told on direct questioning that M.B. was for minor illness, suta was for moderate illness, and capsules for severe diseases. Each tablet was 20 cents and a capsule 40 cents, irrespective of type.
>
> The suta and M.B. 760 tablets we found to be authentic obvious drugs. We were able to buy seven different types of capsules which we later identified as containing ampicillin, tetracycline, chloramphenicol, and one gelatin capsule which was sold to us as a penicillin capsule but which we found to contain multivitamin syrup.
>
> Apart from the multivitamin capsule, all the drugs offered for sale were those drugs included under Parts I and II: Poisons (and should therefore be obtainable

only from authorized sellers). Apart from the suta tablets and one form of tetracycline capsule, all the other drugs were of brands not usually available in Government hospitals of this country, suggesting that they must have been obtained from the private sector. All these drugs were sold at less than half their retail value.[132]

Apart from the competition, theft, and possibility of poisoning, drug-selling alarmed doctors chiefly because it bred drug resistance. It was claimed in 1992 that the dose of penicillin needed to cure gonococcal infection had increased over a hundredfold in consequence.[133] But drug-sellers were only part of the spectrum of healers with whom private practitioners competed. In one remote location of north-western Kenya studied in 1980–1 there was one modern practitioner (a male nurse) and seventy-seven indigenous healers, but this pattern was not confined to rural areas: Mathare Valley in Nairobi at the same period had no government health facility but sixty-seven indigenous healers, located on average 70 metres apart, for towns were as much the growth areas for indigenous medicine as for the modern variety, and for the same reasons.[134] Most healers in Mathare had no schooling, were typically in their forties, operated as full-time general practitioners, and were evenly divided between men and women. Rural practitioners tended to be older and more specialised.[135] Children were generally taken to modern medical facilities wherever possible, but otherwise patients chose indigenous therapy, modern treatment, or often both in an increasingly individualistic, eclectic, and pragmatic manner according to complex considerations including proximity, cost, reputation, type of disease, religion, education, and personal experience.[136]

By comparison with Uganda, indigenous medicine in Kenya was treated with even less respect by modern doctors but experienced the same commercialisation as they did. Although a handful of politicians championed indigenous medicine, more Kenyan leaders were openly hostile than was normal in tropical Africa, probably because of the country's strong Christian and modernising ethos. In 1969 Kenyatta publicly described 'medicine men' as 'lazy cheats, who wanted to live on the sweat of others'. The powerful provincial administration was especially hostile, as was the Ministry of Health, whose policy was defined by a senior official in 1970 as 'to discourage the use of native medicines as far as possible; but there is no law to enable us to stop such practice'.[137] Some districts licensed healers, at a price, but generally government did almost nothing to recognise or encourage them, choosing instead 'a silent dismissal of traditional medicine as useless'.[138] Doctors generally took much the same view, apart from academics who studied indigenous practitioners or, like Kihumbu Thairu, saw them in terms of cultural nationalism.[139] 'One wants to ask these [foreign] experts which herb they would give to their own child if he was suffering from pneumonia or gastroenteritis', *Medicus* once complained.[140] Modern doctors were particularly concerned to stop indigenous healers from advertising improbable cures. Paramedics, who competed most directly with indigenous healers, were especially hostile to them.[141]

As always, the main exception to this negative view was the modern doctors' desire to test whether indigenous medicines contained anything worth incorporating into the modern pharmacopoeia. Research began in the 1970s at the University of Nairobi's School of Pharmacy, while John Kokwaro of the Botany Department published a major study of *Medicinal Plants of East Africa*.[142] KEMRI took up this work from 1984 at its Traditional Medicines and Drugs Research Centre. The only practical result seems to have been anti-malarial tablets made from leaves of the *mwarobaini* tree, but that was the South Asian *neem* tree, introduced into East Africa after being used for medicinal purposes since at least the time of the Buddha.[143] In addition to testing drugs, from the late 1970s the authorities adhered verbally to the WHO policy of attempting to incorporate indigenous healers and birth attendants into community-based health care programmes. Some birth attendants and circumcisers were trained in hygienic methods, but the few approaches made to healers had little apparent effect.[144] One reason, as in Uganda, was that government viewed the several rival associations of healers chiefly as mechanisms of control, while many healers saw them as expensive swindles run by urban entrepreneurs. Another was that although indigenous healers were often eager to acquire modern skills, what they most wanted was recognition and security, not incorporation into a modern medical system in a subordinate capacity less rewarding than their existing practice.[145]

Indigenous medicine had long been divided between purely local healers and experts with wide reputations and sometimes itinerant practices. Urbanisation, modern communications, and commercialisation benefited the wide-ranging expert. The most striking was Jack Githae, a former agricultural extension officer from a family with medical skills who set up as a herbalist near Naivasha in 1974, treated both people and livestock, expanded to Nairobi in 1984, opened other branches in and around Central Province, and claimed to have treated 18,720 patients in 1989–90, chiefly for asthma, bronchitis, hypertension, epilepsy, paralysis, ulcers, sexually transmitted diseases, and infertility. Githae claimed to utilise new technology to create a professional modern herbalism:

> We have incorporated a number of full-time as well as part-time professionals in our undertakings. They include a specialist in the analysis of chemical components of various herbs using the gas liquid chromatography machine, who also assists in the encapsulation of our herbal medicines, for use by some of our patients abroad; and a data analysis consultant (he is currently pursuing a Ph.D. in mathematics at

Harvard University) handling all data at K[arati] R[ural] S[ervice] C[entre]. Others are; two trained clinicians in charge of clinical work; a forester responsible for herbal nurseries and agromedical gardens; a botanist responsible for identification of herbal plants; a senior clinical laboratory technologist working in conjunction with a trainee at the Kenya Polytechnic; and, a biochemist pursuing a Ph.D. degree at the University of Nairobi.[146]

The interesting parallel was between the Karati Centre and the Masaba Hospital as products of Kenya's transition to capitalism.

Doctors and the state after 1981

During the sixteen years after the unsuccessful strike of 1981, Kenyan doctors shared many experiences with their counterparts in Uganda. They too became increasingly the purveyors of preventive medicine and of skilled and literate treatment within a spectrum of medical choice in which the core was self-medication with modern or indigenous drugs. The differences from Uganda were that far more of Kenya's doctors were full-time private practitioners and that the minority of government employees related to a state which, although weakened, was distinctly more powerful than Uganda's. Kenya's doctors were therefore particularly divided, with a minority in especially hostile relations with the state. This appeared in attempts during the 1980s to reorganise the profession and in the protracted medical strike of 1994.

Kenya's medical system continued to expand throughout this period, although not at the breakneck speed of the 1960s. Hospital beds increased between 1978 and 1994 from 26,922 to 37,271, much of the increase coming from self-help wards added to existing hospitals.[147] The number of doctors, similarly, rose to about 4,000 in the mid-1990s and a growing number were women, who in 1983 formed an active Kenya Medical Women's Association.[148] There was more emphasis on preventive medicine, especially while Koinange was DMS, with stress on immunisation and community-based projects. Yet expansion took place without comparable increase in funding, for between 1980 and 1993 Kenya's per capita Gross National Product barely grew, at 0.3 per cent per year. According to one estimate, annual per capita public expenditure on health fell between 1980–1 and 1996–7 from \$9.5 to \$3.5. Yet Kenya's situation remained better than Uganda's, for government took more than twice as large a proportion of GDP as tax. Moreover, during the 1980s Kenya's fertility rate, hitherto the world's highest, fell rapidly in response to economic pressures and family planning.[149]

Financial stringency severely damaged medical institutions. Referral and outreach depended on transport, but in 1996 it was eleven years since the

Ministry of Health had last purchased an ambulance. Institutions habitually overspent their budgets and corruption was widespread, culminating in a bizarre scandal in 1996 when the Ministry's Permanent Secretary was dismissed for signing a provisional tender for anti-malarial chemicals costing 79 per cent of his Ministry's entire annual budget.[150] In 1982 the government at last attacked the drug-supply problem by regularly providing health units with essential drug kits and banning the import of unregistered drugs. Drug supply undoubtedly improved but remained the major public grievance.[151] Other criticisms concentrated especially on overcrowding – bed occupancy rates exceeded 200 per cent in some hospitals[152] – the deterioration of buildings and equipment, and neglect or callousness by staff.

These were the conditions of work for the doctors who attempted after the 1981 strike to reorganise the Kenya Medical Association (KMA) and the medical profession. Although designed at independence to put leadership into African hands, the association had attracted little African interest during the 1970s, when its leaders were mainly Asians and its activities largely confined to Nairobi and Mombasa.[153] Its revival began in 1979 when two young doctors from Kisumu attended an Annual General Meeting, were disgusted by its apathy, returned to organise their local colleagues, and began to stimulate branches at other up-country centres. At a further Annual General Meeting at Kisumu in March 1981, amid interracial tension, the activists took control.[154] Most were early graduates of the Nairobi Medical School, and especially Bwibo's paediatricians, who in a sense now took leadership of the medical profession for the first time. One prominent activist was Vincent Orinda, a former chairman of the Nairobi Medical Students Association, pupil of Bwibo, and author of an MMed thesis on how to involve mothers in the operation of a paediatric ward.[155] Another, J.W. Nyikal, also a paediatrician, dedicated his MMed thesis on kwashiorkor 'to all those children of peasants and workers of the developing and underdeveloped countries who strive to survive under the yoke of starvation and want in a world technologically capable of producing enough food for all mankind. With these children I share roots and perhaps destiny.'[156] As secretary they chose Mohammed Abdullah, a Makerere graduate who had been part of Nelson Awori's renal transplant team.[157] Bwibo became vice-chairman, while the new chairman, Yusuf Ali Eraj, was a Kenyan paediatrician of Pakistani ancestry who wanted the KMA to become a trade union:

> We may call ours a 'profession', a 'vocation', a 'calling', or a 'trade' but it is just another type of hard work. The days of professional mystique, vocation, and status are gone, destroyed by the very society we serve . . . Only the power of collective bar-

gaining will enable doctors to demonstrate their superior knowledge of human misery and affliction and to promote their objective of harnessing their professional skills to solve the many problems that confront us.[158]

The new leaders took control on the eve of the 1981 strike, in which they tried to arrange a settlement. Failing, they discussed how to advance the profession, and especially the position of junior doctors, in order to make further strikes unnecessary. They wanted to expand the association's membership, which in November 1981 was only about 700, and to cooperate with Koinage, who was equally concerned about the state of the profession.[159] At meetings with Koinange and the Medical Board in July and September 1981, both agreed to encourage doctors to join the KMA and even to consider making membership compulsory (as it was for the Law Society of Kenya), but they also pressed the KMA leaders to assist in 'maintaining discipline amongst junior doctors' and 'over-seeing and maintaining ethical and professional care of patients'. Koinange wanted to use the association as a disciplinary body, but the leaders saw it more as an embryonic trade union. As Abdullah wrote, 'We intend to improve our lot, improve our standards of practice, improve our ethics, improve our education and remain the watch-dogs of our affairs.'[160] They published a journal, *Medicus*, arranged a local insurance scheme for doctors, met President Moi and were allocated land in Nairobi for a cooperative housing project, set up an ethical committee, organised an annual scientific conference, attempted to launch a continuing education scheme for doctors and a school health service, and planned to build a headquarters.[161]

Difficulties began in 1984. First personality conflicts led to Eraj's replacement by the emollient Bwibo.[162] Then the association was drawn into a dispute at KNH when Koinange transferred two doctors for 'gross negligence', only for the KNH doctors to denounce his 'dictatorial attitude' and declare no confidence in him. The Minister revoked Koinange's decision and *Medicus* urged him to resign. He remained in office for another three years, but the possibility of reforming the profession in alliance with the state had faded. In its place the bitterness which had reigned before 1981 returned, while the young radicals established private practices and the KMA resumed the introverted conviviality so characteristic of the profession.[163]

Crisis arose in 1994, once more at the initiative of a new generation of junior doctors. On 18 March 1994 a group at KNH applied to register the Kenya Medical Practitioners and Dentists Union, which had many similarities to the earlier Uganda Medical Workers Union except that it was confined to professionals. The union's leader, Givens Ateka, claimed that it represented the 1,000 of Kenya's 4,000 doctors and dentists in the public service.[164] Their chief grievance – that government doctors earned only one-fifth as much as private practitioners – had been exacerbated by a report prepared in 1993 by a Ministry official, Willy Muya, who had recommended that a doctor's minimum earnings should rise from Shs.11,435 to Shs.41,400 a month, a proposal based on comparisons with private practice but so unrealistic in the prevailing economic depression that government had refused to discuss it.[165] Conditions of work were a further grievance: describing his experience of watching a patient die of meningitis for lack of drugs, Ateka said, 'The inadequacies were so common that they were practising something next to "battlefield medicine".'[166] Junior doctors' living conditions were also appalling and educational standards at medical schools were declining. Behind these grievances, a spokesman explained, lay the sense that 'Doctors have ceased to be role models and they want their rightful place in society.'[167] 'If there is one factor that totally demoralises doctors', the *Weekly Review* commented,

> it must be what they perceive as the erosion of their authority as the nucleus or team leaders of the medical profession. Somewhere along the line, it seems, there has been a role reversal in the power stakes in hospitals, with nurses, and especially matrons, largely gaining precedence over doctors even though they can only execute instructions given by the doctors. In relation to administrators, it would appear that doctors are often not consulted over priorities.[168]

These were long-standing grievances. A new element was the political opposition to Moi's regime which had grown during the 1980s and culminated in 1990 with the decision to permit opposition parties.[169] Doctors were divided in their party allegiances, but they came predominantly from the large and educationally advantaged Kikuyu, Luo, and Luyia ethnic groups who formed most of the opposition to Moi. The KMA was represented on the Professional Committee for Democratic Change and was concerned about state violence against dissidents, including some doctors, and the complicity of medical men in concealing violence.[170] Doctors also shared the general discontent of Kenyan professionals at the state's refusal to let them organise trade unions, a discontent which in November 1993 had caused university lecturers to launch a strike still in progress when the KMPDU applied for registration. When that application received no positive response, some 160 doctors from hospitals in many parts of the country met at KNH on 26 May 1994 and resolved to strike on 16 June unless government recognised their union. Ateka acknowledged that the public would suffer, but argued that the long-term effects would be beneficial. The Minister of Health replied that union organisation and strike action were unthinkable for professionals – 'They signed for this when they qualified as doctors' – and that they should instead join their welfare association, the KMA, whose chairman, William Lore, publicly dissociated the association from the strike threat. In return Ateka dismissed the KMA as 'a welfare association with its membership drawn from doctors in private practice'.[171] The division within the profession was there to be seen and exploited.

Knowing that they were breaking the law, KMPDU members at major hospitals struck on 16 June 1994. Some 200 doctors failed to report at KNH, services came nearly to a halt, many patients were sent away, most other major government hospitals joined the strike,[172] and the press carried grim reports:

> Nearby, a young woman with a toddler strapped to her back grimly held onto the hands of another woman who was writhing in pain on a stretcher. She explained that her friend's six-month pregnancy had apparently developed some complications. Idle, seemingly bored nurses watched as the guard told the pair to try their luck at the Pumwani Maternity Hospital at the opposite end of the city.[173]

Opposition politicians quickly supported the doctors – 'If they want a union, give them, it will cost nothing' – but the strikers urged them not to interfere,[174] for Moi promptly denounced the strike as political, saying it cost Shs.1,500,000 to train a doctor 'and now the same doctors have gone on strike leaving the taxpayer to die'. Newspaper opinion was divided but mainly hostile, recognising that the doctors had legitimate grievances but insisting that their action 'is too painful for this country and morally indefensible'.[175] Medical opinion outside the union was divided. On 2 July the chairman of the KMA's social responsibility committee, Joseph Aluoch – who had been among those prosecuted during the 1971 strike – issued a statement urging members not to undertake strikers' work and warning that if government did not negotiate the KMA would have to ask all doctors to withdraw their labour.[176] Moi insisted that 'professionals the world over never engaged in trade unionism'[177] and the KMA committee disowned Aluoch, calling on the strikers to return to work. Amid allegations that government was threatening to review licences of private clinics and that security officers were harassing KMA officials, Aluoch resigned, saying, 'I'm not commenting. I'm doing my medicine because that is where I get my daily bread . . . News come and go. When you talk, you confirm it, when you keep quiet people think you are a fool. So let me see my patients.' The union promptly accused Lore of acting unprofessionally.[178]

Meanwhile negotiations had begun privately on 6 July. Two days later government announced a 16 per cent pay increase. But with the union still demanding registration and the implementation of the Muya Report, negotiations faltered and the government threatened dismissals.[179] In reply, some 100 consultants at KNH withdrew their services until the strike was settled, claiming that they could 'no longer render meaningful service to the patients', although others, who opposed this action, claimed that the real reason was inability to combine emergency work with private practice.[180] A week later Moi told doctors they would be dismissed if they did not resume work within three days. Describing their demands as 'impossible, unrealistic and politically motivated . . . inconsiderate of the economic situation and the needs of other civil servants',[181] he ordered the Public Service Commission to take disciplinary action against them while also preparing a new scheme of service. On 2 September armed police began to evict strikers from flats and houses at KNH in a dawn raid. During the following weeks strikers trickled back to work, which involved applying for reinstatement. By 19 September KNH was returning to normal.[182] But great bitterness remained. When new pay scales raised a medical officer's starting salary only from Shs.8,170 to Shs.9,490 and gave the same responsibility allowance to paramedics as to doctors, Ateka denounced them as 'an insult not just to doctors but to all professionals in Kenya'.[183] He was still trying to hold the strike together, but on 29 September he announced its indefinite suspension because 'the Government did not care about human suffering'. The doctors, he said bitterly, had been 'humbled' and 'felt betrayed throughout the strike as the opposition was impotent and no overt support came from the public'.[184] The strike had lasted 105 days, allegedly the longest doctors' strike in the world.[185]

The medical profession's recovery from this confrontation took place in a changed situation. From the moment that government medical services were made free in 1965, doctors had warned that Kenya simply could not afford such provision and that only the reintroduction of fees could check the medical system's decline. In 1979 government announced its intention to restore fees, but it took no action until the World Bank pressed the issue in 1987. After much debate, cost-sharing was introduced simultaneously at all government hospitals and health centres in December 1989, mainly as a flat-rate charge for outpatient attendance. Most fees were abolished again in September 1990, chiefly because attendances had fallen by up to 45 per cent while the fees collected had been too small to justify the attendant political unpopularity. But financial necessity and pressure from international donors obliged government to make a second attempt late in 1991. This time charges were introduced gradually, were levied only when treatment was available, and were quite quickly accepted. By 1993–4 they covered 20–40 per cent of non-staff expenditure at hospitals and health centres, although there were complaints that institutions did not receive their proper share and that the system became an excuse to reduce central government allocations.[186] Cost-sharing was only one element in a larger policy shift during the 1990s to revitalise the Health Ministry, rely more on the private sector, and decentralise hospital management.[187] This was the context within which doctors reflected on the condition of their profession.

They were a divided body, dominated by a commercialised private sector, with the junior hospital doctors of the KMPDU an isolated special-interest group who in the mid-1990s were for the first time leaving the country in numbers.[188] Too few to aspire to a medical monopoly, which the state was in any case incapable of enforcing, doctors were no longer even the sole professionals within the health system, as clinical officers and nurses increasingly asserted claims to status. Yet doctors still controlled medical policy, designed public health initiatives, and provided the most skilled forms of treatment. Moreover, they still cherished the ideal of professional status, as had been so clearly displayed during the strike, when the KMA had accused the KMPDU of lacking professionalism, the union had thrown the charge back at Lore, doctors had claimed that Moi's Kenya had less respect for professionals than any other state in the world, and Moi had replied by contrasting the strike with an idealised notion of professional altruism. Senior doctors often agreed with the President, but many younger men rejected his model as archaic:

> There should be an end to calling for medical personnel to show self sacrifice. Doctors and other medical workers, despite the nature of their jobs are like all other Kenyans. They have families with school going children, and also wish for comforts enjoyed by other Kenyans. They are in their jobs like professionals and employees. The work demands hard work and dedication to duty. Most of them realise this and work hard at their jobs. However, they are not missionaries and did not join medical services because of a divine calling or as a holy vocation![189]

Between these polarised positions, some thoughtful doctors sought another basis for professional claims in technical expertise and efficiency. When Moi publicly attacked government medical institutions in 1996, the KMA Chairman, Khama Rogo, replied that only professionalism could solve the problem:

> It is the contention of KMA that if today Kenyans had the enormous resources of say the United States or the European Union, but such resources were left in the hands of the current health care management, our health services would get worse, not better . . . We have seen senior officers with no more than high school education rise to terrorise professionals. We have seen directors of medical services tremble before almighty Permanent Secretaries . . .
>
> This is the disaster we have in our hospitals today. And until we are mature enough to respect and reward professionalism, no amount of financing, not even importation of expatriates, will provide lasting changes and benefits to Kenya's health care system.[190]

The debate moved back and forth, but in the Kenya of 1997, as elsewhere in East Africa, there was no sign of consensus.

9 Tanzania: doctors and a socialist experiment

Tanzanian doctors after independence had a different experience from those in Uganda and Kenya. Too few to determine medical policy, the doctors also faced first a revolution in Zanzibar and then a relatively powerful mainland government anxious to transform the medical system in a socialist direction. Just as violence in Uganda and capitalism in Kenya presented doctors with dilemmas which divided the profession, so did socialism in Tanzania. After two decades of idealism and conflict, however, the socialist experiment failed and Tanzania's doctors faced instead what the experiment's architect, Julius Nyerere, called 'the relentless weakening of government and community, and the equally relentless globalisation and marketisation of our economies'.[1] Consequently the outcome was much the same in Tanzania as in Uganda and Kenya, although the route to it was strikingly different. Unfortunately, much about that route is not yet known, for public documents and the press are less revealing in Tanzania than in the other countries.

The origins of the experiment, 1961–71

The first Tanzanian doctors to face a radical challenge after independence were those in Zanzibar, where a revolution in January 1964 replaced an Arab-led government by an African regime looking to communist states for aid. Since almost all Zanzibar's indigenous doctors before independence appear to have been Arabs[2] – although that was often hard to define – the revolution devastated the medical system. It is not clear whether any doctors died in the revolution, but many fled to the Middle East or Britain. Even after the union with Tanganyika, Zanzibar retained its own Ministry of Health and looked chiefly for communist aid. At first this was generous. East Germany staffed the main hospital (renamed the V.I. Lenin Hospital), four new district hospitals were planned, the number of health clinics increased between 1964 and 1973 from thirty-two to sixty-seven, and hospital fees and private medicine were abolished. A training course for doctors opened in 1970, although it subsequently met difficulties, and another forty-five doctors were trained abroad during the first twenty-three years after the revolution.[3]

On the mainland, by contrast, the shift towards a socialist medical strategy did not take place until the late 1960s and early 1970s. For most of the decade after independence in 1961 the priority for Mtawali and the other senior doctors who took over the Ministry of Health was continuity. In September 1965 there were 127 government posts for medical officers, of which 30 were held by Tanzanians and 35 were vacant.[4] The skeleton staff was fully occupied maintaining basic services, especially when demand for medical attention was expanding rapidly and enthusiastic villagers were building self-help dispensaries which the Ministry could neither staff nor supply. As in Uganda, health had low priority in development planning during the 1960s, although its share of government spending rose. Real per capita GDP grew at 1.5 per cent per year between 1960–1 and 1967–8, preventing any major breakdown of services.[5]

Pressures for radical change in medical policy had existed even before independence. Nyerere's impatience with the glacial speed of medical training had inspired Bryceson's plan, as Minister of Health, to train a sub-professional category of rural practitioners, while discontent among medical assistants led to the more successful scheme to upgrade many to Assistant Medical Officers. External pressures for change also existed. Although Tanganyika's medical planners had long favoured preventive medicine, rural health centres, and the doctor's role as team leader, there was a more radical current in international medical opinion which held that these goals could be achieved only by shifting resources away from 'disease palaces', such as the new Muhimbili Hospital in Dar es Salaam, and from Western patterns of medical education. Bryceson tried to tap this current in 1961 by inviting a team of British medical planners led by Richard Titmuss to study the health system. In the event the Titmuss Report counselled realism, warning that Tanganyika was 'a veritable graveyard of health plans'.[6] It stressed preventive medicine, rural health centres, training of rural medical aids, a new category of doctor with four years' training after school certificate, two new referral hospitals, and a balanced articulation between rural and hospital medicine through an effective referral system.

Mtawali and his advisers who drafted the medical section of Tanzania's development plan for 1964–9 probably sympathised with the Titmuss Report, apart perhaps from its advocacy of sub-professional doctors. They too stressed rural health centres, to be built under Ministry control but chiefly with local funds, while central government financed urban hospitals and staff training.[7] In the event two new referral hospitals at Moshi and Mwanza were begun with church aid and 80 per cent of planned hospital beds were provided, but the referral system did not function; of those admitted to Muhimbili, for example, 91 per cent were normally resident within 16 kilometres of Dar es Salaam. Rural health centres also drew 80 per cent of their attendances from the same radius, but only five of the eighty planned centres were completed by 1969 because local governments had little money for health and spent it on dispensaries, which cost less than one-tenth as much.[8] With regard to specific diseases, the national campaign to eradicate smallpox began in 1968 and there was much emphasis on tuberculosis but rather little attention to malnutrition or to measles, reported cases of the latter increasing between 1961 and 1967 from 12,612 to 67,612. The chief priority of the 1960s was to train staff. Between 1961 and 1970 the number of registered Tanzanian doctors on the mainland rose from 12 to 123.[9]

In 1967 Tanzania formally adopted the programme of socialism and self-reliance set out in the Arusha Declaration. Health strategy contributed little to this decision, which was designed to accelerate development, check social differentiation, and produce a new political consensus as purely nationalist objectives faded.[10] The chief priorities for socialist transformation were agriculture, industry, and education, rather than health. But the declaration opened Tanzania to the influence of socialist medical systems elsewhere, especially that of China, which impressed a visiting medical delegation in 1967:

> The Chinese have very large numbers of 'doctors' but they have different grades of doctor, from university doctors with 8 years' training to medical school graduates with 5 years' training, and so on down to what they call 'barefoot doctors' who have only 3–6 months' training and a yearly 10–15 days' refresher course after the harvest. These 'medics' do medical work half the time among the people on their farms, and join them in the farm work the other half of their time. They are usually primary school leavers. They treat common diseases and give First Aid, and also Health Education . . .
>
> We were much impressed by the stage of development of health services, which have been revolutionised and transformed by the new China. In particular the way in which the doctors have to go to the country to serve the broad masses . . . The combination of traditional and modern medicine in order to find out what is good in the traditional methods instead of rejecting them is also something which we might follow.[11]

Many of these ideas were already familiar to medical planners, who had experimented with village health workers since the early 1960s, and they were taken up eagerly by Lawi Sijaona, the Minister of Health in the late 1960s, who proposed free mass immunisation, an essential drugs programme, expanded training of medical auxiliaries, and the training of villagers to provide elementary health care where dispensaries were lacking.[12] The five-year plan for 1969–74 proposed that central government should take responsibility for rural health centres and add eighty new centres to the existing fifty by 1974, while expanding the training of medical assistants, rural medical aids, and village health workers. But the plan also proposed to spend twice as much on hospitals as on health centres, including two further referral hospitals at Iringa and Mtwara, and to accompany paramedical training by roughly doubling the intake to the Medical School. The plan envisaged a fivefold increase in capital expenditure over its predecessor, simply adding socialist objectives to previous priorities.[13] In 1971 some 60 per cent of medical expenditure was still in Dar es Salaam, only 7 per cent was on prevention, and roughly half of development expenditure was externally financed, despite commitment to self-reliance.[14]

The major break in health policy came at the TANU party conference of September 1971, which ruled that rural health services should have top priority in socio-economic development plans. As later defined, the new policy was 'to treat people as close to their homes as possible in the smallest, cheapest and most simply equipped rural health units'.[15] This meant shifting expenditure from hospitals and doctors to health centres, dispensaries, village health posts, and auxiliaries. The new policy sought to cultivate egalitarianism and encourage the rapid concentration of the population into villages which would eventually operate on *ujamaa* (socialist) lines. Some doctors were already experimenting on these lines. By 1970 Pius Stambuli, the District Medical Officer in Lindi, had organised a 'revolutionary and more effective public health programme' in which mobile teams toured villages while the district hospital trained medical helpers for village health centres.[16] More influential was Aloysius Nhonoli, Dean of the Medical School, who by the early 1970s was advocating village health posts run by local workers with a few months' training – possibly indigenous healers or birth attendants – who 'should not be paid salaries but looked after by the village in the normal division of labour'.[17] Similar ideas, but with a specifically socialist emphasis, were advocated by expatriate Marxists, notably Oscar Gish, a planner inserted into the Ministry of Health, who stressed the need to shift expenditure away from the modern hospitals, curative treatment, and sophisticated training favoured by the medical profession and to abandon the idea that egalitarian medicine could be achieved through a referral system, which must be replaced by a widespread network of small medical units.[18] Another pressure came from public criticism of medical facilities which were overcrowded and lacked drugs and functioning equipment[19] – a criticism encouraged by party intellectuals as ammunition against doctors believed to oppose the socialisation of medicine. In response to these pressures, the government produced a new medical plan proposing that between 1970–1 and 1980–1 the proportion of recurrent expenditure devoted to hospitals should fall from 75 to 50 per cent while expenditure on dispensaries and health centres rose from 10 to

25 per cent, on preventive services from less than 5 to 10–15 per cent, and on training from 2 to 7 per cent. Training would concentrate on medical assistants, rural medical aids, and maternal and child health aids. The plan assumed real economic growth of between 6 and 7 per cent per year.[20]

Tanzania's doctors took little public part in these debates, while their official contributions remain unknown. There was opposition within the Ministry of Health, where the post of Chief Medical Officer was abolished in 1973 and three doctors in charge of preventive services, manpower development, and hospital services were made directly responsible to a lay Principal Secretary.[21] Among the profession's rank and file, most private practitioners were Asians who were too discreet to speak their minds, while most African doctors were government servants prohibited from making public statements. They were not necessarily hostile to the new course, on which many probably had mixed feelings, but there was discontent. One grievance was pay. The Arusha Declaration imposed new restraints on elite salaries, including those of doctors which the idealistic Nyerere described as 'small in comparison with the remuneration of doctors in other countries' but 'very large in relation to the average pay in Tanzania'.[22] In 1973 a medical officer started at Shs.1,840 a month and could not earn more than Shs.3,200, which was far below parastatal and private salaries or the incomes of less-qualified senior officers elsewhere in government.[23] By 1973 nearly fifty Tanzanian Asian doctors had left government service and often the country, while several senior African doctors were moving to private practice.[24] Yet pay was not the only problem. 'Doctors are frustrated not necessarily because of low salaries or absence of fringe benefits', wrote Philip Hiza, a surgeon at Muhimbili, 'but they are more frustrated professionally when they cannot discharge their skills to the full to benefit the patient'.[25] Not only did they work amidst deteriorating conditions, but they took blame which they believed should fall on their political masters.[26] Doctors entered Tanzania's socialist period divided in their minds and sympathies.

The experiment in practice, 1971–85

The socialist experiment began vigorously. Between 1970–1 and 1973–4 the share of government expenditure devoted to health rose from 5.2 to 8.9 per cent. Thereafter, however, it declined again. During 1974 the new plan was temporarily shelved in response to drought, oil-price rises, and the effects of forced villagisation.[27] Implementation resumed once the immediate crisis ended, but a renewed and lasting crisis struck the economy in 1979 and the resources available to the mainland government never recovered to the levels of the 1960s, whereas in Zanzibar they held up quite well until the

1980s. Between 1977–8 and 1982–3 real mainland government expenditure per person on health more than halved.[28] During the 1970s Tanzanian funds met most recurrent expenditure, but over 70 per cent of the health development budget came from foreign donors. During the 1980s aid became increasingly important to the recurrent budget also; in 1989 government could pay for only 10 per cent of imported drugs and equipment.[29] Government medical services remained free until the early 1990s.

Despite constraints, the share of mainland government health expenditure going to rural areas rose between 1971 and 1981 from 20 to 42 per cent, a shift without parallel in Uganda or Kenya. In 1969–70 hospital services took 63 per cent of development expenditure; in 1980–1, only 34 per cent, whereas in Zanzibar – whose small area dictated a different pattern – the proportion allocated to curative care remained static. In 1972 the mainland had 99 health centres and 1,501 dispensaries; the numbers in 1980 were 239 and 2,600 respectively.[30] The two institutions were in practice similar, for most health centres lacked the funds, transport, or staff to provide more than local curative care, so that Nyerere's aim to treat patients as close to their homes as possible was exactly what happened.[31] In 1983, some 93 per cent of the people lived within 10 kilometres of a health facility, a significantly higher proportion than in most African countries, but many health facilities were of poor quality; a World Bank survey in 1985 found that only 660 of 1,800 government rural dispensaries were in good condition.[32] Dispensaries handled most outpatient attendances, which almost doubled between 1971 and 1980 to reach nearly six per person per year.[33]

Yet in 1980 only 37 per cent of Tanzania's villages had a dispensary.[34] For the others the policy was for district health authorities to provide a temporary aid post staffed by one or two village health workers selected by the community, trained for three months at the district hospital, and then sent home with a first-aid box to serve the villagers part-time and without pay.[35] The plan had similarities to the tribal dresser scheme of the 1920s, but its immediate roots lay in local experiments during the 1960s and the Chinese model. Initially the scheme was left to local initiative and largely failed. As their trainees most villages chose young primary school leavers seeking an entry to paid employment. Their training was often haphazard, they received little supervision and inadequate supplies of drugs, they were regarded with suspicion by older neighbours, and they were seldom paid by villagers who saw no reason for it when the government paid dispensary staff. By the early 1980s most village health workers had probably ceased to function, although nobody knew even how many there were. In 1983, however, the Ministry of Health took over their training, instituted a standardised six-month course, and tried to improve drug supply. Payment was still left to communities, so that some of those trained continued to abandon their work, but by 1990 some 5,000 had been trained.[36] In the meantime, however, China's barefoot doctors were themselves declining in number and those remaining were evolving into sub-professional doctors or private practitioners.[37] The same process was possible in Tanzania.

Through the training of village health workers Tanzania pre-empted one component of the WHO's primary health care programme. Other elements were also taken up. Mass immunisation against six main childhood diseases (measles, tuberculosis, poliomyelitis, tetanus, diphtheria, and whooping cough) began on the mainland in 1975 and was remarkably successful, achieving figures variously estimated at between 70 and 86 per cent of infants in the early 1990s, while in Zanzibar, where full immunisation was at times a requirement for entering school, the coverage in 1990 was said to be over 90 per cent.[38] Tuberculosis control was also successful, as were maternal and child health clinics, which were said to have provided antenatal care to 96 per cent of expectant women during 1987–91.[39] All these were services provided by bureaucratic means. Nutritional work, by contrast, was less successful; in the early 1990s about 5 per cent of all infants suffered from severe protein energy malnutrition.[40] Some 56 per cent of the population had access to safe water in the late 1980s, compared to 30 per cent in Kenya and 21 per cent in Uganda, but equipment was often broken, helminthic complaints were common (especially in Zanzibar), and the most serious epidemic disease of the period was cholera, which arrived in 1972, caused 5,207 recorded deaths by 1987, and still recurred sporadically in the mid-1990s. Nevertheless, mainland life expectancy rose by some 50 per cent during the first thirty years of independence.[41]

Despite this progress, many problems worsened during the 1970s and became acute during the following decade. One was medical administration, including control of district hospitals, which was 'decentralised' in 1972 to local officials and party leaders, producing much confusion and local conflict. By the early 1990s District Medical Officers were responsible to six different authorities.[42] A second problem was that drug supply could not match the expansion of services in the face of transport breakdown, administrative disorder, and shortage of foreign exchange. By the early 1980s only 15 per cent even of the drugs available reached rural facilities and many people ceased to attend them, until Denmark launched an essential drugs programme which gave Tanzania one of tropical Africa's better supply systems.[43] Transport, however, remained a major weakness in so vast a country. In 1984 only 17 per cent of rural health centres and 4 per cent of dispensaries had a working vehicle,[44] dislocating distribution, supervision, and referral systems and leaving each unit to perform whatever curative functions it could.

Socialist medicine sought to shift expenditure away from referral hospitals where doctors were concentrated. Muhimbili inevitably suffered, although it never experienced Mulago's appalling lack of resources, enjoyed greater autonomy as a parastatal, and was fortunate to have two able Medical Superintendents, Nhonoli and Philemon Sarungi, the latter an orthopaedic surgeon trained in Austria and Hungary. Between the two, however, there was a period of disorder when the number of inpatients increased between 1977 and 1986 from 42,157 to 211,547, outpatients rose from 241,949 to 534,344,[45] the budget was frozen, and equipment and morale deteriorated. It was compared unfavourably with the new church-sponsored referral hospitals at Moshi and Mwanza, but they had to be restored to church control in 1986, when the Mwanza hospital had gravely deteriorated.[46] A fourth referral hospital at Mbeya in the south was formed in 1985 by combining existing units,[47] but otherwise the ban on major hospital construction was maintained against political protest. Many district hospitals also deteriorated for lack of funds. A study of 150 caesarean deliveries at Kilosa District Hospital in 1981–5 found that 8 per cent of the mothers had died, compared to 1.2 per cent at Muhimbili, itself a high proportion.[48]

The chief victims of rural-focused health policy were the towns, for while expenditure was being channelled into the countryside, people abandoned it in response to the physical uprooting and economic disorder caused by forced villagisation. During the 1970s Tanzania's urbanisation rate, 11.4 per cent per year, was the highest in the world after the United Arab Emirates and Mozambique.[49] The population of Dar es Salaam grew between 1967 and 1988 from 272,515 to 1,360,850, swamping local health services and helping to abolish differentials in health status between town and country.[50] By the 1980s immunisation rates in the city's shanty towns were often below those in the countryside, tuberculosis rates were much higher, and urban clinics were notoriously long on queues and short on drugs.[51] One victim of independence, decentralisation, and socialist medicine was control of malaria, which spread in both urban and rural areas, as did resistance to chloroquine. The proportion of mainland hospital admissions due to malaria rose between 1968 and 1985 from 13 to 25 per cent.[52] Malaria was also a major problem in Zanzibar, which abandoned the WHO's very successful malaria eradication project in 1968 and saw infection rates soar until a new American-financed programme began in 1981, only itself to end in 1990.[53]

All these problems stimulated public complaints. They emerged strongly in Zanzibar in the early 1980s,[54] while on the mainland there was a steady undercurrent throughout the 1970s and 1980s, although Nyerere had taken steps to end the clamour against doctors which had arisen in the early 1970s, fearing that it would further damage morale.[55] Corruption, a fertile source of grievance elsewhere, was relatively rare in Tanzania until the later 1980s, when complaints of dirt and negligence in hospitals also escalated again.[56] Illicit drug-selling and medical practice seem to have become important problems only during the 1980s.[57]

From the present evidence it is hard to assess how Tanzania's doctors reacted to the socialist experiment of the 1970s and 1980s, beyond saying that their responses were predictably diverse. In 1982 the mainland had 1,060 doctors, 52 per cent of them officially serving in rural areas (as against 34 per cent in 1972), although since about 85 per cent were based in hospitals, 'rural' must have included many small administrative or trading centres. In 1984 some 72 per cent of doctors were Tanzanians.[58] Doctors surveyed in 1979 said that they worked an average of forty-six hours a week, compared to the average of fifty hours claimed by all health workers, and spent 40 per cent of their time on inpatients, 29 per cent on outpatients, and 19 per cent on administration.[59] A proportion, led by Nhonoli and the Minister of Health during the 1980s, Aaron Chiduo, were committed to the socialist programme. A few even exported it by working in independent Mozambique, notably Saleh Ali Mgawe, who died there after ten years of service, much of it at a hospital on the Beira railway several times attacked by Renamo guerrillas.[60] More doctors probably viewed socialist medicine with ambivalence, respecting its concern for social justice but misliking the sacrifices it claimed to justify. 'The question of service to other human beings was in fact the sole justification for medical training', Vice-President Kawawa had declared.[61] Nyerere was sensitive to the professional costs he imposed on doctors:

> We have to maintain our priority of providing basic care near to the people rather than providing expensive treatment and facilities for the smaller number who suffer from less common diseases. This policy is rational and necessary. But for those who work in our hospitals it is not easy. The doctors of Tanzania, like those elsewhere in the world, are naturally reluctant to see people die in their hospitals when they know the treatment which could cure them but lack the facilities or the modern drugs to do it.[62]

Nyerere was less sensitive, however, to the doctors' material concerns. In 1981 a medical officer's starting salary rose to Shs.2,555 a month, against Shs.1,840 in 1973, but the Dar es Salaam price index had increased by 137 per cent between 1973 and 1976 alone and inflation in the early 1980s approached 30 per cent per year. Further salary increases later in 1981 benefited chiefly the lower-paid medical workers favoured by the government's egalitarianism, which was in reality a levelling down. Doctors protested that their meagre earnings should be compensated by the right to practise privately.[63]

Private practice was a particular point of conflict between doctors and the state, as so often in East Africa. At independence, when doctors were so scarce, Bryceson had proposed to license and tax private practitioners in order to press them out of Dar es Salaam into up-country centres or government service. This had produced a storm of criticism, some claiming that victimised doctors would simply leave, others denouncing 'unpleasantly veiled attempts at total Government domination of the profession'. Even the normally quiescent local branch of the British Medical Association had described the proposal as 'utterly iniquitous'.[64] Bryceson had been obliged to refer the matter to a committee whose report, if any, never became public, but in 1962 government doctors had lost the right to practise privately outside working hours.[65] As the socialist policy took shape, the number of private practitioners in Tanzania fell between 1968 and 1973 from 141 to 73 as foreigners departed, but some senior African doctors resigned from government service to practise privately, notably Mtawali, who bought a small hospital in Dar es Salaam in 1968.[66] When the exodus from government service accelerated during 1975, Nyerere replaced the Minister of Health by Leader Stirling, an austere former mission doctor who was also Tanzania's Chief Scout and had publicly demanded the abolition of private practice.[67] 'What we want to do is to take the profit motive out of people's heads', Stirling explained. 'It is not good that anybody should make private profit out of human suffering.'[68] Stirling found, however, that government could not afford to take over all existing private facilities and operate them without charge. In April 1977 he proposed, therefore, that private clinics and hospitals should be run solely by approved institutions which might employ doctors and charge fees at rates fixed by the state. The proposal aroused unusual opposition in parliament and the press on the grounds that it would merely reduce medical care without improving its quality, to the disadvantage of ordinary people.[69] The Medical Association of Tanzania, which had been reactivated by African doctors in 1975, took the cautious line that 'Government had good reasons for the decision', but warned that government institutions must not become more crowded, scarce funds could be spent better on improving government services, and doctors must not be provoked to leave the country.[70] The grounds for caution appeared in the language employed by the party newspaper:

> A small minority of petty-bourgeois doctors who uphold private ownership of the means of production as against collective ownership have smuggled out of circulation their qualifications and expertise so that they can dance along in private business . . . Such a trade is similar to that of a coffin maker whose festival is an earthquake.

It was because these miscreants neglected their duty, the editor argued, that public health services were so poor.[71]

Stirling's bill passed but proved difficult to implement because only the most efficient private institutions registered and the alternative was to close all the others, many of which proved to be clinics run by paramedics 'covered' by qualified doctors. Eventually, in July 1980, twenty-one private doctors were allowed to continue practice under public or religious institutions, three (including Mtawali) were permitted to continue private practice on account of 'the good services they have rendered over the years', and forty-seven were required to close down, although it was later said that many went underground so that 'even cataract extractions . . . were done in people's homes on kitchen tables'.[72] It appears to have been during the late 1970s that the first Tanzanian African doctors left the country for better conditions elsewhere. The numbers increased during the 1980s, although never on the Ugandan scale.[73]

Control of private practice was virtually Stirling's last political act, for 'the opposition from crypto-capitalists among our minor political leaders was so severe as to cost me my seat in Parliament'.[74] Under his successor, Aaron Chiduo, private dispensaries covertly reappeared and the Ministry had to reregister all practices in 1983 in an attempt to prevent evasion.[75] It continued, however, and in 1986 Philemon Sarungi, as President of the Medical Association of Tanzania, took advantage of Nyerere's recent retirement to urge, amidst applause, that the policy should be reconsidered because it had in practice been fraudulent. A year later the government agreed to reopen the issue.[76]

Chiduo held office throughout the 1980s. The first modern doctor from his Kilosa District, he saw himself not as an innovator but as a technician to implement the *ujamaa* programme which agreed so closely with the community medicine he had learned at Makerere:

> Our ultimate aim is to achieve total coverage of the population, to distribute equitably the basic health services throughout the country and to put more emphasis on preventive programmes. What is required is:
>
> – Courage to define the social goals of health development. This has been effectively done by our political party.
>
> – Courage to break away from conventional methods of delivering health care based on the hospital with its bias on curative services.
>
> – Courage to mobilise the political will to effect the necessary change. Fortunately we have CCM to rely on.[77]

A man of reason and good sense, Chiduo shared with his Kenyan counterpart, Karuga Koinange, an alarm at the decline of the medical profession, which he blamed on poor working conditions and salaries, intellectual laziness, and a lack of leadership from senior doctors.[78] But like Koinange he was frustrated by the continued decline of the economy and public morale, plus in Chiduo's case the underlying impracticability of the *ujamaa* strategy. During the late 1980s Chiduo, as a realist, initiated the reversal of socialist health policy. In 1990 he was held politically responsible for the notorious corruption in his ministry and was replaced, although he was not himself tainted.[79]

The attack on private practice was the most doctrinaire aspect of socialist health policy. The other area of strong political intervention concerned indigenous medicine. As in Kenya and Uganda, most modern Tanzanian doctors treated indigenous medicine with reserve, wishing to appropriate any scientifically proven remedies, often encouraging healers to organise themselves so that they could be controlled and possibly incorporated in a subordinate capacity, but generally showing less enthusiasm than populist politicians like Museveni. The difference in Tanzania was that the politicians were more powerful and that some tried to use indigenous medicine both as an expression of racial pride and as a weapon against the professional claims of modern doctors. The model was China, where, especially during the Great Leap Forward of 1958 and the Cultural Revolution of 1966–76, Reds had compelled Experts to accord indigenous medicine an equal place in hospitals and training centres.[80] Tanzania's first medical delegation to China in 1967 brought back news of this and subsequent exchanges fostered the interest.[81] In 1969 the Ministry instructed Regional Medical Officers to collect material, but they were too busy and the matter was referred instead to the university, which opened a Traditional Medicine Research Unit at Muhimbili in 1974. By 1991 it had identified over 40,000 healers and tested 3,000 herbs.[82] Publications included substantial lists of medicinal plants and interesting but negative studies of treatments for particular complaints,[83] but no practical products, despite annual assurances to parliament of hopeful remedies for diabetes, peptic ulcers, malaria, cancer, asthma, epilepsy, skin diseases, and mental ailments.[84] A study of forty-two Regional or District Medical Officers in 1982 found that most of them favoured research and also, in principle, collaboration with indigenous healers,[85] which in practice mainly took the form of teaching hygiene to traditional birth attendants and incorporating healers into village health programmes in Zanzibar and coastal areas.[86] But the National Union of Indigenous Healers formed in 1971 had to be banned after disputes over money and accusations of 'dabbling in witchcraft',[87] while the study of medical officers found that the collaboration they contemplated 'would not be on an equal footing, with the allopathic [i.e. modern] health workers taking the more domineering position'.[88] In China the Reds eventually lost to the Experts and indigenous medicine passed into conscious decline as a subordinate speciality within a modern system.[89] Moves in that direction could be seen in Tanzania in the early 1990s when Sarungi, as Minister of Health, announced that government would include indigenous healers in the modern health service, urged them to cooperate 'so that their discoveries are scientifically proved harmless to human beings', and told them that government would compile a book of herbs which could legally be administered and would issue each healer with a licence showing which herbs he might prescribe or sell: 'Even if you have 100 types of medicine, if we authorise only two, you will only be allowed to sell the two.'[90] Little more was heard of the policy. Tanzania's abortive cultural revolution did not in the long run enable indigenous medicine to threaten the modern doctors' professional dominance.

By the late 1980s the socialist medical experiment was close to failure. Health facilities had multiplied, as had staff at all levels, but the facilities were often dilapidated and the staff demoralised, chiefly for lack of money in a country whose real Gross National Product per capita had fallen by an average of 0.5 per cent a year between 1965 and 1988.[91] Lack of money explained why poverty-related conditions like malnutrition, malaria, and diarrhoea were those that Tanzania had treated least effectively. Poverty explained why the main complaint against health facilities was lack of drugs, for poverty not only prevented their procurement and distribution but corrupted the medical staff who sold them for their own profit.[92] Corruption was now widespread:

> When we consulted a doctor, he said 'The ink in my pen is finished'; when we asked again he said 'My lamp at home has no kerosene.' We didn't get discouraged but went to another doctor who said 'Do you think the service is free of charge? Do you think it is possible?'[93]

Such neglect was the public's other major grievance. These were the problems that politicians and doctors faced when Nyerere retired from the presidency in 1985.

Medical education and research

The Medical School launched at Muhimbili Hospital in 1963 was integrated into the University College, Dar es Salaam, five years later and upgraded to degree level. Thereafter it began to play the same role in shaping a national medical profession as its counterparts in Kampala and Nairobi.

Since the Medical School was a university faculty but located several kilometres away at the Ministry of Health's chief referral hospital, the relationship between academic and administrative authorities had to be defined. At one point the academics urged construction of a separate teaching hospital, but the ban on hospital building in the 1970s vetoed that.

Instead, in 1977 the whole Muhimbili complex became a parastatal Medical Centre, on the American model, with extensive autonomy and teaching supplied by the Medical Faculty.[94] Nhonoli, who had been Dean of the Medical School since 1969, became also Director of the Medical Centre. After he left in 1981 the two offices were generally divided, with the Dean acting after 1984 as chief academic assistant to the Director-General. During the next seven years the Centre increasingly separated from the university and there was talk of the Medical School becoming a separate University of Health Sciences, but instead it was reconstituted in 1991 as a College of Health Sciences with extensive autonomy within the university.[95]

The socialist health experiment of the early 1970s had little impact on the Medical School's syllabus and teaching, for its aim was already to produce future District Medical Officers rather than urban hospital doctors, and its syllabus provided an integrated course with a strong practical bias, including nearly 20 per cent of study time devoted to community medicine and an additional twenty-two weeks of field work.[96] Nhonoli's appointment as Dean had put control in African hands and his successful personal synthesis of medical science, nationalism, democratic socialism, and Catholicism enabled him to demonstrate that there was no contradiction between professional quality and political commitment:

> We tend to be confused about standards as often standards are equated to systems which is wrong. You can have very high standards in different systems. International prestige and recognition are important, but in my view *not* as important as the relevance of the institution to the problems and conditions in its own country. It should develop its own highest standards under its own system and international prestige and recognition will follow.[97]

This implied, as Nyerere also emphasised, that Africans must have the courage to think for themselves and innovate:

> Medical Schools . . . have produced graduates with a competent capacity to adapt to change, but they have been too conservative and hence the graduates have not been equipped to identify places where the system of Health Delivery itself needs changing in order to produce significant social change. In other words the medical graduates can and have used new knowledge to the benefit of the individual patient but rarely to the direct benefit to society in general.[98]

This made the Medical School an exciting place and its students engaged eagerly in research, publishing it in their own periodical, the *Dar es Salaam Medical Journal*. In one case, twenty-four students immunised 80 per cent of the population of Mafia Island against four major communicable diseases.[99]

Nevertheless, the socialist programme had a profound impact on Muhimbili and the Medical School. Its economic repercussions led to overcrowding, the deterioration of buildings and equipment, and worsening conditions for teaching and research. But the chief impact was on the student body, and not only because policy froze the undergraduate intake at fifty a year. In 1974–5, when Alanagh Raikes surveyed the medical students, they were an elite group selected from a rapidly expanding and state-funded education system.[100] Only 22 per cent had fathers or guardians with secondary education, although the figure for a control group of students in other faculties was even lower, at 10 per cent, and for the student-age population as a whole it was probably less than 1 per cent. Entry to medicine was thus still relatively open, but the high entry qualifications required already favoured those from educationally privileged backgrounds, a point strongly reinforced by the fact that 35 per cent of medical students (and 25 per cent of the control group) came from the most privileged region, Kilimanjaro, which had only 8 per cent of Tanzania's population. Only 34 per cent of medical students were children or wards of farmers, who were 91 per cent of the general population. One-quarter of medical students had a relative who was an indigenous healer, but so did 19 per cent of the control group, while only 8 per cent of medical students said that it had influenced their choice of career, whereas 23 per cent had a parent or close relative who was a modern doctor. Some 42 per cent said medicine was the only career they wanted, 53 per cent that it was one of several they would be happy with, and 5 per cent that they had chosen wrongly. As Raikes commented, 'The importance of a specific course is subordinate to success in gaining access to a profession.' She also found that new medical students made idealistic judgments on issues like the qualities needed in a doctor or the desirability of upgrading sub-professionals, whereas senior students were more conscious of professional distinctions and interests. About half of the students wanted to specialise after graduation, the proportion rising as they neared the end of the course. Raikes concluded:

> The data supports the thesis that the values and attitudes socialised into medical students in the West have been duplicated in Tanzania and that the ambitions of the majority of students by the time they are in their fifth year, are to specialize with a significant number stating that they intend to go into private practice (13%). This is problematic in a situation where the goals of the Faculty are to train students as District Medical Officers to work mainly in rural areas.

Yet these students were the last of their kind. In 1975 TANU abolished direct entry from school to university, required that entrants must first have completed National Service and work experience together totalling three years, and facilitated the entry of mature students.[101] This caused much alarm among academics, for mature students' ability to cope with the medical course declined with the number of years they had been in employment. Between 1975 and 1980 their failure rate rose from 22 to 66 per cent,[102] and although many eventually passed by retaking the examinations, their impact on pass rates and the intellectual quality of the Medical School was disastrous. When only seventeen of the forty-one candidates passed the first part of their final examination in 1983, an enquiry blamed the lack of incentives for teachers, staff shortages, poor teaching, under-qualified students, family distractions, and scarce transport, equipment, housing, and books. Students protested that they learned anatomy with one cadaver for dissection by forty students in a room where those at the back could not see. The decline continued into the early 1990s.[103] Plans to double the annual intake to 100 were frustrated by lack of accommodation and facilities, so that by 1991 the School had produced only about 700 doctors in 28 years.[104] Its most vehement critics were private practitioners, notably Hubert Kairuki, proprietor of Dar es Salaam's main African-owned private hospital, who blamed the academic staff for an outdated syllabus, non-intensive use of existing facilities, and unsympathetic treatment of students, and the government for not providing the Medical School with a proper teaching hospital and for failing to use other referral hospitals for teaching purposes. The Medical Association of Tanzania promptly appointed him to head a committee of enquiry into medical education.[105]

The impact of socialism on medical research is more difficult to assess. Within limits, the Medical School had a research profile distinct from those at Kampala and Nairobi. Research began slowly, technical facilities were limited, and priorities were shaped by political insistence on practicality and relevance, as mediated chiefly through the influence of Nhonoli, who on leaving Muhimbili in 1981 also spent a decade as Chairman of the National Institute of Medical Research. 'As our economic capacity is limited, and the majority of our people live in rural areas where medical facilities are minimal', Nhonoli wrote in 1976, 'it is essential that our research at the moment be heavily weighted in favour of applied research aimed at solving our common problems'.[106] He practised what he preached. As a student he had written a penetrating analysis of infant mortality in his home Nzega district, stressing not 'racial proclivity' but the effects of poor hygiene and environmental stress.[107] As a young doctor he wrote on anthrax, malnutrition, infantile anaemia, and duodenal ulcers – all complaints confronting him as a clinician.[108] His doctoral thesis, presented in 1969, was a study of anaemia, the most common cause of admissions to Muhimbili's medical wards, and the role of hookworm disease in causing it and the resultant cardiovascular complications. 'The principle adopted', he wrote, 'is that both the pilot scheme and the main project to be essentially clinical in approach and not wholly laboratory based. In this way it is hoped that whatever facts are established by this thesis, they will be of practical use here and now.'[109] The interest in helminthic complaints expanded into surveys of rural infections, the effects of malaria in childbirth, the sickle-cell trait, and attempts to define what was physiologically normal in East Africans.[110]

It was this greater concern with common complaints and public health – rather than 'diseases of civilisation' – that gave Tanzania's medical research a special emphasis. Anaemia was a lasting interest.[111] Malaria was a major concern at Muhimbili, especially in the 1980s when the breakdown of control measures led to a rapid increase in the cerebral form, and it became the first priority for the National Institute of Medical Research, whose first Director, Wenseslaus Kilama, was a malaria specialist.[112] Bilharzia, also widespread, was long the chief concern of the Medical Research Centre at Mwanza.[113] Perhaps the most productive researcher at Muhimbili, along with Nhonoli, was Valerian Kimati, a dedicated paediatrician who specialised on measles, malnutrition, and sickle-cell disease before leaving to work for UNICEF.[114] Tanzania's most prolific surgeon, Joseph Shija, was also a paediatrician who established a specialised surgical unit at Muhimbili in 1975 and published extensively on conditions facing paediatric surgeons in tropical environments.[115] Much research was also stimulated by epidemic diseases, notably plague and cholera, which broke out in Muhimbili's overcrowded children's ward three times between 1977 and 1983 and led to important research on its transmission by Fred Mhalu, who also specialised on venereal diseases.[116]

This concern with common diseases and relatively simple technology was not uncontested. Nhonoli's work had in part concerned cardiovascular complaints,[117] but the leading specialist in that field was his successor as Dean of the Medical School, William Makene, a Makerere graduate who had worked at Harvard, published on hypertension and cardiac conditions,[118] established a cardiac clinic at Muhimbili, and criticised exclusive concentration on primary health care:

> As a contrast to the rapid [medical] advances of the affluent West, we are behind by centuries . . . There is an all-prevailing malaise and lethargy in the development of our health care facilities. The reasons for this are not far to seek – we have our priorities, we are a developing country and much of our time and money has to be spent in combating our health care priorities. I do not deny this but there is also another reason for our lethargy. It was Oscar Wilde who said 'nothing succeeds like excess'. The more often you repeat a thing, the more likely it is to be believed. This is exactly what some of the pundits have done . . . They have repeatedly pronounced loudly that we in the developing countries should look to our health care priorities, to the exclusion and detriment of all else. Some of our health administrators have turned a deaf ear to our pleadings for improved health facilities, especially in areas of curative medicine which are in urgent need of development.
>
> Ladies and gentlemen, it is time we physicians stood up with our demands to

improve the services in our teaching hospitals, we cannot lie idle. This is the time for action. Let not the future doctors blame us for neglecting our duties to our community.[119]

In 1984 Makene established a Tanzania Heart Foundation which sought overseas funds to build an open-heart surgery unit at Muhimbili. Kidney transplants were also contemplated hesitantly in the early 1990s. There had been somewhat more success with cancer treatment, thanks to the establishment in 1980 of a Tanzania Tumour Centre, largely with financial aid from German sources anxious to collaborate in research on African viral cancer.[120] But the main weight of Tanzanian research was on communicable and environmental diseases.

The new course, 1985–97

Nyerere's retirement as president in 1985 removed the chief obstacle to liberalisation of the mainland economy. A structural adjustment agreement with the International Monetary Fund was signed in August 1986.[121] Zanzibar's economy was in severe decline at that time owing to a dramatic collapse of clove prices and output, so that health expenditure there, which had held up well during the 1970s, was severely curtailed.[122] On the mainland, GDP grew between 1985 and 1989 at 3.9 per cent a year, barely 1.0 per cent faster than population and sufficient to permit only gradual change in the health system.[123] In 1986 Sarungi, as President of the Medical Association of Tanzania, called on the government to re-examine the 'non-economic' and 'impractical' ban on private practice, but there was opposition to change within the party and bureaucracy, so that although private practice resumed in Zanzibar in the late 1980s, on the mainland it was not until late in 1991 that the Prime Minister promised to repeal the ban, which he described as 'out of tune with the current situation in the country'.[124] Cost-sharing was also pressed on the government during 1988 by the World Bank and was briefly accepted, but it was abandoned without being introduced, probably owing to opposition from Nyerere and his committed socialist supporters.[125]

The change of policy in 1991 followed Sarungi's appointment as Minister of Health. He promptly expressed disgust at the condition of government hospitals and ordered a nationwide cleanliness competition. He also denounced the corruption pervading the health system.[126] Professional ethics had suffered during the 1980s, when doctors had been implicated in assisting or concealing the torture of suspects and the Medical Council had heard highly publicised charges of negligence, drunkenness, and misconduct.[127] Doctors' morale was low. In 1991 Hubert Kairuki claimed that some 200 Tanzanian doctors were working abroad. Zanzibar too was losing doctors at an alarming rate.[128] On the mainland a commission in 1988 made a new attempt to meet financial grievances by proposing a special salary scale for 'rare professions', headed by doctors, and a number of new allowances were promised to mainland doctors during 1990 and to Zanzibari doctors during 1991.[129]

These grievances, and piecemeal attempts to resolve them, lay behind a series of strikes and stoppages which dislocated several Tanzanian hospitals between 1990 and 1992. They culminated on 22 January 1992 when some sixty members of the Junior Doctors Association at Muhimbili struck over allowances and the transfer of four of their leaders to up-country posts, which the Centre's Director insisted was routine staff deployment. Threatened with dismissal by the hospital trustees and denounced by senior colleagues for breach of ethics, the striking doctors won the support of university students and tried to extend their action to other hospitals. On 28 January they were dismissed and three days later the paramilitary Field Force Unit evicted them very roughly from staff housing in defiance of a court order. This immediately restored public sympathy. Senior Muhimbili staff and the trade union organisation expressed support, while several hundred hospital workers and students marched to the Prime Minister's Office, where negotiations ended with the reinstatement of those dismissed, an inquiry into the situation at Muhimbili, a return to work, and eventually the conviction of the Hospital Director for disobeying a court order.[130]

The sequence of strikes probably damaged Sarungi's position – he was replaced in October 1992 – but it accelerated change within the health system. During the early 1990s privatisation became a central element in mainland health policy, as in other fields. Restrictions on private practice were removed in 1992.[131] Clinics run by doctors or less qualified proprietors appeared first in major towns. In 1995 Dar es Salaam had some 300 private clinics and hospitals, plus pharmacies and drug sellers; taken together, they were used nearly twice as often as government facilities. By the mid-1990s private clinics were also appearing in villages.[132] Government hoped initially to separate official employment from private practice, but in reality government doctors continued to practise part-time at private institutions and the government decided in 1997 to sanction this, barring them only from owning hospitals.[133] In the early 1990s certain private institutions in Dar es Salaam like Hubert Kairuki's Mission Mikocheni Hospital began to approach their counterparts in Nairobi in scale and sophistication of facilities, although fees were said to be lower in Dar es Salaam. An Association of Private Hospitals was established in 1994.[134]

Another aspect of liberalisation, cost-sharing, remained controversial. Zanzibar rejected it until 1997,[135] but on the mainland it was introduced in

1993, under strong external pressure, after studies had suggested that 'free' services were equally expensive to patients and that people were prepared to pay fees provided services improved. Collecting institutions were meant to keep most fees and use them to improve facilities. The system did not apply to the primary care level.[136] It was initially unpopular in many quarters, sufficiently for the opposition in the 1995 election to promise to abolish it, but that may well have been impracticable.[137]

With privatisation went indications that doctors were gaining a degree of power within the health system which they had not previously enjoyed. The post of Chief Medical Officer was recreated within the Ministry in 1986. Legislation was planned to free the Medical Council from ministerial control. The new allowances introduced in the early 1990s made Tanzanian doctors distinctly better rewarded than those in Uganda and were partly blamed by the Minister of Finance for causing serious budgetary overspending.[138] The levelling down of the socialist years was reversed in favour of 'rare professions', among others. Perhaps, too, the number of Tanzanian doctors – probably about 1,000, although figures varied[139] – was sufficient to give the profession a substantial collective influence, especially because most shared experience at a single medical school, much as former medical students at the University of Nairobi had begun to exercise a collective influence in Kenya in the early 1980s. Yet Tanzania in 1997 did not yet have a new medical system. The country was littered with the debris of past systems, with the remains of socialism lying thick and the surface patches of private practice still spreading. As in Uganda, medicine had begun to follow the Kenyan path. But it had only begun.

10 AIDS

The AIDS epidemic of the 1980s and 1990s gave East Africa's doctors and their history a global significance. It was they who first recognised AIDS in the region and, with expatriate collaborators, chiefly uncovered the epidemiology of the disease when transmitted by heterosexual contact, as it was to be in most of the world. This epidemiological research drew on a tradition established at Makerere in the 1940s, while the inability of East Africans to contribute significantly to basic research into the microbiology of AIDS, for lack of specialised equipment and skills, echoed Trowell's frustration that he could never take a problem beyond a certain point. Further, East Africa's doctors were largely responsible for devising national AIDS control programmes which became the models for other regions of heterosexual transmission. In formulating these programmes, doctors were hindered by the dilapidated condition of national health systems as a result of the weakening of economies and states. Different patterns of medical evolution also to some extent distinguished Kenyan policies from those in Uganda and Tanzania. But control programmes were shaped also by the combination of rationalism and nationalism which was the doctors' distinctive intellectual inheritance and their contribution to the compassion with which East Africans generally met the calamity. Finally, modern doctors bore the chief responsibility for the care of AIDS patients. They did not bear the chief burden, for the doctors' role, as it had evolved during the previous century, had given them a much-criticised detachment and consultant status which left most hands-on care to other medical workers and especially to patients' families. But it fell to the doctors to plan, to diagnose, and to prescribe. The task was awesome and their responses to it ranged from devotion to charlatanism. Their inability to cure AIDS weakened the claims of their medicine and strengthened the challenge of alternative therapies. But their common responsibility perhaps reinforced the cohesion of a profession which was otherwise fragmenting. And if the expansion of AIDS could be slowed and a vaccine developed to prevent it – both conceivable in the later 1990s – then modern medicine and its practitioners would gain immeasurably in prestige.

The coming of AIDS

Anthony Lwegaba had recently arrived as the first District Medical Officer in Rakai District, a backwater on Uganda's south-western border with Tanzania, when, in mid-1984, he observed a local epidemic which turned his mind to what he had read or heard about AIDS. Some months later, in November 1984, 'with little *analysis* and *hypathesis* [sic] formation', he reported his findings to the Ministry.[1] Local people called the epidemic 'Slim' because it was a wasting disease. Lwegaba's enquiries suggested that it had caught local attention early in 1982. 'In late 1983 and much of 1984, the patients seeking treatment in Kyotera town with complaints of "slim" increased tremendously so were those claimed to have died of the same.' Most victims were young adult males engaged in trade along the lakeshore with Tanzania, often in insanitary conditions: 'poor food handling, poor dwellings and improper waste disposal'. The first symptoms experienced by victims of the disease were general malaise and sporadic fever, which they usually treated with self-medication. After six months they began to suffer periodic diarrhoea and lose weight and colour. At this stage they generally consulted indigenous healers, 'as the disease to many is attributed to witchcraft'. Thereafter the patient developed an ugly and irritating skin rash and a dry cough. 'Earlier on or after a year, the patient may be so weak that even when taken to hospital (not much can be done due to late reporting), goes into chronicity and death.' Transmission to family members seemed to be rare: 'it appears to be "one-person-disease"', unless the incubation period was long. Some patients recovered, but no cure was known and sufferers 'may be isolated or forbidden from the public places'. Lwegaba then made his only reference to AIDS (in his own words):

What is the possible mode of transmission of slim?

The insanitary and behavioural conditions prevailing at the lake-landing sites would among other diseases favour the transmission of diseases which are well known: (a) water/food borne disease – diarrheal diseases, enteric fevers (typhoid etc); (b) contact diseases/air borne – poor housing; respiratory diseases, t.b. inclusive and skin diseases: (c) poor waste disposal – as in (a) worms, etc. (d) sexually transmitted diseases (STD) occur in abundance. Syphilis can and does cause varied forms skin disease. The currently feared AIDS may not be new in Africa. Some authorities think that it originated from Africa. (Acquired immune deficiency syndrome is known to be sexually transmitted and parentally by blood transfusions etc. It appears that a virus similar to Hep[atitis] B is involved. Characteristically there is fever, hympoodemopothy and wasting.

It is known to be complicated by Pneumocyctis pneumonia and Kaporas sarcoma.

In all these malaria fever wouldn't be an exception. All these are contagious and would be expected to spread beyond those visiting the lake landing sites. Therefore they are probably not true causes of 'slim'. But in view of the fact that all long standing diseases enevitably cause wasting or 'body weight loss' a cardinal sign in 'slim', then 'slim' might not be one disease, but a collection of diseases.

Thus Lwegaba did not suggest that Slim was AIDS or a symptom of AIDS, but that it was a wasting disease which might have multiple causes of which AIDS might be one. Cases of Slim had been observed in southwestern Uganda since at least 1982,[2] when Kitovu Hospital is said to have recorded eighty-four,[3] but reports to the Ministry of Health were later said to have been discounted, 'thinking that the disease would go away since it would not yield to any medicine',[4] probably more because the Ministry was in disorder than from any deliberate attempt at concealment. AIDS had probably existed as a rare disease in equatorial Africa by 1959 and perhaps for some decades before that,[5] but because it had no distinctive symptoms (since it attacked the immune system and allowed other diseases to penetrate) and the technology needed to recognise its causative agent (a retrovirus) did not exist until 1978, there was no way of recognising it as a disease.[6] In 1982 physicians at Mulago noted cases with the diarrhoea, wasting, and other symptoms characteristic of Slim. Later they observed young men with aggressive Kaposi's sarcoma, a cancer hitherto thought to be slow-acting and found in elderly men, but now gaining notoriety as a common symptom of AIDS in young homosexual men in America.[7] Indeed, the first speculation that AIDS might be present in Uganda probably came from the cancer expert, Charles Olweny, who published it in 1984 as a possible implication of the prevalence of Kaposi's sarcoma.[8]

Meanwhile, the isolation of the AIDS virus (HIV-1) in 1983 made blood testing possible.[9] When Wilson Carswell, an expatriate surgeon, was alerted to the cases of Kaposi's sarcoma at Mulago in 1984, he sent blood samples for testing in Britain. In October 1984 he learned that they showed HTLV-3 (as the HIV-1 virus was then known).[10] A month later Lwegaba's report arrived from Rakai, and this time it was not ignored. On Obote's instructions, a research team visited Masaka and Rakai. In addition to Carswell and two other expatriates, it included three Ugandan doctors from Mulago who took leading parts in subsequent research and policy formulation: David Serwadda, a family-planning expert then working at the Cancer Institute; Nelson Sewankambo, who had specialised in cardiology; and Roy Mugerwa, also a cardiologist. The team took blood samples showing that most patients with Slim also had HTLV-3, which the researchers believed was probably transmitted mainly by sexual contact and perhaps exacerbated by poor hygiene. But they thought that the chief symptoms of Slim, 'extreme weight loss and diarrhoea', distinguished it from AIDS as then known in the United States,[11] so they concluded that it was 'a manifestation of enteropathic AIDS'. Early in 1986 Carswell, Mugerwa,

Sewankambo, and two others, now known as the Clinical Committee on AIDS, published the view 'that both Slim and atypical Kaposi's sarcoma are part of the spectrum of the Acquired Immunodefiency Syndrome (AIDS) which is caused by the HTLV-III virus'. They added that it was spreading at frightening pace, with seropositivity rates in the general population already about 10 per cent. Their finding that married couples were often both infected suggested that heterosexual contact was the chief means of transmission. Data from Mulago also indicated that AIDS patients had on average been more promiscuous than others. Blood transfusion was a major risk and the Clinical Committee were alarmed that Mulago might be infecting many patients by this means. They recommended public education against promiscuity, blood screening, avoiding the use of contaminated needles, but no discrimination against infected patients or health workers.[12]

Uganda in 1985 was in the midst of civil war. News of AIDS did not reach the press until Obote was overthrown, when the *Weekly Topic* reappeared and publicised it during September 1985.[13] Two months later the Undersecretary in the Ministry of Health visited Mulago and was briefed on the extent of the disease there. Instructions to prepare a Cabinet paper on the subject with plans to seek donor assistance were directed to Samuel Okware, the Ministry's epidemiologist and expert on international negotiations.[14] Politics now intervened again when Museveni's National Resistance Army took Kampala in January 1986, but the new Minister of Health, Ruhakana-Rugunda, almost immediately grasped the danger, appointed Okware to head an AIDS Surveillance Sub-Committee (including Mugerwa and Carswell), and told the press of his anxiety.[15] By September 1986, when the Sub-Committee had begun to organise public education, the supply of protective condoms, and the screening of blood donors, Museveni's personal concern had been aroused, apparently by a visit to Rakai,[16] and he met the Sub-Committee to discuss strategy. It was decided to adopt a policy of openness, to stress 'zero-grazing' (i.e. faithfulness to one sexual partner), and to accelerate blood-testing.[17] A month later Okware was appointed Chairman of a National Committee for the Prevention of AIDS to formulate and implement a national programme.[18] Incisive, objective, but with a strong nationalist sensitivity, Okware became the most important figure in the formulation of AIDS strategy in East Africa. 'It all started as a rumour', he later reflected. 'Then we found we were dealing with a disease. Then we realised it was an epidemic. And, now we have accepted it as a tragedy.'[19]

In the meantime the authorities in Tanzania and Kenya also became aware of AIDS. Villagers in the Kagera Region of north-western Tanzania, bordering Rakai, first noticed the wasting disease in 1982. Two years later they reported it to the government. By then three cases had been observed but not recognised at a local hospital.[20] It was not until October 1984 that doctors at Bukoba Regional Hospital became aware of the syndrome and not until one of their patients died after transfer to Muhimbili in March 1985 that AIDS was diagnosed serologically.[21] Three months later the Ministry sent an investigation team to Kagera. In January 1986 the government announced a national AIDS survey and a three-year programme, chiefly educative.[22] Zanzibar's first cases were reported in 1986 and a task force was appointed to contain the disease.[23] In Kenya, Jack Githae later claimed to have been approached during 1982 by patients suspecting they had contracted AIDS, but the first certain case, a Ugandan, was identified in 1983 and described in 1984 by Arthur Obel of the Nairobi Medical School.[24] Newspaper reports began in January 1985 and became urgent in September when the Nairobi *Weekly Review* quoted a rumour that over half the city's prostitutes were infected. In response to press and parliamentary pressure, the government appointed a National AIDS Committee late in 1985 to draft guidelines for professionals and the public.[25]

All three governments had to decide whether and how to control investigation and discussion of the epidemic. At first much reporting was ill-founded and offensive to national sensitivities. One foreign-led research group in Kenya, using faulty reagents, reported in 1985 that over half the pastoral Turkana people were infected with HIV. Another, in Uganda, claimed that frozen blood from West Nile showed 67 per cent seropositivity in the early 1970s, which Carswell, Sewankambo, and others refuted.[26] Claims that AIDS originated in Africa, however probable, could not be proved and were bitterly resented. At WHO meetings, so Okware claimed in 1989, 'We managed to out-argue the theories about the Monkey origin and no scientist now talks about the Africa origin of AIDS these days.' He also denied that Africans were exceptionally promiscuous, as was widely alleged, and he insisted that the weakening of traditional values allowed the epidemic to spread.[27] Others went further to claim that AIDS was a Western disease or even a form of germ warfare.[28] Foreign research was resented, especially where, as in Kenya, much consisted initially of testing prostitutes for seropositivity. As Vincent Orinda wrote in *Medicus*, 'We wonder why we should allow "Corridor experts" to sneak around our streets and wards and publish whatever they lay their hands on.'[29] Research was in fact controlled in all three countries, but expatriates were not banned, partly because their money and equipment were needed, partly because sensible African doctors recognised the value of good research. When Western newspapers garbled the first findings and reported in 1985 that 10 or 20 per cent of all Kenyans had AIDS, the government suspected a 'hate campaign' to destroy the tourist industry and thereafter Kenya remained more secretive than the other regimes, probably thereby permitting the disease to spread more quickly.[30] Uganda's leaders, too, resented sensationalisation of the information they released, but they remained relatively frank, for against national sensitivities had to be set the fact that, as the Permanent Secretary to the Ministry of Health explained, 'in the absence of any known drugs or vaccines, Education – public education – . . . is still the only method open to the world in the effort to combat the dreaded disease'.[31] There were limits to openness. Okware banned his staff from speaking to the press. Carswell was deported in February 1987, officially for an unguarded remark to a journalist, but perhaps also because he occupied too pivotal a place for an expatriate. The task, as Okware put it, was to 'give approved inoquous [sic] information in a most pro-Uganda, Pro-Africa profile'.[32] Yet Okware did not allow his nationalist sensitivities to interfere with serious policy decisions, not did Tanzanian decision-makers like Chiduo and Sarungi, who kept their heads when many others were losing theirs amid a crisis which might have bred appalling irrationality and cruelty. That it did not, anywhere in East Africa, was perhaps the greatest debt that the region owed to its doctors.

Research

East Africa's first major contribution to the global campaign against AIDS was to take a large role in uncovering its epidemiology in a region of largely heterosexual transmission, given that previous research in America and Europe had concentrated on homosexual transmission. Epidemiology was a field in which East African doctors had a long research tradition. Each country made a distinctive contribution to the research.

In Uganda, once it had been confirmed that Slim was in fact a local manifestation of AIDS, research initially focused on three issues. One was to investigate the clinical aspects of the disease and especially to identify other opportunistic infections, notably aggressive Kaposi's sarcoma and tuberculosis.[33] A second was to demonstrate that heterosexual contact was the chief means of transmission by studying the household contacts of twenty-three AIDS patients, which showed that of the twelve contacts with HIV, ten were sexual partners, implying that other possible means of transmission – by chance contact, non-sexual secretions, insect bites, and the like – were at most of secondary importance.[34] Thirdly, Carswell began to identify high-risk groups, finding 68 per cent seroprevalence in barmaids and 32 per cent in long-distance drivers and turnboys, which suggested social mechanisms of transmission.[35] Taken together, these findings located AIDS as a sexually transmitted disease and indicated the two main directions which further research must follow.

One was to gain a detailed understanding of the epidemiology, which was the work chiefly of two teams working in south-western Uganda. One, which began work in Rakai District in 1988, grew out of the original research team headed by Serwadda and Sewankambo, with a medical sociologist, Joseph Konde-Lule, and finance and participation from Columbia University. A longitudinal study continuing into the early 1990s, it aimed 'at determining an average incubation period of the disease, its progression and the social behaviour that cause the increase or decrease in AIDS incidence, as well as risk factors'.[36] After much initial suspicion and political difficulty, the team reported in 1989 that the chief risk of infection was to have multiple sexual partners, and that this risk was highest in main road trading settlements (where 26 per cent of adult men and 47 per cent of adult women were HIV positive), less in small trading villages (22 and 29 per cent respectively), and least in agricultural villages (8 and 9 per cent).[37] Subsequent study showed that transmission to the countryside was chiefly by male villagers with sexual partners in trading centres, that young adults were especially at risk, that both infection and risky sexual behaviour initially increased despite the team's education programme, and that by 1991 AIDS was responsible for 52 per cent of adult mortality in the district.[38] The second epidemiological team started work in 1989 in fifteen villages of the neighbouring Masaka District, continued its work deep into the 1990s, and became the most elaborate programme of its kind in the world. Organised jointly by the British Medical Research Council and the Uganda Virus Research Institute, it was led by senior expatriates and trained a number of Ugandan researchers. Its broad findings confirmed those of the Rakai team, but it examined additional issues, including sexual mixing patterns between town and country and the prevalence of other sexually transmitted diseases. The team found that seroprevalence did not correlate with education but with personal mobility, that urban–rural transmission was less rapid than had been thought, that HIV was especially common among those with genital ulcers, and that the progression from HIV infection to death was very rapid.[39]

Alongside these epidemiological studies went sociological research on knowledge, attitudes, and practices. The pioneer was Joseph Konde-Lule, who, having written a public health thesis demonstrating the continuing prevalence of syphilis and the lack of public understanding of the disease,[40] transferred his techniques in 1987 to study AIDS in the Kasangati area outside Kampala. He found that public education was reaching villagers, but that many false ideas (e.g. that AIDS was due to insect bites, witchcraft, or casual contact) also prevailed, as did stigmatisation of sufferers, and that there had as yet been little change of behaviour. Returning to the area five years later, he found much less casual sex, not much more use of condoms, and huge economic consequences for the community.[41] Between these two studies, Konde-Lule worked with the Rakai team, where he found higher levels of AIDS awareness, little interest in knowing whether one had the disease, reduced promiscuity, a growing but still limited use of condoms, and generally compassionate attitudes to AIDS sufferers.[42] Summarising his findings, Konde-Lule wrote an explanation of the epidemic, as due to the impact of urbanisation on a distinctive sexual system, which was coloured by Ganda conservatism but was perhaps the most thoughtful African analysis yet proposed:

> It is fairly evident that while sexual mobility appears to have increased with urbanization, it is not a new phenomenon in the African cultures. It was, however, traditionally practised with a lot of discretion and within some accepted norms for each culture. Urbanization has combined with the influence of Western civilization to bring to an end the habit of sexual networking within the extended family circles but has promoted commercial sex and prostitution, previously unknown in rural Africa.[43]

A similar programme of sociological research was part of the Masaka project but focused especially on coping mechanisms and the impact of AIDS on families and orphans.[44]

Whereas Ugandan research on AIDS concentrated on extensive rural surveys, Kenyan research focused to an extraordinary extent on Nairobi and the high-risk groups among its population. The continuity of research from STDs to AIDS, seen in Konde-Lule's work, was especially clear here. The University's Department of Medical Microbiology was a WHO Collaborating Centre for Research and Training in STDs. Its professor, Herbert Nsanze, a refugee from Makerere, had studied STDs there in the 1970s and was engaged during the early 1980s in research into drug regimens for chancroid, a form of genital ulceration.[45] Together, it appears, with other members of the department – notably Frank Plummer, a Canadian, and Jackoniah Ndinya-Achola – he launched in 1985 an investigation into STDs among prostitutes in the Pumwani red-light district, in collaboration with expatriate researchers and Elizabeth Ngugi, the Deputy Chief Nursing Officer in the Ministry of Health with much experience of Pumwani and STD work. They were astonished to find that over 60 per cent of the women tested had HIV.[46] The finding gave a crucial direction to AIDS research and prevention, demonstrating that in Africa, as in America, 'identifying core groups . . . is key to STD/HIV control'.[47] While Ngugi organised a remarkably successful programme to popularise condoms among Nairobi's prostitutes, further research suggested that risk of HIV infection was especially high among those suffering genital ulcers and among uncircumcised men and their partners. As Plummer told a journalist, 'We're doing the best work in Africa, bar none.'[48] During the

1990s their focus on other STDs as the best short-term technique to combat heterosexual AIDS became the new orthodoxy, especially when advanced further by work in Tanzania.

In Dar es Salaam, as in Nairobi, AIDS research grew out of work on other STDs. In April 1984, before the new epidemic was perceived, doctors at Muhimbili opened a referral clinic for STDs, reporting that 47 per cent of their initial patients had genital ulcers.[49] One of the researchers, Fred Mhalu, was a Makerere-trained microbiologist specialising in the control of communicable diseases, and it was he who became Tanzania's leading authority on AIDS. During 1986 the Dar es Salaam group found high HIV seroprevalence among the city's barmaids, whom they continued to study as a reference group, and especially among the general population in Kagera Region, where Mhalu participated in 1987 in a team led by Japhet Killewo of Muhimbili which revealed a pattern of transmission similar to that in Rakai and Masaka.[50] Given Kagera's long reputation for STDs and the export of prostitutes (which Mtawali had studied in the 1950s) the doctors quickly concluded, as Mhalu put it, 'that areas of the country which have had a big problem with sexually transmitted diseases . . . are also emerging as HIV problem areas'.[51] At a time of wild schemes – a seminar in Dar es Salaam in 1986 advocated the sterilisation of AIDS sufferers and Mhalu himself was despatched to Congo to investigate a local miracle drug – Mhalu advocated scientific caution.[52] 'Effective therapy', he wrote in 1991, 'is most likely going to emerge from utilisation of good scientific approaches resulting from knowledge of the molecular biology and biochemistry of the HIV. Haphazard clinical trials using remedies without scientific bases are of doubtful value.'[53] He was also quick to see that the prevalence of other STDs in sub-Saharan Africa was both a major reason for the heterosexual HIV epidemic and an important way to counter it.[54]

Tanzania's two initial foci of AIDS, Dar es Salaam and Kagera, were a thousand kilometres apart. That dispersal continued to characterise both the epidemic and research into it. Contributions came especially from the new referral hospitals at Moshi and Mwanza, both as research centres and as collaborators in larger projects with external participants and, in Mwanza, with the National Institute for Medical Research. The epidemiological pattern in both areas was much like that in Kagera, with infection spreading outwards from high-risk urban groups via main roads and trading centres to the countryside.[55] In Mwanza, however, an epidemiological survey in twelve matched communities was followed by treatment of STDs in six of them, resulting in a 42 per cent lower seroprevalence of HIV.[56] This was the first successful HIV intervention with a general population. It was widely interpreted as the most effective control technique yet discovered for Third World populations and similar programmes were formulated for other parts of East Africa.[57] Ironically, however, the public often saw other STDs as shameful symptoms of AIDS, rather than causes, and were deterred from seeking treatment for STDs by the fear of learning that they had AIDS.[58]

Almost all this research fell into the Makerere tradition of epidemiology. It was essential work, but by the late 1980s and early 1990s its findings often seemed predictable. Peasants in Kagera Region told one team, 'We want help not more research.' Of 1,382 long-distance drivers approached by interviewers outside Mombasa in 1991–2, 1,099 refused to respond, some complaining that 'they had been screened earlier on in other studies but nothing useful was done about their results'. Donors, too, grew impatient with AIDS studies.[59] In fact their value was soon to be demonstrated, for in 1994 they suggested that the expansion of the epidemic was slowing in the worst-affected areas.[60] Nevertheless, East African research was almost entirely epidemiological and contributed little to fundamental study of AIDS or its treatment. There was research on the course of the disease, its opportunistic infections, and its effects on other conditions such as pregnancy, but East Africans lacked the equipment and, often, the skills for more fundamental work. 'Uganda's contribution to the pool of AIDS information is negligible', a specialist complained in 1988, adding that without an electron microscope the staff of the Virus Institute could not even see a virus.[61]

This constraint appears to have rankled especially at KEMRI, the most ambitious and best-equipped institution in the region with a determination that East Africans should contribute actively to international science. Its director, Davy Koech, participated in the early research on AIDS among Nairobi prostitutes. In 1988 he was joined at KEMRI, as Chief Research Officer, by Arthur Obel, an experienced physician who had identified Kenya's first AIDS case and treated many AIDS patients. KEMRI began to test an interferon drug apparently developed in America but denied approval for testing against AIDS there. KEMRI's only contribution seems to have been to reduce the drug's normal concentration,[62] but at KEMRI's tenth anniversary celebration in December 1989 Koech announced the discovery of a drug – later christened Kemron – which did not cure AIDS but 'successfully reverses all the signs and symptoms of aids within a matter of days'.[63] In their results published in July 1990, Koech and Obel claimed that eight of their forty HIV-positive patients treated with Kemron were seroconverted and another twenty-nine experienced substantial reduction of symptoms, although the mechanism was not yet understood.[64] Welcoming 'a miracle drug against AIDS – at last!' Nairobi's respected *Weekly Review* hailed it as potentially 'a triumph which will signal that African science has finally come of age'.[65] *Medicus* was equally excited – 'At this rate, a cure can't be far off' – and dismissed Western scepticism as predictable: 'To them nothing good ever comes from the third world except raw and cheap resources.'[66] Even the sober *East African Medical Journal* rejoiced.[67] 'We wanted to believe so much that Africans, and Kenyans, in particular, too, could be counted amongst the best in medical and scientific research', the *Weekly Review* later recalled.[68] Tanzania's Ministry of Health, under pressure, hoped that Kemron might be on sale in the country by the end of 1990, while Uganda undertook to test the new drug. In July 1990 President Moi launched the product with much publicity.[69] By then, however, the American origin of the drug was becoming clear. Mhalu expressed scepticism. In October Kenya's DMS said KEMRI had merely tested the drug, which needed further trials. By December the *Weekly Review* was calling it 'the year's biggest let-down'.[70] Despite this, many desperate patients apparently spent large sums on it. Trials at Makerere and elsewhere found Kemron ineffective,[71] but Koech remained defiant. 'History is yet to vindicate these investigators', he wrote in 1994.[72] Obel, by contrast, had resigned from KEMRI in January 1991.[73]

Yet that was not the end of Professor Obel. Early in 1996 he announced a new drug, Pearl Omega, claimed to have seroconverted seven patients.[74] This time the press, led by the *Weekly Review* in an article headed 'Preying on a Holocaust',[75] was almost unanimous in its denunciation, dissent coming chiefly from a periodical, apparently in sympathy with the group around KEMRI, which argued, 'In Africa those inflexibly concerned about nineteenth or twentieth century procedures or protocols will simply keep the continent waiting to consume products manufactured elsewhere . . . The upheaval caused by professor Obel's Pearl Omega is at least a sign that Africans are also trying to do something about HIV and not just waiting for others to move or innovate.'[76] The drug was said to be selling at Shs.30,000 or even Shs.150,000 for a course of treatment, but this time the medical establishment was determined to assert itself. Challenged by the Dean of the Medical School to defend his claims in public, Obel described Pearl Omega as a protease inhibitor, a type of drug then under investigation in many quarters as a remedy for AIDS. He also claimed to be Chief Government Scientist in the Office of the President, where he had enjoyed the patronage of the former Head of the Civil Service.[77] Unconvinced, the Health Minister disowned the drug, the Pharmacy and Poisons Board banned it, and the Society of People With AIDS in Kenya announced that it was suing Obel.[78]

Control

Once AIDS had been identified and national committees appointed in 1985–6, all three East African countries (and Zanzibar) formulated national AIDS control programmes during 1987 in collaboration with the WHO, the recognised international coordinating body. Uganda's programme, the world's first, was presented to a donors' conference in Kampala in May 1987 and provided for a thirty-six-member National Council for the Prevention of AIDS (including Okware as Chairman, Lwegaba, Carswell, Sewankambo, Serwadda, Mugerwa, and Konde-Lule) with an executive organ, the AIDS Control Programme (ACP), also headed by Okware, based in the Ministry of Health and with a staff (by 1989) of nearly eighty. At the donors' conference, Okware listed seven main activities for the ACP: health education, blood screening, rehabilitating blood transfusion services, surveillance of infection, distribution of condoms, research, and patient care. The scheme won wide praise and became a model for national programmes not only in Africa but as far away as Thailand, the Yemen, and the Solomon Islands. It also persuaded donors to pledge $21,676,000 in support for the first five years, which was more than Uganda had asked. The funds were channelled through the WHO, with which the ACP established a profitable working alliance.[79] The Tanzanian programme was drawn up with Okware's aid and was presented to a conference two months later; it called for $13,810,000 over five years and, after some delay, received the necessary pledges.[80] Kenya's National AIDS Control Programme, also launched in 1987, was on paper almost identical.[81]

Of the seven activities listed by Okware, the stress on health education, with the open public discussion of AIDS which it implied, won special praise, for it was seen as the only weapon yet available against the epidemic. The ACP organised an elaborate programme of seminars and training courses, introduced AIDS education into school science syllabuses from the upper primary level onwards (with an AIDS knowledge test in the examinations), and encouraged leaders from Museveni downwards to propagate 'zero-grazing'. As Okware told a conference in 1993, 'We have demystified AIDS and given it a face.'[82] Tanzania's approach was largely open, although religious and conservative opposition prevented the introduction of AIDS education in schools. By 1990 knowledge of the disease had spread rapidly there, but, as in Uganda, consequent changes in behaviour were not observed until the 1990s.[83] Perhaps because party politics were more contentious in Kenya and Christian involvement in them especially strong, its approach, after an initial phase of openness, was more reticent, with President Moi remaining virtually silent on the issue, but much education nevertheless took place through the media, schools, and seminars, although again without much immediate impact on behaviour.[84] Condom promotion, an element in Okware's programme, was especially contentious because it offended both the religious and the conservative. Tanzania distributed them through the health system but met much opposition, Kenya preferred to make them available through its family planning programme, while Museveni's doubts about the wisdom of government provision ensured that this aspect of Uganda's programme was confused. Cultural resistance was in any case very strong: in 1993 only 3 per cent of Ugandan men regularly used condoms, despite millions of dollars spent on promotion.[85]

The screening of blood before transfusion was one of the most urgent priorities. The first ELISA machines for the purpose arrived in 1986, but they were expensive. By January 1988 Uganda had fourteen screening centres, but most of its hospitals were still transfusing unscreened blood. Tanzania, similarly, could only slowly supply its hospitals; fifteen had blood-screening equipment by December 1988 but they included only one in the worst-affected Kagera Region. By 1992, however, about 80 per cent of transfused blood was screened. Kenya had equipped thirty-eight of its forty-one district hospitals by mid-1989.[86] Sentinel surveillance sites to monitor seroprevalence levels at antenatal clinics and blood-donor centres were established in Uganda during 1989 and at much the same time in the other countries. By 1993 Uganda had eighteen.[87]

The chief, although understandable, weakness of these early control programmes was that they concentrated almost entirely on checking the spread of AIDS but made little provision for the care of those who already had it or of widows and orphans. With necessary ruthlessness, Uganda's ACP ruled in 1987, 'As soon as possible the AIDS patient should be referred to outpatient care, preferably in the extended family setting.' 'Counselling is a must, but there is as yet no manpower', the National Committee observed later that year, while a discussion with Museveni concluded that orphans should normally be left to relatives to support. By 1988 physicians were complaining that patient care was gravely neglected.[88] In Uganda it grew up initially from the bottom, with individual doctors at Mulago and the major Catholic hospitals creating special AIDS clinics and counselling services, assisted by voluntary societies like TASO (The AIDS Support Organisation). Tanzania began to train counsellors in 1987, but care was left largely to families and voluntary organisations. Kenya was particularly slow to act in this field. In 1996 Okware still saw patient care as one of the least effective parts of the control programme.[89]

The need to strengthen care was one reason why national programmes were reformulated in the early 1990s, although not the most important reason. In Tanzania, for example, the new programme adopted in January 1990 emphasised the training of counsellors and health workers at all levels, but also laid more stress on target groups, especially the young, and more emphasis on countering STDs other than AIDS.[90] Behind this programme lay the belief that indiscriminate public education had proved expensive and ineffective, while the most efficient method of checking the epidemic might be to tackle other STDs which facilitated infection, as research was beginning to suggest. The latter policy was adopted especially by the World Bank, which had hitherto left international coordination of AIDS programmes to the WHO but was increasingly dissatisfied with their effectiveness, as indeed were many WHO officials.[91] The details are not yet clear, but it was the World Bank that in 1990 pressed for a reorganisation of Uganda's programme, claiming that under the Ministry of Health's control it treated AIDS purely as a medical problem rather than as a social disease whose control needed a multi-sectoral programme embracing all ministries under presidential leadership.[92] After intensive lobbying, in 1992 the Uganda Government replaced the National Council for the Prevention of AIDS by the Uganda AIDS Commission (UAC), based in the Prime Minister's Office, thereby downgrading the executive ACP to a purely ministerial organ of the Ministry of Health alongside similar ACPs to be established in other ministries. This in turn meant, as a newspaper put it, that Okware 'was kicked upstairs to Commissioner of Health', the coveted post of UAC Director-General going instead to Stephen Lwanga, a Ugandan medical statistician from the WHO who had helped to model the epidemiology of AIDS.[93] Okware's dominant position had undoubtedly alienated many, but he remained responsible within the Ministry of Health for control of AIDS and other communicable diseases. In 1995 it was he who chaired the Ninth International Conference on AIDS and STDs in Africa when it met in Kampala.[94]

Uganda's new arrangements were slow to prove their value. Financed at international salary levels – Lwanga was alleged to earn a thousand times more than Okware's salary – the UAC initially displayed great extravagance and little experience of medical administration. The ministers summoned to its monthly meetings did not attend. It exceeded its competence by apportioning tasks to ministries, planning an elaborate field staff, and interfering in medical issues like vaccine trials which properly belonged to the Ministry of Health. A feud developed between Commission and ministries.[95] Eventually, with little accomplished and donors exasperated, Lwanga's contract was not renewed, the ACP programme manager in the Ministry of Health was transferred, and the UAC developed a new strategy emphasising decentralisation, community responsibility, and the targeting of youth, women, and high-risk groups, while the ACP (now combined with the Health Ministry's STD programme) focused especially on controlling other STDs, patient care, and preparing for vaccine trials.[96] By 1996 each of Uganda's thirty-nine districts had an AIDS Coordination Committee, twelve ministries had ACPs, and cooperation between UAC and ACP was becoming more effective.[97]

Similar problems existed elsewhere in East Africa. Tanzania's National AIDS Control Programme, also regarded by donors as bureaucratic and extravagant, received only two-thirds of the funding sought for its 1992–6 plan and was pressed to concentrate on STDs, its programme manager expressing the anger felt by many East African medical administrators at such interference.[98] Zanzibar raised only a quarter of its planned expenditure for 1991–6 and also expanded its concern with STDs.[99] Kenya accepted advice to establish a National AIDS Control Council, but the Ministry of Health resisted subordination and the donors, led by the World Bank, often channelled their funds in the 1990s away from the Ministry and towards STD care, NGOs, and decentralisation.[100] Meanwhile the number of East Africans infected with HIV was by 1997 probably about four million, or some 5 per cent of the entire population.[101]

Amidst this criticism of control programmes as profligate and ineffective, the discovery in 1994 that the epidemic's expansion appeared to be slowing in the worst-affected areas of Uganda and possibly in parts of Kenya came as an unexpected boost to morale.[102] The Ugandan data, from women attending antenatal clinics, were confirmed by evidence from both the Rakai and Masaka inquiries.[103] The government there quickly attributed the findings to the success of its control programme.[104] Others were sceptical. Some suspected that the antenatal tests were becoming less efficient. Other possible reasons were that the epidemic had saturated high-risk groups, that it was losing some virulence, or that new cases remained as numerous as before but were outweighed by deaths of older cases. A study of Ugandan military recruits suggested no comparable decline in rates of infection.[105] But the data from the meticulous Masaka study showed that the decline in prevalence had taken place among the young people who were probably most susceptible to public education.[106] Not only did this appear to justify the policy of open persuasion which governments had adopted when the epidemic was first recognised, but, as Okware reflected, it 'gives us hope that intensified awareness campaign against AIDS targeted at the future generations, will save this country'.[107]

Care

With over 500 HIV sufferers for every modern doctor in the mid-1990s, East Africa's medical profession might have been overwhelmed by the epidemic. In some senses that was true, but its impact was complex and intelligible only in the context of the profession's historical evolution. As elsewhere in the Third World,[108] many doctors, especially private practitioners, probably spent less time with AIDS patients than might have been expected. Early in the epidemic some doctors were said to refuse to treat them and hospitals to admit them,[109] but that was probably rare. More importantly, 95 per cent of the population did *not* have HIV and most of those who did were unaware of it. A study in Kenya in the mid-1990s showed that some 30 per cent of AIDS patients died without ever contacting the health system.[110] Moreover, busy modern doctors had come to be seen, and often resented, as impersonal figures from whom patients sought treatment in serious illness rather than assistance in distress. In Kenya, for example, only a doctor was supposed to diagnose HIV, but in one study of 127 subjects, only 44 per cent had heard of their diagnosis from a doctor. 'The doctors, they thought, were only important for making the initial diagnosis, after that they did not seem to have a clearly defined role', an experienced counsellor reported of one group of AIDS sufferers.[111] A survey in northern Tanzania found not a single respondent who would have turned to a modern doctor on contracting AIDS, except for specifically medical treatment.[112]

Nevertheless, many doctors did spend much time treating AIDS patients, especially in large hospitals. In 1996 over half of the adult beds in Ugandan hospitals were occupied by patients with HIV-related diseases, with higher proportions in medical wards in the worst-affected regions. The figures were somewhat lower in Kenya and Tanzania.[113] Most of these patients were young adults. Of admissions with HIV to Mulago in 1991, for example, 46 per cent were in their twenties and 32 per cent in their thirties. 'Today it is common to see great numbers of younger people (between ages 20–40 years) waiting in the out-patients and the clinics, and on the wards whereas previously the great majority were either children or the elderly', Nsambya Hospital reported in 1988.[114] David Okello, who studied 740 AIDS-related admissions to Mulago in 1991, found that their most common opportunistic complaints were diarrhoea and vomiting and that 134 died in the hospital, 97 of them (including 41 aged 0–9) within 24 hours of admission. The average inpatient cost the hospital $25 for a median stay of only five days, for, as a Senior Nursing Officer at Muhimbili explained in 1987, AIDS patients 'were looked after for sometime before their relatives were asked to take them home as there was no cure for the disease'.[115] The exceptions were patients with tuberculosis, to which AIDS gave great vulnerability. New cases of tuberculosis in Kenya trebled between the 1980s and 1995, while a study of adult medical admissions to KNH found that between 1984 and 1995 most opportunistic infections related to AIDS (including tuberculosis and respiratory infections) had roughly trebled, while non-infectious conditions not related to AIDS declined slightly, thus reversing the entire twentieth-century 'health transition'.[116] Cancer wards experienced an influx of patients with Kaposi's sarcoma. Pregnant women with HIV at Mulago were 50 per cent more likely to suffer complications in delivery. Complications of AIDS became the commonest organic states seen by psychiatrists.[117]

Some AIDS sufferers expressed resentment at the detachment and even brutality with which doctors had conveyed their diagnoses. 'He just said, "Well there you are, you're positive. You've got AIDS, so there is nothing I can do. Too bad,"' one patient recalled.[118] Most doctors, of course, knew that if they were to reveal the dreaded information at all, they must do it gently and slowly, but, as one asked, 'How can you inform them in the course of a supportive interview, when you see from 70 to 150 people with HIV or AIDS each week?'[119] Quite apart from the emotional strain of conveying what was in effect a death sentence, it was hard to explain the difference between HIV and AIDS or to convince desperate patients that they had a fatal illness with, as yet, no symptoms.[120] 'It is not easy to tell any one that he or she has got AIDS and that he is going to die in the next few months', wrote Uganda's most experienced AIDS specialist, Elly Katabira:

> Yet some of the patients need to know and some ask to be told. This is not the type of news you can pass on in hurry. You need to be prepared to explain the gravity of the news and be able to offer comfort and support to the patient, and be able to answer some of the questions which are likely to be asked, related to the fate of the victim.
>
> This is counselling and it starts with the one who breaks the ice, who is usually the doctor. Unfortunately counselling is a lengthy process. It cannot all be done in a few minutes or hours. It needs follow up to guide the patient through the various stages of shock, denial, anger, bargain, acceptance and hope. Such counselling is also extended to the family and relatives looking after the victim to enable them to cope with the situation.[121]

Katabira's colleague, Richard Goodgame, estimated that the initial explanation alone needed at least forty-five minutes. Few doctors had such time or believed that they should spend it on a task which did not require their medical skills. Goodgame thought the only answer was 'an army of counsellors who will be able to handle 99 percent of the support of the patients. We basically need a brand new category of health care people who have never existed in the African context.'[122]

Doctors therefore generally transferred – and *had* to transfer – as much as possible of the burden of explanation, counselling, and care to nurses, auxiliaries, counsellors, voluntary workers, or the patients' families and friends. As the training of counsellors took shape from the late 1980s, it became the general principle that the patient should have counselling before the HIV test, after it if the test proved positive, and regularly thereafter with the aim of helping him to accept his status and live as positively as possible with it. Although all health workers were supposed to receive training, the task was commonly left mainly to those who showed ability and willingness to undertake it, often in addition to their routine work. Many health workers charged with counselling resented this lack of training, support, or reward.[123] Yet most counselling was done not by health workers but by volunteers – often themselves people with AIDS – trained and administered by religious organisations or NGOs like TASO in Uganda, WAMATA (Walio Katika Mapambano na AIDS Tanzania – People Struggling Against AIDS in Tanzania), and KAS (Know AIDS Society) in Kenya.[124] Moreover, even these organisations provided only a small part of the care for AIDS sufferers. Most came from their families, which meant chiefly from mothers, daughters, and sisters.[125]

There has been no study of the impact of AIDS on East African doctors, although surveys have been made of dentists and dental auxiliaries in Nairobi and of nurses in the Nyeri District of Kenya and at four Tanzanian hospitals.[126] Medical care of AIDS has been harrowing everywhere, although not necessarily more demanding than caring for other incurable patients.[127] Some of the special characteristics of AIDS which weighed on carers elsewhere[128] may have been less burdensome in East Africa. Its epidemic character was no novelty there, nor was it unusual, as it was in the West, for many deaths to take place among young people, although, as the report quoted from Nsambya suggests, in the past children rather than young adults had been numerous among the dying. That, as one health worker put it, AIDS patients 'die such hideous deaths'[129] was no less true in East Africa but perhaps more familiar, and in addition most victims there either did not die in hospital or died soon after admission. By contrast, the fear of contracting AIDS from patients was especially acute in East Africa, because AIDS patients were so numerous and doctors and nurses so often worked without even the most elementary protective equipment. Many medical workers died of AIDS. Even by 1986 six Ugandan doctors were said to have been victims.[130] Subsequent press notices of deaths of doctors in the prime of life throughout East Africa suggest that the pattern continued. It was reported in 1993 that over 30 per cent of Uganda's District Medical Officers were infected with HIV. Reports of high death rates among other health workers were also common.[131] Yet there was little evidence that these workers had contracted the disease from *patients*[132] rather than in the ordinary course of life, for an important study of the main hospital in Kinshasa had shown that levels of infection among exposed health workers were no higher than in the general community.[133] Yet that could not silence fears. 'Sixteen workers of the Bukoba Regional Hospital have died of AIDS within four years', it was reported in 1990, 'and remaining workers attribute their deaths to mainly lack of protective gear for attending AIDS patients'. A study of northern Tanzanian hospitals in

1993 showed that prick and splash accidents were alarmingly common among surgeons and nurses, the latter being especially ill-protected when handling maternity cases. Doctors threatening to strike in Kenya in 1994 complained of 'working in appalling and risky conditions such as lack of basic facilities as gloves which exposed them to many risks like AIDS and hepatitis'. Studies of nurses showed that many feared to contract AIDS from objects like patients' food remains which were in fact harmless.[134] Doctors probably had fewer irrational fears but are unlikely to have been completely without them. It is not easy to imagine the impact on a student who learned his medicine in wards where over half the patients had AIDS.

Another special characteristic of AIDS in the West, that it was a 'dirty' disease associated with homosexuality, was not true in East Africa where transmission was predominantly heterosexual, but a similar stigma attached to it, for it was instead associated with promiscuity, especially in women. One study in northern Tanzania 'found that the subjects were more concerned with the social consequences of the disease than with the technical facts about AIDS, and that AIDS was associated with death, sex, misbehaviour (sin), blame, shame, rejection, and stigma'.[135] These attitudes came partly from traditional values – as Charles Nzioka wrote, AIDS was a godsend to traditional moralists[136] – and partly from the Christian values which were especially strong among health workers. Thecla Kohi's study of Tanzanian nurses found that about half blamed AIDS on the patients and their promiscuity, while 21 per cent agreed that if they had the choice they would refuse to nurse AIDS patients – this figure being only half that found by some studies in the West.[137] Nurses found some AIDS patients especially troublesome: 'They are a nuisance. You can't manage them. They are violent, maybe because they know they are going to die soon.' But generally African AIDS victims were unassertive when compared with those in the West.[138] The moralising so prevalent among health workers and the general public may have been less common among doctors, but it existed. A Ugandan woman, infected by her husband, recalled that, after a caesarean operation, 'One elderly doctor scolded her: "Now your baby might die." An orderly hissed: "Look at you. You've got AIDS."'[139] Although, given the scale of the epidemic, East African attitudes to AIDS victims were mostly generous, there was also discrimination and cruelty.[140]

A final special characteristic of AIDS was that it demoralised medical workers by displaying the impotence of their medicine. 'The effects of AIDS and HIV infection in the society we live, have started eroding our confidence and ability to cope with the situation', Samson Kisekka reflected in 1991.[141] The impact may have been muted in East Africa by the fact that modern medical systems were already in decay and health workers were inured to inadequacy and failure. But a disease totally unresponsive to drugs was especially alarming in a region which had for so long thought of health care overwhelmingly in terms of drugs. The scepticism and suspicion with which ordinary people regarded modern doctors – as seen, for example, during the Ugandan disturbances of 1949 – surfaced again in beliefs that doctors deliberately killed off AIDS patients and their children, beliefs sufficiently widespread for the District Medical Officer in Masaka to deny them publicly.[142] The sense of impotence, however, probably affected health workers most deeply where it meant that their lack of drugs and equipment prevented them from alleviating the sufferings of AIDS patients in ways which they knew to be possible.[143]

In addition to these burdens shared by all health workers, doctors faced especially difficult ethical questions of confidentiality. As in many parts of the world, it had not been customary in East Africa for doctors to tell patients they had incurable diseases. 'Psychologically', a Tanzanian declared, 'a doctor should always tell a patient of his/her immediate recovery, and not of the seriousness of the disease'.[144] Indigenous healers often did not tell patients that they suspected AIDS, for healers were expected to fight disease to the death, not abandon cases as hopeless. 'Why are you telling me this? You must not be a real doctor!' was said to be a frequent response to bad news.[145] Many modern doctors were accustomed to the older British practice of giving a hopeless prognosis to the relatives rather than the patient. Okware warned that patients told they had AIDS might commit suicide, go mad, or maliciously spread the disease, and although other physicians insisted that these fears were doctors' excuses for avoiding a painful duty,[146] there was some evidence of high rates of suicide or attempted suicide among AIDS patients,[147] although there was little more than rumour of malicious infection.[148] Reactions to positive HIV tests varied from prostration through disbelief to resolution, often giving priority to the survival of the family.[149] Equally diverse is the evidence as to whether people wished to know their HIV status. Only 10 per cent of Kenyan blood donors wanted the information, but most of their counterparts at Kitovu in Uganda asked for the result and the AIDS Information Centre established in Uganda in 1990 tested over 270,000 applicants during its first six years.[150] Okware saw no point in telling patients the painful truth – 'What are you going to do with them?' – and Uganda's initial policy was to remain silent. Other doctors, however, held, with Katabira and Goodgame, that 'All mentally competent people should be informed of their results', and this view came to predominate as counselling facilities expanded and confidence grew in patients' ability to handle the truth.[151] Kenyan guidelines issued in 1988 stated, 'After confirmatory testing, every HIV seropositive person should in principle be informed unless the individual explicitly does not want to know.' Tanzania adopted the same policy in 1989, except for blood donors lest they should be deterred. As Elizabeth Ngugi stressed, the main reason for openness was to stop sufferers from spreading the disease unknowingly.[152]

The more difficult ethical dilemma was whether people other than the patient should be informed. There was general agreement that employers did not need to know and should not be told, although some doctors apparently breached this rule. It was agreed, too, that insurance firms could be informed because it would by definition be with the patient's consent. Some doctors avoided recording AIDS on death certificates.[153] One especially delicate problem was to inform the parents of children with AIDS, for this implied that the parents were probably also infected.[154] But the most difficult issue, as many doctors testified, was whether to inform a victim's spouse, who could otherwise so easily become infected. Some doctors insisted that it was for the sufferer to pass on the information: 'that is what patient confidentiality is all about!'[155] But sufferers often found this a harder task than receiving the news of their condition, so that many (probably especially husbands) did not tell their partners or families.[156] Doctors disagreed about what to do in this situation. Alexander Odonga espoused one view in his textbook of medical ethics:

> If the infected partner refused to tell the other partner, the doctor has moral duty to the other partner and this is a deadly disease, to tell the other partner and to ask him to come for examination and if found negative to be advised accordingly. By doing so the doctor runs the risk of court action for damages as a result of breaching the confidentiality, but this will be regarded as privilege information.[157]

Official pronouncements were more cautious. The Uganda Medical Association went no further than counselling 'that there should be a degree of confidentiality but where necessary a relative should be told'.[158] Kenya's guidelines were obscure and evasive:

> Strict confidentiality is a constraint because it contradicts the Kenyan cultural set up where all is shared by the community, and where sometimes a burial may be refused unless the cause of death is known. Thus strict individual confidentiality could jeopardize the community support required in counselling and increase the myths surrounding AIDS. If the patient himself wishes to disclose his HIV status, it is his responsibility. The advantages of confidentiality versus community sharing in the Kenyan environment should be studied.[159]

In the West, the constellation of stress surrounding AIDS caused among doctors and other health workers the emotional and moral exhaustion known as burnout.[160] Remarkably little is known about this in East Africa, despite the greater scale of the epidemic there. Some suggested that circumstances in poor countries were so different that Western experience of burnout might be irrelevant, but Sewankambo warned that the phenomenon was to be expected and there were reports of health staff leaving or refusing to work at places of special stress, such as the AIDS clinic at Mulago.[161] In 1991 a Ugandan doctor described his experience:

Who will help the helpers? In my area, the people who are suffering most from AIDS are the ones without the disease – as yet – but with the burden of supporting those who do. I must confess that I am here on the run from AIDS. In addition to being a doctor in my remote village, I am also a pastor, and I had gone two years without a funeral until several years ago when mystically I began burying uncles and aunts from the large extended family dependent on me. I was called upon for counselling this whole community reeling under the fear of the unknown as I began holding funerals first at the rate of one, then two, now three per month. This is occurring as AIDS sweeps through my people in the countryside in an area said to have developed community support programmes for dealing with this plague, but when I turn for support in my own exhausting efforts, I find my colleagues numbed and any hope for outside support 'burned out'.[162]

Probably AIDS had quite different consequences for, on the one hand, the bulk of doctors obliged to treat cases as they appeared, and, on the other, a small minority who chose to make the disease their vocation. The most distinguished specialist was Elly Katabira, who established the first AIDS clinic at Mulago in April 1987, helped to found TASO, and served as its medical adviser and chairman of trustees.[163] Together with Richard Goodgame, Katabira published in 1989 an account of AIDS treatment written in the full tradition of Albert Cook. Its principle was that although AIDS was then incurable, patients could nevertheless be helped by health workers at all levels without elaborate diagnostic tests or therapeutic methods: '*Use what you have*.' Where possible, specialised AIDS clinics should be established at hospitals, even if initial response was slight: 'Eventually patients will come.' Clinics could treat opportunistic infections, restore morale, and conduct research. The important point was to do all that could be done:

The diagnosis of AIDS should not be the main feature determining admission or non-admission. Rather, the health worker should consider the specific clinical condition of the patient. Many treatable conditions requiring hospitalization occur in AIDS patients. No patient should be denied admission because the diagnosis is AIDS or presumed AIDS . . . The notion among health workers, patients and families that AIDS patients are mainly admitted to the hospital to die needs to be eliminated.

The truth was that, if properly treated, most AIDS patients improved before leaving hospital, and they should be released to family care when the hospital could do no more:

Hospital care is a useful link in the total management of AIDS patients. It should not be looked on as the last resort or as the mainstay of care. It should be used appropriately to improve the quality and longevity of life and should be integrated with home care, clinic care and counselling.

Although AIDS was incurable, chronic, infectious, and widespread, they argued, it was also treatable, long-survived, hard to transmit, and widely shared. That reversal of attitude was crucial to its management.[164] The same message was propagated by Katabira's colleague at Mulago, Donna Kabatesi, by his counterpart at Masaka, Sam Kalibala, by Nelson Sewankambo, and in Tanzania by Fred Mhalu.[165]

For these doctors AIDS was an intellectual and professional challenge giving purpose to their lives, much as leprosy had attracted similar dedication earlier in the century. As a missionary physician confessed, 'I love the challenge, both as a priest and a doctor.' Other health workers probably gained satisfaction from the care they gave, as was reported in the West.[166] There were material rewards: international salaries or WHO supplements for a few, the higher pay generally available from NGOs, misappropriation which led many ordinary people to regard AIDS work as yet another pork-barrel for the elite,[167] an influx of private patients, and especially the many employment opportunities created for a generation of young educated people unable to find the civil service posts available to their fathers. Miracle workers like the Apostle Deo Balabyekubo of the Prayer Palace Christian Centre could drive to healing sessions in white Mercedes.[168] Indigenous healers could profit, both the mercenary claiming cures, whom the authorities sought to suppress,[169] and the dedicated seekers of herbal remedies who for the first time found support from governments which recognised that anything was worth trying where nothing worked.[170] In Uganda the epidemic stimulated many attempts at collaboration between modern and indigenous medicine, with Museveni's strong support.[171] Dr Lukwago, diagnosed HIV-positive and apparently required to retire, opened several herbal clinics to treat other sufferers. Bwogi Kanyerezi, private practitioner and former Professor of Medicine at Makerere, collaborated with herbalists, experimented with herbal remedies, claimed to have seen seroconverted patients, and had to defend himself, successfully, before the Medical Council.[172] Most controversy focused on Charles Ssali, a gifted ear, nose, and throat specialist who fled Uganda during the violence following Amin's overthrow and returned with a drug, Mariandina, said to consist mainly of herbal substances freely available in Britain, with which he claimed to treat the opportunistic infections of AIDS patients and to retard the course of the disease. In 1996 some 13,500 patients were said to be taking Mariandina.[173] One Tanzanian doctor with postgraduate training was reported to charge a maximum of $500 for treatment with a mixture of twelve local herbs claimed to cure 40 per cent of AIDS cases.[174]

Yet the most important service that modern doctors could give was to display the objective rationality at the heart of their profession. Many did so throughout the growth of the epidemic, but perhaps particularly during the mid-1990s when Ugandan doctors had to defend their desire that the country should participate in trials of an HIV vaccine. As early as 1988 Okware had urged that 'Uganda with its high incidence of HIV infection, good surveillance for disease and wealth of experienced clinicians is the perfect place to test vaccines for HIV.'[175] During the following years hopes of preparing a vaccine against a virus so mutable as HIV had often waned and international research funds had been spent overwhelmingly on basic microbiology and the search for curative drugs.[176] In principle, however, a vaccine was the most effective – possibly the only effective – counter to a viral disease, as had been demonstrated with smallpox and poliomyelitis.[177] In holding to this principle, Uganda's leading doctors displayed their continuing faith in the modern medicine they had learned at Makerere. A national plan for vaccine research, development, and education was prepared in 1992,[178] but the vaccine itself did not become available until 1997. The strain to be tested (strain B) was not that common in Uganda, but the doctors were nevertheless keen that preliminary trials should take place, for there might be cross-immunity between strains, other strains were in preparation, the trials were a contribution to the general good of humanity, and, as the government newspaper put it, 'Uganda has led the way in the war against HIV and Aids in the past and it should continue to do so today.'[179] Nevertheless, trials involved risks and the plan to begin them met much resistance, some of it within the medical profession but most from members of the public, who feared that Ugandans were being used as guinea-pigs by foreign interests with sinister motives. At one point there were street demonstrations against the proposal.[180] The main burden of responsibility and justification lay on Roy Mugerwa, Chairman of the Vaccine Organising Committee, who had been at the heart of AIDS research since the first investigation in 1985. The first young military volunteers were to be vaccinated in mid-1997.[181] If, in the long term, a vaccine proved successful, the modern doctors' faith would be justified and the prestige of their profession would rise immeasurably.

11 Conclusion

This book has ended, as it began, with AIDS. The concern of Uganda's leading doctors that their country should participate in the testing of an AIDS vaccine was a declaration of their commitment to the global community which distinguished modern medicine from all its predecessors and justified its claim to be described, uniquely, as modern. East African doctors had been especially loyal to this international medicine, not least because they lacked a rival literate tradition and had come to maturity as contemporaries of the WHO. AIDS had encouraged a few to collaborate with indigenous treatments, but they had done so for the most part along scientific lines. Moreover, modern doctors – especially in Uganda, where African medical education had begun – had taken a leadership role of international importance in East Africa's response to AIDS, both in research, where they had drawn on a tradition of epidemiological enquiry at Makerere dating back for half a century, and in the planning of control programmes. To these they had brought both the rationality of their scientific training and the drive for national and racial dignity which had informed their research, their pursuit of professional equality during the colonial period, and their earlier struggle to escape from menial apprenticeship. All this had taken place within the 120 years separating James Ainsworth's first experience of modern medicine from Samuel Okware's chairmanship of the International AIDS Conference.

Yet the doctors who planned AIDS Control Programmes were only the most visible members of the modern profession. Diagnosis and treatment of AIDS rested chiefly with hospital doctors, half of whose beds were often occupied by victims of the disease. Some, like Elly Katabira, made AIDS their speciality and treated it with a compassion inherited from the missionary tradition of Albert Cook and Adrien Atiman. Most struggled to give what help they could amid the dilapidated conditions and minimal rewards which had turned hospital doctors towards a trade union style of professionalism. Divisive as this was, it was a logical response to a situation where weak states did not provide the support which other forms of professionalism needed in order to flourish outside the Anglo-American context – and perhaps, by the late twentieth century, even within it.

However, most East African doctors in the time of AIDS were not confined to hospitals but were private practitioners, either full-time or part-time. They were the heirs to the entrepreneurial strand in East African medicine, displayed by the free-for-all competition among pre-colonial healers, the eager pursuit of advancement by tribal dressers and early medical students, and the pioneering practices of private European and Asian doctors. African private practitioners had emerged in the 1950s and multiplied in the 1980s and 1990s alongside urbanisation, class differentiation, economic privatisation, and state decline, most vigorously in Kenya's transition to capitalism but even in Tanzania, where a strong ruling party and a weak medical profession had at independence set the country temporarily on a socialist course. This book has said little about the private practitioners' role in the treatment of AIDS, or indeed about any aspect of private practice. It is the most obvious of the many gaps in knowledge of East African doctors and their history which it is hoped that the book may at least have revealed. Sociological studies of the contemporary medical profession are especially needed, but so is a programme – which must be conducted by East Africans – to collect the life histories and papers of modern doctors. It is worth repeating that the last to publish his memoirs was Adrien Atiman.

The three branches of the modern medical profession – medical administrators, hospital doctors, and private practitioners – occupied only part of the spectrum of medical provision and cared for only a proportion of those who suffered from AIDS. The great area of growth during the generation after independence had been sub-professional practice by medical auxiliaries and especially the sale of modern pharmaceuticals. The East African medical profession had grown up alongside modern chemotherapy, had been shaped by it, and was now in turn threatened by it. Yet AIDS, paradoxically, revealed the limitations of self medication, which had hitherto seemed to hold the medical future. A fatal disease completely unresponsive to the drugs available to East Africans, it could be countered only by public health policies and sophisticated vaccines which needed professional skills and authority. The doctors who advocated vaccine trials and mass education could hope not only, as Okware said, that they 'will save this country', but also that they might restore professional status.

The final components of East Africa's medical spectrum in the 1990s were indigenous healers, whose medicines were as ineffective against the new epidemic as those of their modern rivals. Yet indigenous healing had survived, chiefly as a residual activity[1] but with elements of transformation to meet modern conditions, partly because of the great gaps in modern medical systems but also because it met two of the primary needs which pre-colonial medicine had sought to satisfy but the modern variety had not adequately met: the desire for patient power to choose among a range of therapies, and the desire for holistic treatment which provided concern and reassurance as well as medication. AIDS intensified those needs, but if modern medicine could find an effective counter to AIDS, indigenous therapy might be its chief victim.

This medical spectrum, as it existed in the 1990s and is sadly oversimplified here, cannot be understood as a failure to create a modern medical profession in East Africa along Anglo-American lines, still less as the product of a process of deprofessionalisation since independence. It was a distinct form of medical pluralism,[2] still in formation and with no trend of future development yet marked out. It was the product of a distinctive history which could only be obscured – and often was obscured – by negative contrasts with stereotyped and misleading notions of professionalisation in the West and by oversimplifications of the ambiguity inherent in professionalism itself. The role of modern doctors in this plural medical order was not diminishing, nor was their medicine blending to any significant extent with other therapies. Rather, East Africa desperately needed the technical efficiency which medical professionalism implied, just as the AIDS epidemic had revealed how much East Africa needed its modern doctors.

Notes

1 THE ARGUMENT

1 The main study is Alexander Mwa Odonga, *The first fifty years of Makerere University Medical School and the foundation of scientific medical education in East Africa* (Kisubi [1990?]).
2 The idea for this book came partly from reading David K. Leonard, *African successes: four public managers of Kenyan rural development* (Berkeley, 1991).
3 See Simon Ndirangu, *A history of nursing in Kenya* (Nairobi, 1982).
4 This is the argument of Thomas Neville Bonner, *Becoming a physician: medical education in Britain, France, Germany and the United States, 1750–1945* (New York, 1995).
5 See Amira elAzhary Sonbol, *The creation of a medical profession in Egypt, 1800–1922* (Syracuse, 1991).
6 Talcott Parsons, 'Professions', in *International encyclopaedia of the social sciences*, vol. XII (1968), pp. 540–2.
7 A.M. Carr-Saunders and P.A. Wilson, *The professions* (Oxford, 1933), pp. 284–5.
8 Eliot Freidson, *Profession of medicine: a study of the sociology of applied knowledge* (New York, 1972), pp. xvii, 53, 69, 205.
9 Terence Johnson, 'Imperialism and the professions', in Paul Halmos (ed.), *Professionalisation and social change* (Keele, 1973), pp. 281–309.
10 See esp. Geoffrey Cocks and Konrad H. Jarausch (eds.), *German professions, 1800–1950* (New York, 1990), p. 4.
11 Eliot Freidson, *Professional powers: a study of the institutionalization of formal knowledge* (Chicago, 1986), pp. xiii, 130.
12 Freidson, *Profession of medicine*, p. 73.
13 Gerald L. Geison (ed.), *Professions and the French state, 1700–1900* (Philadelphia, 1984), pp. 8–9, 225–6.
14 Charles E. McClelland, *The German experience of professionalization* (Cambridge, 1991), p. 10.
15 William E. Steslicke, 'The political life of the Japan Medical Association', *Journal of Asian Studies*, 31 (1971–2), 815–8.
16 R. Jeffery, 'Allopathic medicine in India: a case of deprofessionalization?' *SSM*, 11 (1977), 561–73.
17 See the essays in Sjaak van der Geest and Susan Reynolds Whyte (eds.), *The context of medicines in developing countries: studies in pharmaceutical anthropology* (Dordrecht, 1988).

18 See Byron Good and Mary-Jo DelVecchio Good, 'The comparative study of Greco-Islamic medicine', in Charles Leslie and Allan Young (eds.), *Paths to Asian medical knowledge* (Berkeley, 1992), ch. 11; Kenneth G. Zysk, *Asceticism and healing in ancient India* (New York, 1991), ch. 4.

19 For this usage of 'modern', see Anthony Giddens, *The consequences of modernity* (Cambridge, 1991), esp. pp. 51–2.

2 PIONEERS

1 Albert R. Cook, *Uganda memories (1897–1940)* (Kampala, 1945), p. 264, quoting his diary for 28 February 1909.

2 D.J. Bradley, 'The situation and the response', in E.E. Sabben-Clare, D.J. Bradley, and K. Kirkwood (eds.), *Health in tropical Africa during the colonial period* (Oxford, 1980), pp. 6–7.

3 David F. Clyde, *Malaria in Tanzania* (London, 1967), esp. ch. 1; Albert R. Cook, 'Notes on the diseases met with in Uganda', *Journal of Tropical Medicine*, 4 (1901), 175.

4 Cook, 'Notes', pp. 196–7; Dr Wolff, 'Bilharzia in Deutsch-Ostafrika', *Archiv für Schiffs- und Tropen-Hygiene*, 15 (1911), 224–30.

5 C.J. Hackett, 'On the origin of the human treponematoses', *Bulletin of the WHO*, 29 (1963), 8–10, 29.

6 *Kikuyu News*, 101 (September 1927), 6; 'Gesundheitsverhältnisse in Deutsch-Ostafrika im Jahre 1902/1903', *Arbeiten aus dem Kaiserlichen Gesundheitsamte*, 21 (1904), 566.

7 Cook, 'Notes', pp. 176–7.

8 Marc Harry Dawson, 'Socio-economic and epidemiological change in Kenya: 1880–1925', PhD thesis, University of Wisconsin-Madison, 1983, pp. 71–83.

9 K.R. Dumbell and Farida Huq, 'Epidemiological implications of the typing of variola isolates', *Transactions of the Royal Society of Tropical Medicine and Hygiene*, 69 (1975), 303–6; Marc H. Dawson, 'Smallpox in Kenya, 1880–1920', *SSM*, 13B (1979), 245–50.

10 James Christie, *Cholera epidemics in East Africa* (London, 1876).

11 J.N.P. Davies, 'The history of syphilis in Uganda', *Bulletin of the WHO*, 15 (1956), 1041–55; Dawson, 'Socio-economic', ch. 4; Megan Vaughan, 'Syphilis in colonial East and Central Africa', in Terence Ranger and Paul Slack (eds.), *Epidemics and ideas* (Cambridge, 1992), ch. 11.

12 David O. Nyamwaya, 'Societal response to illness – the Pokot of Kenya', University of Nairobi Institute of African Studies paper no. 127 (December 1979), p. 3.

13 Ferdinand Walser, *Luganda proverbs* (Berlin, 1982), no. 2990; J.S. Lwanga and C. Kisamba-Mugerwa, 'Ugandan traditional healers study: indigenous knowledge and management of childhood diarrhoeal diseases', duplicated (1991), p. 3 (UMOH library).

14 A. Karasek, 'Beiträge zur Kenntnis der Waschambaa', *Baessler-Archiv*, 1 (1911), 197.

15 Gerhard Lindblom, *The Akamba in British East Africa* (Uppsala, 1920), p. 319; Mark W.T. Bura, 'The Wairaqw concepts of causation, diagnosis and treatment of disease', *Dar es Salaam Medical Journal*, 6 , 1 (November 1974), 59.

16 Diane Leinwand Zeller, 'The establishment of Western medicine in Buganda', PhD thesis, Columbia University, 1971, p. 53; John Roscoe, *The soul of central Africa* (London, 1922), p. 189; John Roscoe *The Banyankole* (Cambridge, 1923), p. 136.
17 Roscoe, *Banyankole*, p. 137; Nyamwaya, 'Societal response', pp. 12–14; Michael G. Whisson, 'Some aspects of functional disorders among the Kenya Luo', in Ari Kiev (ed.), *Magic, faith, and healing* (New York, 1964), p. 304.
18 Lindblom, *Akamba*, pp. 254–6; Zeller, 'Establishment', pp. 22–3.
19 Roscoe, *Soul*, p. 189.
20 Susan Reynolds Whyte, 'Social implications of the interpretation of misfortune in Bunyole', PhD thesis, University of Washington, 1973; Steven Feierman, 'Therapy as a system-in-action in northeastern Tanzania', *SSM*, 15B (1981), 353–6.
21 Karasek, 'Beiträge', p. 196; Steven Feierman, *Peasant intellectuals* (Madison, 1990), pp. 102–3.,
22 Fridolin Bösch, *Les Banyamwezi* (Münster, 1930), pp. 171–9.
23 *Ibid.*, p. 169; Lindblom, *Akamba*, p. 269; Karasek, 'Beiträge', p. 196.
24 See, e.g., Mayunga H.H. Nkunya, H. Weenen, and D.H. Bray, 'Chemical evaluation of Tanzanian medicinal plants', in Keto E. Mshigeni and others (eds.), *Proceedings of an international conference of experts from developing countries on traditional medicinal plants* (Dar es Salaam, 1991), pp. 103–5.
25 Zeller, 'Establishment', p. 54; L.S.B. Leakey, *The southern Kikuyu before 1903: volume II* (New York, 1977), pp. 933–5; M. Merker, *Die Masai* (Berlin, 1904), pp. 181–8.
26 Robert W. Felkin, 'Notes on labour in central Africa', *Edinburgh Medical Journal*, 29 (1884), 928; J.N.P. Davies, 'The development of "scientific" medicine in the African kingdom of Bunyoro-Kitara', *Medical History*, 3 (1959), 47–57; N.C. Roles, 'Tribal surgery in East Africa during the XIXth century', *EAMJ*, 43 (1966), 579–94, and 44 (1967), 17–30.
27 John Roscoe, *The Bakitara or Banyoro* (Cambridge, 1923), p. 290; G.S.P. Freeman-Grenville, *The French at Kilwa Island* (Oxford, 1965), p. 121; Eugenia W. Herbert, 'Smallpox inoculation in Africa', *JAH*, 16 (1975), 547–58.
28 Lindblom, *Akamba*, p. 271; John Roscoe, *The Baganda* (2nd edn, London, 1965), p. 310.
29 Roscoe, *Bakitara*, p. 34; Davies, 'Development', pp. 54–5; David F. Clyde, *History of the medical services of Tanganyika* (Dar es Salaam, 1962), p. 13.
30 L.P. Gerlach, 'Some basic Digo conceptions of health and disease', in East African Institute of Social Research, 'One-day symposium on attitudes to health and disease among some East African tribes', duplicated (1959), p. 28.
31 Feierman, *Peasant intellectuals*, p. 237; Bruce Berman and John Lonsdale, *Unhappy valley: conflict in Kenya and Africa* (2 vols., London, 1992), vol. II, p. 340.
32 Yuet-wah Cheung, *Missionary medicine in China* (Lanham, 1988), pp. 94–5.
33 Karasek, 'Beiträge', pp. 196–7; [Otto] Peiper, 'Der Suaheli-Arzt', *Archiv für Schiffs- und Tropen-Hygiene*, 14 (1910), 562.
34 E.g. W. Scoresby Routledge and Katherine Routledge, *With a prehistoric people: the Akikuyu of British East Africa* (reprinted, London, 1968), p. 250.
35 Feierman, *Peasant intellectuals*, p. 104.

36 Robert B. Edgerton, 'A traditional African psychiatrist', in Z.A. Ademuwagun, John A.A. Ayoade, Ira E. Harrison, and Dennis M. Warren (eds.), *African therapeutic systems* (Waltham, 1979), p. 93.
37 Karasek, 'Beiträge', p. 196; 'General-Sanitätsbericht über die Kaiserliche Schutztruppe für Deutsch-Ostafrika für das Berichtsjahr vom 1. April 1895 bis zum 31. März 1896', *Arbeiten aus dem Kaiserlichen Gesundheitsamte*, 14 (1898), 650, 665; Feierman, *Peasant intellectuals*, p. 114.
38 Feierman, *Peasant intellectuals*, pp. 103–4; Diane Leinwand Zeller, '*Basawo Baganda*: the traditional doctors of Buganda', in Ademuwagun and others, *Therapeutic systems*, p. 138.
39 See, e.g. Dorothy Porter and Roy Porter, *Patient's progress: doctors and doctoring in eighteenth-century England* (Cambridge, 1989), pp. 19–27, 113; Paul U. Unschuld, *Medicine in China: a history of ideas* (Berkeley, 1985), p. 223.
40 *CMS Monthly Reporter*, January and May 1875.
41 A.J. Temu, *British Protestant missions* (London, 1972), pp. 8–12.
42 Price to Wright, 23 February 1876, CMS C.A5/O.23/48.
43 Forster, 'Report of the medical work done at Mombasa', 1 January–30 April 1876, CMS C.A5/O.10.
44 Price, journal, 28 April 1876, in *Church Missionary Intelligencer*, 1 (1876), 670.
45 Forster, 'Report of the medical work done at Mombasa', 1 January–30 April 1876, CMS C.A5/O.10.
46 *Ibid.*
47 See Adelola Adeloye, *African pioneers of modern medicine: Nigerian doctors of the nineteenth century* (Ibadan, 1985).
48 David and others to ?, 28 February 1881, CMS G3/A5/O/1881/30.
49 Taylor to Lang, 6 July 1883, CMS G3/A5/O/1883/89.
50 Lang to Handford, 26 October 1883, CMS G3/A5/L3/56.
51 Handford to Lang, 24 December 1883, CMS G3/A5/O/1884/3.
52 Quoted in Samuel K. Arap Ng'eny and others, *Rabai to Mumias: a short history of the Church of the Province of Kenya 1844 to 1944* (Nairobi, 1994), p. 14.
53 Ardagh to Lang, 15 November 1887, CMS G3/A5/O/1887/402.
54 Ardagh to Lang, 10 February 1888, CMS G3/A5/O/1888/76.
55 Ardagh to Lang, 5 April 1888, CMS G3/A5/O/1888/160.
56 Edwards to Lang, 1 January 1892, CMS G3/A5/O/1892/39.
57 Frere Town Finance Committee minutes, 17 January 1895, CMS G3/A5/O/1895/48.
58 Minute on *ibid.*, CMS G3/A5/P5/1895/48.
59 'The Native Agents Committee, Mombasa' [1900] CMS G3/A5/O/1900/89; C.S. Edwards, 'East African patients', *Mercy and Truth*, 1 (1897), 132.
60 *Mercy and Truth*, 17 (1913), 56.
61 R.K. Shepherd, 'About native doctors', *ibid.*, 14 (1910), 13–14.
62 CMS log-book, Freretown station, 13 October 1896, KNA CMS 1/624.
63 'Freretown Estate', list (1928) in KNA CMS 1/677.
64 François Renault, *Lavigerie, l'esclavage africain, et l'Europe, 1868–92* (2 vols., Paris, 1971), vol. I, pp. 158–61, 225, 233, 235.
65 *Ibid.*, pp. 221, 226, 232–4; [Roger] Fouquer, *Le docteur Adrien Atiman, médecin-catéchiste au Tanganyika* (Condé-sur-Escaut, 1964), pp. 35–6, 116–17.

66 This account is based on Adrien Atiman, 'Adrien Atiman, by himself' (trans. L.B. Cave), *TNR*, 21 (June 1946), 46–76; Adrien Atiman, 'The dispensary at Karema', *The White Fathers in Africa*, November 1940, pp. 114–15; Fouquer, *Adrien Atiman*.
67 Atiman, 'Adrien Atiman', pp. 50–1.
68 *Ibid.*, p. 51.
69 *Ibid.*, pp. 50–1.
70 *Ibid.*, p. 51.
71 Fouquer, *Adrien Atiman*, p. 155.
72 Atiman, 'Adrien Atiman', p. 55.
73 *Ibid.*, p. 61.
74 Atiman, 'Dispensary', p. 115.
75 Renault, *Lavigerie*, vol. I, p. 233.
76 Friedrich Karl Kleine, *Ein deutscher Tropenarzt* (Hannover, 1949), p. 133.
77 Atiman, 'Dispensary', p. 114.
78 See Roland Oliver, *The missionary factor in East Africa* (2nd edn, London, 1965).
79 Horace R.A. Philp, *A new day in Kenya* (London, 1936), p. 83.
80 Especially in *Kikuyu News*.
81 Terence O. Ranger, 'Godly medicine: the ambiguities of medical mission in southeast Tanzania, 1900–1945', *SSM*, 15B (1981), 263.
82 A. Le Roy, quoted by Nicolas Ossama, 'Pratique médicale missionnaire lors de la première évangélisation', in M. Hebga and others, *Croyances et guérison* (Yaoundé, 1973), p. 75.
83 M. Louis O'Hara, OSF, 'An unfinished canticle: the story of the Franciscan Missionary Sisters for Africa', typescript, 1980, pp. 27–8 (St Joseph's College Archives, Mill Hill).
84 Margaret Mary Nolan, MMM, *Medical Missionaries of Mary, 1937–1962* (Drogheda, n.d.), p. 36.
85 *Uganda Argus*, 4 November 1965.
86 Quoted in Kenneth Richardson, *Garden of miracles: the story of the Africa Inland Mission* (reprinted, London, 1976), p. 124.
87 Furley, journal, 22 March 1897, CMS G3/A5/O/1897/157; Cook to Baylis, 29 June 1898, CMS G3/A7/O/1898/168.
88 Cook, *Uganda memories*, p. 311. For similar Catholic experience, see O'Hara, 'Unfinished canticle', p. 28.
89 *The Mission Hospital*, 30 (1926), 27.
90 E.g. CMS Embu Medical Mission log-book, 22 February 1911, KNA CMS 1/637.
91 *Target*, 27 June 1976.
92 Cook, *Uganda memories*, pp. 311–12.
93 *Mercy and Truth*, 18 (1914), 300.
94 Cook, *Uganda memories*, p. 312; *Report of the CMS Mengo Medical Mission, Kampala, 1933*, pp. 30–1 (RH Micr. Afr. 609 (1)).
95 Quoted in E. Baihireyo Turya, 'Which way medical assistants of Uganda?' MSc thesis, University of London, 1980, p. 30.
96 *Kikuyu News*, 133 (September 1935), p. 5, and 90 (December 1924), pp. 6–7.
97 *Mercy and Truth*, 19 (1915), 399; Gustav Menzel, *Die Bethel-Mission: aus 100*

Jahren Missionsgeschichte (Neukirchen-Vluyu, 1986), p. 137; Brian G. McIntosh, 'The Scottish Mission in Kenya, 1891–1923', PhD thesis, University of Edinburgh, 1969, p. 395 n126.

98 *The Mission Hospital*, 30 (1926), 29.

99 A.R. Cook, diary, 16 December 1902, Wellcome Institute for the History of Medicine, London.

100 CMS Hospital, Mengo: Operation Book, 1919–28, MP.

101 *Kikuyu News*, 46 (January 1914), 20.

102 *Mercy and Truth*, 13 (1909), 209; James Ndung'u Mburu, 'The dissemination of Christianity in Nyeri District (1903–1963) with special reference to the work of African teachers and evangelists', MA thesis, University of Nairobi, 1975, p. 32; *Kikuyu News*, 81 (September 1922), 7.

103 *Kikuyu News*, 133 (September 1935); 5; *ibid.*, 46 (January 1914), 20–1; *ibid.*, 61 (October 1916), 10.

104 Ndirangu, *History*, p. 25.

105 *Ebifa mu Buganda*, 1920, pp. 51–2; Cook, *Uganda memories*, p. 312.

106 CMS Hospital, Mengo: Monthly wages book, Matron's office, 1916–44, MP; *Mercy and Truth*, 7 (1903), 263.

107 *Mercy and Truth*, 4 (1900), 112.

108 CMS Hospital, Mengo: Monthly wages book, Matron's office, 1916–44, MP; Annual report for Buganda Province, 1913–14, UNA A.46/438.

109 A.R. Cook, diary, 12 January 1898 and 16–20 December 1898, Wellcome Institute for the History of Medicine, London: *The Mission Hospital*, 38 (1934), 20; W.D. Foster, *The Church Missionary Society and modern medicine in Uganda* (n.p., 1978), pp. 165–9, 204.

110 CMS Hospital, Mengo: Monthly wages book, Matron's office, 1916–44, MP.

111 *Kikuyu News*, 25 (January 1911), 7–8.

112 *Ibid.*, 78 (November 1921), 15.

113 *Mercy and Truth*, 17 (1913), 202.

114 E. Kuwokulya in *Ebifa mu Buganda*, September 1911.

115 Arthur to his mother, 25 January 1907, Arthur papers, EUL.

116 Mrs Savile, 'Among the Maragoli Hills', *Mercy and Truth*, 10 (1906), 230.

117 *Kikuyu News*, 49 (June 1914), 20.

118 *Ibid.*, 71 (January 1920), 19.

119 *Mercy and Truth*, 6 (1902), 70, 246.

120 Quoted in Foster, *Church Missionary Society*, p. 110.

121 Musajawaza to Stones, 12 March 1935, MP 17.

122 There is an intriguing parallel in Wu Lien-teh, *Plague fighter: the autobiography of a modern Chinese physician* (Cambridge, 1959), p. 282.

123 *Mercy and Truth*, 14 (1910), 12–13.

124 Yosef Afrika in *Rafiki Yangu*, November 1913.

125 Apolo Kagwa, *The customs of the Baganda* (trans. E.B. Kalibala, New York, 1934), p. 128; Zeller, 'Establishment', p. 269; *Mercy and Truth*, 16 (1912), 307.

126 *Mercy and Truth*, 5 (1901), 212.

127 Diocese of Uganda, Medical Sub-Conference minutes, 25 November 1908, MP.

128 *Uganda Notes*, July 1916.

129 Quoted in W.D. Foster, *The early history of scientific medicine in Uganda* (Nairobi, 1970), p. 72.

130 'Report of the Medical Sub-Conference' [?1909] MP 9.
131 Diocese of Uganda, Medical Sub-Conference minutes, 7 April 1911, MP 9.
132 *Mercy and Truth*, 18 (1914), 302–3; CMS Medical Committee, 12 November 1914, noted by W.D. Foster, Foster papers, RH; H.T.C. Weatherhead, 'Re. Medical education', 4 February 1914, MP 4; Keane to Cook, 23 October 1913, MP 5; W.D. Foster, 'The Mengo Medical School, Uganda', in Sabben-Clare and others, *Health*, ch. 18; Shaw to Cook, 11 March 1914, MP 4.
133 Diocese of Uganda, Medical Sub-Conference minutes, 11 January 1916, MP.
134 *Mercy and Truth*, 22 (1918), 76.
135 Henri Brunschwig, *Noirs et blancs dans l'Afrique Noire Française* (Paris, 1983), pp. 198–200.
136 J. Farley, 'Bilharzia: a problem of "native health", 1900–1950', in David Arnold (ed.), *Imperial medicine and indigenous societies* (Manchester, 1988), p. 189.
137 Generally, see John Iliffe, *Africans: the history of a continent* (Cambridge, 1995), pp. 208–11.
138 Sabben-Clare and others, *Health*, p. 14.
139 See Stanley Joel Reiser, *Medicine and the reign of technology* (Cambridge, 1978); W.F. Bynum, *Science and the practice of medicine in the nineteenth century* (Cambridge, 1994).
140 Clyde, *History*, pp. 20, 28.
141 Juhani Koponen, *Development for exploitation: German colonial policies in mainland Tanzania, 1884–1914* (Helsinki, 1994), p. 464.
142 Uganda, *AMR* 1912 p. 5; Kenya, *AMR* 1913 p. 11, 1916 p. 14.
143 Uganda Medical Registration Ordinance, 31 May 1913, in Charles Griffin (ed.), *Laws of the Uganda Protectorate* (3 vols., Entebbe, 1924), vol. I, p. 485. The same wording was used in Kenya and (after 1918) in Tanganyika.
144 Poonam Bala, *Imperialism and medicine in Bengal* (New Delhi, 1991), pp. 40–53; Adelola Adeloye, 'Some early Nigerian doctors and their contribution to modern medicine in West Africa', *Medical History*, 18 (1974), 275–93; Anne Digby, '"A medical el Dorado"? Colonial medical incomes and practice in the Cape', *Social History of Medicine*, 8 (1995), 475.
145 Wallis to S. of S., 24 December 1912, UNA A.46/935/59.
146 E.g. South Africa, *Blue book on native affairs*, 1910, pp. 105–9.
147 Rechenberg to Bezirksamt Wilhelmstal, 26 June 1910, TNA G.54/1/96.
148 See the valuable reports in 'General-Sanitätsbericht über die Kaiserliche Schutztruppe für Deutsch-Ostafrika für das Berichtsjahr vom 1. April 1895 bis zum 31. März 1896', *Arbeiten aus dem Kaiserlichen Gesundheitsamte*, 14 (1898), 647–67.
149 Clyde, *History*, pp. 4, 10; Dr Glatzel, '3 Monate im Sewa Hadji Hospital zu Dar es Salaam', *Archiv für Schiffs- und Tropen-Hygiene*, 10 (1906), 263–87; 'Wirtschaftsbericht des Sewa-Hadji-Hospitals in Daressalam', 1 April 30 September 1905, TNA G.3/26/76.
150 Ann Beck, *Medicine and society in Tanganyika 1890–1930* (Philadelphia, 1977), p. 48; David F. Clyde, 'Tanzania', in Sabben-Clare and others, *Health*, p. 99; Owen to Partridge, 3 March 1934, TNA SMP 22068/I/4.
151 R. Stanley, 'How the natives of the British East Africa and Uganda Protectorates are medically provided for', *Journal of the RAMC*, 8 (1907), 447; Kenya, *AMR* 1913 p. 62; Uganda, *AMR* 1912 p. 31.

152 Milne to Lumb, 8 January 1913, KNA Health 1/1182.
153 Milne to CS, 21 November 1913, KNA Health 1/8531/2.
154 Uganda, AMR 1910 (typescript in RH Micr. Afr. 609 (4)).
155 Zanzibar, *Annual reports*, 1909–10 p. 42, 1911 p. 79, 1912 p. 10, 1913 p. 13; Ardagh to Lang, 10 February 1888, CMS G3/A5/O/1888/76; 'Freretown Estate', list (1928) in KNA CMS 1/677.
156 August Hauer, *Kumbuke: Erlebnisse eines Arztes in Deutsch-Ostafrika* (Berlin, 1922), p. 100.
157 Clyde, *History*, p. 20.
158 Otto Panse, 'Die Malaria unter den Eingeborenen in Tanga', *Archiv für Schiffs- und Tropen-Hygiene*, 6 (1902), 423.
159 Dr Engeland in *Medizinal-Berichte über die deutschen Schutzgebiete 1909–10*, pp. 41–3.
160 Dr Schörnich in *ibid.*, p. 43.
161 Koponen, *Development*, p. 473; Zanzibar, *Annual reports*, 1909–10 p. 266, 1911 p. 178.
162 Generally, see Harvey G. Soff, 'Sleeping sickness in the Lake Victoria region of British East Africa, 1900–1915', *African Historical Studies*, 2 (1969), 255–68; John Ford, *The role of the trypanosomiases in African ecology* (Oxford, 1971); T. Koerner, P. de Raadt, and I. Maudlin, 'The 1901 Uganda sleeping sickness epidemic revisited', *Parasitology Today*, 11 (1995), 303–6.
163 Zeller, 'Establishment', pp. 163–72; *Medizinal-Berichte über die deutschen Schutzgebiete 1905–6*, p. 64.
164 F.X. Lwamgira, 'The history of Kiziba and its kings', duplicated translation by E.R. Kamuhangire, 1969, part B, pp. 137–8. See also Kleine, *Ein deutscher Tropenarzt*, p. 59.
165 Cook, 'Notes', p. 176.
166 See Ilana Löwy, 'Testing for a sexually transmissible disease, 1907–1910: the history of the Wasserman reaction', in Virginia Berridge and Philip Strong (eds.), *AIDS and contemporary history* (Cambridge, 1993), ch. 4; Richard Gonder, 'Paul Ehrlich und die Tropenmedizin', *Archiv für Schiffs- und Tropen-Hygiene*, 19 (1915), 509.
167 F.J. Lambkin, 'An outbreak of syphilis in virgin soil', in d'Arcy Power and J. Keogh Murphy (eds.), *A system of syphilis: volume II* (Oxford, 1908), pp. 339–55 (quotation on p. 343). See also A.R. Cook, 'Venereal diseases', 14 December 1907, MP 1.
168 G.J. Keane, 'An account of the reform and development of the native hospital organisation of the Uganda Protectorate' [1926] CO 536/140/613.
169 John P. Mitchell, 'Colonial medical schools, III. Makerere College, Uganda', *Health Horizon*, April 1948, p. 9.
170 Uganda, *AMR* 1913 p. 80; Nizaralli Abdulalli Motani, 'The growth of an African civil service in Uganda, 1912–1940', PhD thesis, University of London, 1972, pp. 94–5.

3 THE AGE OF THE TRIBAL DRESSER

1 John Iliffe, *A modern history of Tanganyika* (Cambridge, 1979), pp. 240–50; Ludwig Boell, *Die Operationen in Ost-Afrika: Weltkrieg 1914–1918* (Hamburg, 1951), pp. 158, 427–8.

2 Quoted in Blasius Undole, 'Habari za Wandamba', typescript [?1965] pp. 47–8 (in my possession).
3 Iliffe, *Modern history*, pp. 269–70; J.H. Driberg, *The Lango* (London, 1923), p. 55; Dawson, 'Socio-economic change', ch. 3.
4 Uganda, *AMR* 1915 p. 8, 1914 p. 14.
5 E.g. Uganda, *AMR* 1916 p.17.
6 For one patronising cameo, see Hauer, *Kumbuke*, p. 147.
7 *Military Labour Bureau handbook* [?1917] pp. 25–6 (H.B. Thomas papers, RCS collection, Cambridge University Library).
8 G.J. Keane and D.G. Tomblings, *The African Native Medical Corps in the East African campaign* (London [?1920]), pp. 11–14.
9 *Ibid.*, p. 15.
10 *Ibid.*, pp. 15–16, 19; Odonga, *First fifty years*, p. 15; Annual report for Buganda Province, 1917–18, UNA A.46/431.
11 *Ebifa mu Buganda*, 1917, p. 234.
12 *Standing orders for the African Native Medical Corps* (Dar es Salaam, 1917), in CO 691/19/337.
13 Keane and Tomblings, *ANMC*, pp. 19, 33; W.W. Pike, *Report on medical and sanitary matters in German East Africa 1917* (Nairobi, 1918), in CO 691/19/286.
14 Keane and Tomblings, *ANMC*, p. 37; *Uganda Notes*, April 1919.
15 Y.B.K. Nsubuga Nsibirwa in *Ebifa mu Buganda*, 1917, pp. 234–6.
16 *Kikuyu News*, 65 (November 1917), 1–6. Generally, see Geoffrey Hodges, *The Carrier Corps* (Greenwood, 1986), pp. 176–83.
17 *Target*, 27 June 1976.
18 Kenya, *AMR* 1914 p. 46; Uganda, *AMR* 1919 p. 7; Arthur to his father, 22 March 1918, Arthur papers, EUL.
19 *Ebifa mu Buganda*, 1920, pp. 126–30.
20 *Ibid.*, 1935, p. 186.
21 'Medical students of Mengo Medical School, founded 1916', MP; *The Mission Hospital*, 40 (1936), 184.
22 *Kwetu*, 14 July 1938; Iliffe, *Modern history*, pp. 266, 407.
23 N.J. Westcott, 'An East African radical: the life of Erica Fiah', *JAH*, 22 (1981), 86.
24 Clyde, *History*, pp. 105, 114; *East African Standard*, 26 October 1956; Robert V. Dolbey, *Sketches of the East African campaign* (London, 1918), p. 95.
25 T.O. Ranger, *Dance and society in eastern Africa 1890–1970* (London, 1975), p. 52; *Mambo Leo*, January 1942.
26 *Ebifa mu Buganda*, 1919, p. 115; *Matalisi*, 12 November 1930.
27 For meetings, see *Matalisi*, 10 December 1930, 12 April 1937, 15 October 1943; *Gambuze*, 13 November 1936.
28 Harry Thuku, *An autobiography* (Nairobi, 1970), p. 19.
29 S.L. Kalyesubula in *Matalisi*, 10 December 1930.
30 Arthur to Hooper, 24 March 1918, CMS UP 85/F4.
31 *Gambuze*, October 1931.
32 E.M.K. Mulira in *Uganda Argus*, 7 December 1970.
33 *EAMJ*, 18 (1941–2), 161, and 20 (1943), 355–6.
34 Odonga, *First fifty years*, p.16; *Kikuyu News*, 66 (February 1918), 9–10; Kenya, *AMR* 1921 p. 18.

35 Zanzibar, *AMR* 1925 p. 110, 1926 pp. 228 and 232–3, 1927 pp. 152–3.
36 Standing orders for district dispensaries, Zanzibar, 1928, typescript, Young papers, RH.
37 R.J.K. Tallack, 'Aspects of the public health of the Zanzibar Protectorate', DPH thesis, University of London, 1954, p. 33 (copy in Tallack papers, RH).
38 *Kikuyu News*, 73 (July 1920), 14; *ibid.*, 77 (July 1921), 7; *ibid.*, 80 (June 1922), 22; *Mercy and Truth*, 25 (1921), 97, 145; Kenya, *AMR* 1920 p. 17; Bruce Berman, *Control and crisis in colonial Kenya* (London, 1990), pp. 149–50.
39 Stones to Cook, 6 December 1923, MP 12; *Kikuyu News*, 100 (June 1927), 8; Kenya, *AMR* 1932 pp. 44, 46.
40 Kenya, *AMR* 1932 p. 48.
41 Leader Stirling, *Tanzanian doctor* (London, 1977), p. 21.
42 Tanganyika, *AMR* 1921 pp. 57–9, 1922 p. 82; Kenya, *AMR* 1923 p. 10, 1930 p. 8.
43 J. Japhet in *Habari*, July 1929. For suppression, see Dawson, 'Socio-economic change', pp. 6, 190, 276–7.
44 Tanganyika, *AMR* 1923 p. 172.
45 Alonsi Gonzaga in *Mambo Leo*, May 1928.
46 Tanganyika, *AMR* 1930 p. 6; W.K. Connell, 'The origin and development of bismuth therapy in yaws', *Kenya and East African Medical Journal*, 8 (1931–2), 274.
47 Tanganyika, *AMR* 1926 pp. 10–11, 1930 p. 5.
48 Shircore to CS, 4 May 1929, TNA SMP 12602/I/40.
49 See the comparison in Margery Perham, *East African journey* (London, 1976), p. 151.
50 *Mambo Leo*, June 1928.
51 *Ibid.*, February 1937.
52 C.A. Wiggins, memorandum, enclosed in Morris Carter to S. of S., 9 January 1920, CO 536/99/48; Uganda, *AMR* 1932 p. 8; W. Leslie Webb, 'The subdispensary system in Uganda', *Tropical Diseases Bulletin*, 31 (1934), 366.
53 Uganda, *AMR* 1923 p. 8, 1927 pp. 12 and 80, 1930 p. 14, 1939 p. 22, 1947 p. 18, 1949 p. 30.
54 *Kenya Medical Journal*, 2 (1925–6), 325–6; G.A. MacGregor and W.R.G. Thomas, 'A guide to the rural medical stations of the western region of Tanganyika' [?1951] TNA SMP 12602/IV/395.
55 Menzel, *Die Bethel-Mission*, p. 305; Mary Gibbons, 'Medical training at Minaki', *Central Africa*, 57 (1939), 159–60; Timotheus W.J. Schulpen, *Integration of church and government medical services in Tanzania* (Nairobi, 1975), pp. 47–52.
56 Cook, *Uganda memories*, p. 313; *Report of the CMS Mengo Medical Mission, Kampala, 1933*, p. 30 (copy in RH Micr. Afr. 609 (1)); Diocese of Uganda: Medical Sub-Conference minutes, 28 March 1921, 7 December 1921, 7 July 1926, MP; *The Mission Hospital*, 33 (1929), 175, and 34 (1930), 177.
57 Certificate enclosed in Diocese of Uganda: Medical Sub-Conference minutes 1908–1935, MP.
58 *Ebifa mu Buganda*, 1919, pp. 85–8.
59 'Mengo Medical School: syllabus of training' [?1924] MP 12; E.N. Cook to A.R. Cook, 16 November 1920, MP 9; Turya, 'Which way?' p. 40.

60 *Uganda Church Review*, January 1928; *Mercy and Truth*, 22 (1918), 76.
61 *Uganda Church Review*, January 1928; *Mercy and Truth*, 24 (1920), 139.
62 Diocese of Uganda: Medical Sub-Conference minutes, 10 September 1919, MP.
63 'Mengo Medical School: syllabus of training' [?1924] MP 12.
64 Diocese of Uganda: Medical Sub-Conference minutes, 7 June 1917, 6 January 1921, MP; *Mercy and Truth*, 24 (1920), 157; Mengo medical students to Cook, 17 May 1929, MP 15.
65 *The Mission Hospital*, 43 (1939), 294.
66 'Medical students of Mengo Medical School, founded 1916', register in MP.
67 Foster, *Church Missionary Society*, p. 179; Diocese of Uganda: Medical Sub-Conference minutes, 28 April 1932, MP; Cook, *Uganda memories*, p. 313.
68 Archer to S. of S., 23 April 1923, CO 536/125/144; Uganda, *AMR* 1923 p. 12.
69 Uganda, *AMR* 1924 p. 69; Zeller, 'Establishment', pp. 256–7.
70 *Regulations relating to native staff of the Uganda Medical Service* (1925), CO 536/146/14257/10; Keane, 'An account of the reform' [1926] CO 536/140/613.
71 Tanganyika, *AMR* 1925 p. 1, 1926 p. 25; Clyde in Sabben-Clare and others, *Health*, p. 105.
72 Tanganyika, *AMR* 1926 pp. 9–10, 1940 p. 2; E.D. Pridie, 'Report on the medical and health services of Tanganyika Territory' [1949] Sneath papers, RH.
73 P.A.T. Sneath, 'Memorandum on rural medical services for the information of Executive Council', 6 December 1947, and R. de Z. Hall, 'Development of Native Administration dispensaries' [May 1946] TNA SMP 12602/II/8 and 4A.
74 'Memorandum by the Senior Medical Officer, Lake Province, on the Mwanza Medical School and the medical auxiliary scheme' [1940] TNA SMP 27285/I/1c.
75 A.G. Farr, quoted in P.A.T. Sneath, 'Organisation of rural medical work in the Western Province', 29 January 1945, Sneath papers, RH.
76 Sneath to Mahaffy, 19 July 1948, Sneath papers, RH.
77 Sneath, address to Provincial Commissioners' Conference, 3 June 1946, TNA SMP 12602/II/7; Sneath to SMO, Southern Highlands, 18 September 1947, and Sneath, 'Internal organisation of the Department', 29 January 1945, Sneath papers, RH.
78 Hall, 'Development' [May 1946] and Johnston to CS, 13 December 1946, TNA SMP 12602/II/4A and 42.
79 Pridie, 'Report' [1949] and Surridge to Sneath, 6 March 1950, Sneath papers, RH.
80 Kenya, *AMR* 1924 p. 1.
81 'Dr Hugh Trowell', Trowell papers, RH.
82 Ndirangu, *History*, pp. 35–9; A.D. Williams, 'The provision of hospitals for, and the medical training of, Africans in Kenya', *Kenya Medical Journal*, 3 (1926–7), 46–51.
83 There is no evidence of this.
84 Kenya, *AMR* 1932 pp. 50–1, 1933 p. 51; James H. Sequiera, 'The educational aspect of public health work in the tropics (with special reference to Kenya)', *EAMJ*, 9 (1932–3), 71–2.

85 Trowell, transcribed interview, p. 14, and 'Dr Hugh Trowell', Trowell papers, RH.
86 H.C. Trowell, 'The medical training of Africans', *EAMJ*, 11 (1934–5), p. 347; Kenya, *AMR* 1934 p. 28; Trowell, transcribed interview, pp. 21–3, Trowell papers, RH.
87 *Kikuyu News*, 104 (June 1928), 22, and 71 (January 1920), 5; Stirling, *Tanzanian doctor*, p. 50; 'Medical students of Mengo Medical School, founded 1916', register in MP.
88 See the unusually sensitive account in Friedrich Kroeber, *Der Doktor am Viktoriasee* (Stuttgart, 1950), pp. 151–4.
89 *Mambo Leo*, April 1942; *Kikuyu News*, 139 (March 1937), 11.
90 C.M. Goodfellow papers, RH; *Uganda Herald*, 24 February 1949; J.D. Akwiri, 'Kenya African Medical Staff Union: tour of branches' [April 1955] KNA Health BY/3/37/1.
91 *The Mission Hospital*, 40 (1936), 138, and 41 (1937), 210; 'Summary – Conference of Provincial Medical Officers', November 1945, Sneath papers, RH; A.G. Farr, 'Service in Africa', Farr papers, RH; *Inland Africa*, March 1935; *Sunday News*, 6 March 1977.
92 *The Mission Hospital*, 40 (1936), 178 (on Kaloleni).
93 Kenya, *AMR* 1930 appendix pp. 1–2.
94 Uganda, *AMR* 1931 p. 47, 1934 p. 56.
95 F.M. Mzoo, 'Ugonjwa wa malaria', *Mambo Leo*, March 1936; *Kwetu*, 12 March 1940; D.F. Clyde and F.M. Mzoo, 'Malaria distribution in Tanganyika: part III – the south-east', *EAMJ*, 41 (1964), 7–14.
96 Tanganyika, *AMR* 1938 p. 98; Clyde, *History*, p. 138.
97 Raphaeli Kanyempwe in *Mambo Leo*, January 1945.
98 Perham, *Journey*, p. 86.
99 Clyde, *History*, p. 119; *The Mission Hospital*, 27 (1923), 176; *Mercy and Truth*, 24 (1920), 53.
100 J.M.B. Paul in *Mambo Leo*, May 1937.
101 A.C. Stanley-Smith, 'Sir Albert Cook's legacy', duplicated, 1967, Foster papers, RH.
102 *Mambo Leo*, September 1936 and May 1937; N. Chilton, 'Medical Department, Lake Province: annual report, 1947', TNA 450/1423/18.
103 Mitchell and Butler 693, the first sulphonamide.
104 A.G. Farr, diary, 12 October 1942, Farr papers, RH.
105 Daudi Mfuko, 'My job: VI – an African dispenser in the Zaramo', *Central Africa*, 57 (1939), 171.
106 Zeller, 'Establishment', p. 305; *The Mission Hospital*, 33 (1929), 177.
107 Zakaria Mlela in *Mambo Leo*, February 1946.
108 Ranger, 'Godly medicine', p. 273.
109 J.M. Justino Mpinga in *Mambo Leo*, September 1943.
110 *Uganda Herald*, 20 December 1944.
111 *Who's who in East Africa 1967–68* (Nairobi, 1968), s.v. Gethegi; N. Chilton, 'Medical Department, Lake Province: annual report, 1947', TNA 450/1423/18.
112 K.M.A. Komagi Sanza in *Mambo Leo*, May 1939.
113 Ranger, 'Godly medicine', pp. 271–2.
114 Peter C.W. Gutkind, *The royal capital of Buganda* (The Hague, 1963), pp. 77, 79.

115 This must have been Yusufu Musajawaza's son.
116 Paulo Kiwanuka in *Gambuze*, 11 October 1940.
117 *The Mission Hospital*, 40 (1936), 244. See also *Uganda Argus*, 7 April 1956.
118 Maseno Hospital annual report, 1939, KNA CMS 1/24/34.
119 Perham, *Journey*, p. 151.
120 Trowell, transcribed interview, p. 9, Trowell papers, RH.
121 Pat Holden, *Doctors and other medical personnel in the public health services in Africa 1930–1965* (Oxford, 1984), p. 145.
122 Raphael Liapembile Merera in *Mambo Leo*, November 1929.
123 Tanganyika, *AMR* 1923 p. 45; Yorke to Commissioner of Police (Special Branch), 28 October 1946, UMOH 1/A.
124 *The Mission Hospital*, 34 (1930), 147.
125 Halfani bin Omari in *Mambo Leo*, October 1938.
126 George W.K. Waswa in *Matalisi*, 18 August 1950; *Tanganyika Opinion*, 7 May 1928; D.G. Chenga in *Kwetu*, 31 March and 18 April 1941.
127 Anthony Ulambo in *Kwetu*, 5 February 1941.
128 Downes Shaw to General Secretary, 21 December 1948, KNA CMS 1/501/81; E. Wilson papers, RH.
129 Allen to Smith, 2 October 1936, KNA CMS 1/67/433; *Kwetu*, 6 September 1942; Holden, *Doctors*, p. 32.
130 See, e.g., *Uganda Herald*, 29 May and 27 November 1935, 2 September 1942.
131 *Uganda Herald*, 9 April and 21 May 1941.
132 Evidence of Festo Ndiri in transcript of criminal case no. 1531/33, 12 July 1933, KNA CMS 1/458/178.
133 Paterson, circular, 16 May 1933, KNA CMS 1/458/204; Diocese of Uganda: Medical Sub-Conference minutes, 4 July 1933, MP; [Stones] circular, 25 April 1938, MP 17; F.K. Musoke and others to Governor, 22 June 1942, Cook papers 14/L/20, Wellcome Institute for the History of Medicine.
134 See *Kikuyu News*, 112 (June 1930), 33–5; Church of Scotland, 'Memorandum prepared by the Kikuyu Mission Council on female circumcision', duplicated, 1931 (KNA library).
135 A.G. Farr, diary, 16 March 1943, Farr papers, RH.
136 'Dr Hugh Trowell', Trowell papers, RH.
137 R. Mugo Gatheru, *Child of two worlds* (London, 1964), p. 71.
138 *Ibid.*, p. 78.
139 K.G. Kamukulo in *Gambuze*, October 1931.
140 *Ebifa mu Buganda*, 1927, p. 295.
141 *Habari*, July and August 1929; Zeller, 'Establishment', p. 269.
142 Mitchell, minute, 23 October 1933, TNA SMP 21845/I.
143 E.O.G. Mkali Mpunduki in *Mambo Leo*, March 1941.
144 W.Z. Kitusa in *Habari*, July 1931.
145 A. Katumbi in *Mambo Leo*, May 1928.
146 Juma Sefu in *ibid.*, February 1944.
147 T. Aron Mwambu in *ibid.*, June 1942.
148 *Ibid.*, August 1939.
149 B.R. Mbwana in *ibid.*, November 1938.
150 Abdulla Mohamed in *Habari*, July 1931.
151 Mfuko, 'My job', p. 171.

152 L. Andrea Mzirai in *Mambo Leo*, March 1931.
153 For the sense of threat, see Job C.G. Kuchuchu in *Muigwithania*, November 1928.
154 Abbush M. Mtawa in *Mambo Leo*, September 1936.
155 Quoted in Ranger, 'Godly medicine', p. 267.
156 Translated in *Matalisi*, 5 January 1945, from *Mambo Leo*, November 1941.
157 *Mambo Leo*, August 1943,
158 Kornelio M. Ngaweje in *ibid.*, March 1943.
159 H.M.T. Kayamba, 'African medicines' [?1933] TNA SMP 21845/I/10.
160 *Kwetu*, 16 April 1939.
161 *Mambo Leo*, April 1939. For Ali Ponda, see G.G. Hajivayanis, A.C. Mtowa, and John Iliffe, 'The politicians: Ali Ponda and Hassan Suleiman', in John Iliffe (ed.), *Modern Tanzanians* (Nairobi, 1973), ch. 12.

4 MAKERERE AND ITS STUDENTS, 1923–49

1 See Sonbol, *Creation*, *passim*, esp. p. x; Murray Last and G.L. Chavunduka (eds.), *The professionalisation of African medicine* (Manchester, 1986), pp. 9–10.
2 Motani, 'Growth', pp. 78–88.
3 'Report of the committee appointed to consider the terms of service of native civil servants' [December 1919] UNA A.46/1983/1.
4 Uganda, *AMR* 1919 p. 7.
5 Archer to S. of S., 14 August 1923, CO 536/126/332.
6 For the general history of Makerere, see Margaret Macpherson, *They built for the future: a chronicle of Makerere University College 1922–1962* (Cambridge, 1964).
7 CS to Cook, 8 June 1923, MP 17.
8 Hugh Brindley Owen, 'Medical education in Uganda', *Tropical Diseases Bulletin*, 30 (1933), 660.
9 Uganda, *AMR* 1927 p. 59; Hussey to CS, 29 December 1926, CO 536/147/14350/15.
10 E.R.J. Hussey, *Tropical Africa 1908–1944: memoirs of a period* (London, 1959), pp. 65–7.
11 See Bonner, *Becoming a physician*, *passim*.
12 'Report of a committee appointed by H.E. the Governor to consider a proposal for the establishment of a medical school', 11 June 1927, UNA A.46/2629/1.
13 Uganda, *AMR* 1927 p. 60.
14 Uganda, *AER* 1928 pp. 13, 15; Uganda, *AMR* 1934 p. 6.
15 Uganda, *AMR* 1927 p. 8, 1936 p. 67.
16 *EAMJ*, 13 (1936–7), 356; Adeloye, *African pioneers*, p. 213.
17 Isherwood to CS, 19 August 1929, TNA SMP 13658/I/1; Clyde, *History*, pp. 146–7.
18 'Minutes of the Branch Council, Kenya Branch, British Medical Association', 22 February 1933, RH; Trowell, interview transcript, p. 21, Trowell papers, RH.
19 Uganda, *AMR* 1936 pp. 8–9.

20 Heather Bell, 'Medical research and medical practice in the Anglo-Egyptian Sudan, 1899–1940', DPhil thesis, University of Oxford, 1996, pp. 30, 33, 38.
21 Uganda, *AER* 1926 p. 6; Uganda, *AMR* 1929 p. 65.
22 Kayamba to Mitchell, 7 October 1929, TNA SMP 13658/I/17.
23 Mitchell to Bottomley, 10 January 1936, CO 536/189/40120/I/162.
24 There is a brilliant cameo of de la Warr in Maurice Cowling, *The impact of Hitler* (Cambridge, 1975), pp. 321–2.
25 Great Britain, *Higher education in East Africa*, Colonial no. 142 (London, 1937), pp. 118, 99, 95, 97.
26 O'Brien, minute, 24 May 1939, CO 536/204/40251.
27 Davies to CO, 8 August 1939, CO 536/204/40251/40.
28 Richard Needham, 'A note on the visitation of the Schools of Medicine, Uganda and Nigeria' [April 1940] CO 859/31/4/13.
29 Uganda, *AMR* 1940 p. 11.
30 Odonga, *First fifty years*, p. 68.
31 G.C. Turner, 'Comments upon medical education in Uganda with reference to a report by Sir Richard Needham', 13 September 1941, CO 859/62/3/7.
32 Iliffe, *Modern history*, p. 356.
33 J.E. Goldthorpe, *An African elite: Makerere College students 1922–1960* (Nairobi, 1965), pp. 4, 11; Turner to CS, 23 October 1943, UNA S.88/46/1; Uganda, *AMR* 1946 p. 11.
34 'Uganda Medical School: minutes of the examiners' meeting held at Mulago on 17th December, 1943', KNA Health BY/12/100/1A.
35 Macpherson, *They built*, pp. 45–6.
36 Uganda, *AMR* 1944 p. 2, 1946 p. 11; Macpherson, *They built*, p. 42.
37 *EAMJ*, 23 (1946), 65; Kenya, *AMR* 1945 p. 4; 'Summary of training facilities and syllabus at Mulago Medical School, Uganda' [November 1947] Sneath papers, RH; H.S. de Boer, *Report and recommendations on the post-war development of the medical services of Uganda* (Entebbe, 1944).
38 H.S. de Boer, 'The training of Africans in medicine at Mulago' [?September 1943] KNA Health 1/292/273b.
39 Pedler to Treasury, 24 November 1944, and Hall to Cohen, 4 July 1946, CO 536/213/40251/130 and 69.
40 The issues were posed especially in B.A. McSwiney, 'Report on medical education in Uganda', October 1946, CO 822/127/1/2 (also in KNA Health BY/19/45/52a).
41 Great Britain, *Report of the Commission on Higher Education in the Colonies*, Cmd 6647 of 1945 (London, 1945), p. 63.
42 Adams to Lamont, 30 October 1947, BW 90/4; Extract from the report of the IUC delegation, July 1949, CO 822/127/4/18; Kauntze to McSwiney, 27 August 1946, CO 822/144/3/14B.
43 Waterman to Adams, 6 August 1948, CO 859/156/4/16E; Bernard de Bunsen, 'Makerere College: the University College of East Africa', *Universities Review*, 24 (1951–2), 77.
44 Lamont to Adams, 26 August 1948, BW 90/187/34.
45 Holmes to Adams, 15 April 1948, BW 90/188/27.
46 Holmes to Adams, 13 December 1949, BW 90/1190/41; H. Ogilvie, 'Medical School of Makerere College' [?December 1948] BW 90/187/49A.

47 Holmes to Adams, 28 October 1947, BW 90/16.
48 Galloway to Adams, 21 November 1947, BW 90/16.
49 Potter to Wallace, 25 May 1948, and Wallace to Potter, 1 July 1948, CO 822/127/3/16 and 17.
50 *Makerere*, September 1949, p. 3; de Bunsen to GMC, 8 October 1949, BW 90/1190/13.
51 Zeller, 'Establishment', p. 248.
52 For the Kamba, see Mary Tiffen, Michael Mortimore, and Francis Gichuki, *More people, less erosion* (Chichester, 1994), p. 148. None of the three students from north-eastern Tanganyika known to have sought entry to the medical course at this time (Geldart Mhina, Godfrey Kayamba, and Silvester Mdachi) completed it.
53 J. Muhangi, *Psychiatry in Kenya: new horizons in medical care* (Nairobi, 1980), p. 1.
54 Lwamgira, 'History', part B, pp. 134–5, 143–5; *Matalisi*, 24 May 1933.
55 'Makerere College register, vol. I, 1922–58 (confidential version)', manuscript, s.v. R.J. Kafamba (MUL).
56 *Uganda Argus*, 29 March 1962.
57 *Ibid.*, 31 July 1957; *Matalisi*, 2 January 1942.
58 E.g. George Sembeguya (Kemp to DMS, 5 July 1952, UMOH C.379/13) and Frederick Kalibala (*Matalisi*, 7 January 1949).
59 E.g. Samson Kisekka (Delbert W. Baker, *From exile to Prime Minister* (Washington, 1988), p. 31) and Eria Babumba (*New Vision*, 28 July 1987).
60 B.E. Kipkorir, 'The inheritors and successors: the traditional background to the modern Kenyan African elite', *Kenya Historical Review*, 2 (1974), 143.
61 *Kikuyu News*, 149 (September 1939), 274.
62 *East African Standard*, 28 December 1960; Kipkorir, 'Inheritors', p. 153.
63 *Matalisi*, 2 January 1942; *Uganda Argus*, 10 November 1972; *Weekly Review*, 29 June 1979; *Daily News*, 24 May 1986; Mwanjisi family tree in Goldthorpe papers, RH.
64 D.N. Kiremerwa, application for appointment, 29 June 1966, UMOH C.740/23; *Daily News*, 10 April 1976; 'Professor Swedi A. Mwankemwa: transcript of interview by John Iliffe, Dar es Salaam, 25 July 1995', p. 1 (tape and transcript in University of Dar es Salaam library; transcript in RH); Tanganyika, *AMR* 1942 p. 5; *Uganda Argus*, 6 July 1961.
65 *Makerere College Magazine*, May 1941, p. 45.
66 Note in Goldthorpe papers, RH.
67 'Examiners meeting, December, 1941', KNA Health 1/292/184A; Francis to Director of Education, 5 March 1938, KNA Education 1/935/153.
68 CS to DMS, 18 March 1942, UNA 4161/34.
69 Hussey, minute [13 December 1927] UNA A.46/2371/46.
70 *Makerere College Magazine*, July 1936, p. 6; *Makerere College register 1922–53* (Kampala, 1955), s.v. Y. Okulo.
71 *Matalisi*, 14 January 1938; *Who's who*, s.v. A.M. Odonga.
72 Goldthorpe, *African elite*, p. 28.
73 Zeller, 'Establishment', p. 249; Mitchell to Macdonald, 18 July 1938, CO 822/90/2/68.
74 Uganda, *AER* 1929 p. 42.

75 This was the most common motive among medical assistants in the Belgian Congo: Willy de Craemer and Renée C. Fox, *The emerging physician* (Stanford, 1968), p. 11.
76 J.B. Mugwanya in *Makerere College Magazine*, July 1938, pp. 189–90.
77 Quoted in Zeller, 'Establishment', p. 247.
78 *Medicus*, November 1983, p. 23.
79 Above, p. 63; *Daily News*, 10 April 1976.
80 Mwankemwa, 'Transcript', p. 1.
81 Zeller, 'Establishment', p. 248.
82 F.G. Sembeguya, 'Presidential address 1962: the growth of an indigenous medical profession', *EAMJ*, 41 (1964), 39.
83 Baker, *From exile*, p. 44.
84 S.J. Nkinda, 'Fate of a "dream career"', *Makerere Medical Journal*, 8 (May 1965), 16.
85 J.E. Goldthorpe, 'Past Makerere students: a preliminary survey of present position and status', East African Institute of Social Research conference paper, January 1954; *Makerere College Magazine*, August 1939, p. 278.
86 E.F. Mwaisela, 'The nation's strength: mutual service', *Makerere College Magazine*, December 1940, p. 25.
87 *Ibid.*, July 1936, p. 5; Goldthorpe, *African elite*, p. 3.
88 Baker, *From exile*, p. 39; *Daily News*, 10 April 1976; Turner to Woods, 23 May 1945, Turner papers, RH.
89 Uganda, *AER* 1926 p. 18; de Boer to CS, 12 November 1943, UNA S.88/46/6; Joan Vincent, 'Colonial chiefs and the making of class: a case study from Teso, eastern Uganda', *Africa*, 47 (1977), 151.
90 de Boer to CS, 12 November 1943, UNA S.88/46/6; Note [April 1930] in TNA SMP 13658/I/28; 'Report on the inspection of Makerere College, by the Directors of Education', February 1936, CO 536/189/40120/I/41.
91 Owen, 'Medical education', p. 662; Uganda, *AER* 1929 p. 42; CS to Treasurer, 15 June 1934, UNA 4161/14.
92 'Speech by H.E. the Governor at Makerere on the 21st December, 1935', CO 536/189/40120/I/163.
93 'Student agreement', 3 August 1937, FCB papers 121/1/47, RH; Keane, minute, 17 December 1927, UNA A.46/2371/46.
94 Goldthorpe, *African elite*, p. 54; B.E. Kipkorir, 'The Alliance High School and the origins of the Kenya African elite 1926–1962', PhD thesis, University of Cambridge, 1969, p. 168.
95 Goldthorpe, *African elite*, p. 56.
96 Wilkin to CS, 2 March 1944, TNA SMP 32489/1.
97 D.M. Wako, 'Makerere from many angles', *Makerere College Magazine*, August 1939, p. 278.
98 Simon Senkubuge, 'The work of an African Assistant Medical Officer', *Uganda Teacher's Journal*, 1 (1939), 99
99 *Medicus*, May 1983, p. 1; Kauntze to CS, 31 January 1934, UNA 4161/1; Odonga, *First fifty years*, p. 48.
100 See 'Report on the inspection', February 1936, CO 536/189/40120/I/41.
101 Uganda, *AER* 1925 p. 12.
102 Turner to Woods, 23 May 1945, Turner papers, RH.

103 *Makerere College Magazine*, May 1940, p. 342.
104 Amon J. Nsekela and Aloysius M. Nhonoli, *The development of health services and society in mainland Tanzania* (Nairobi, 1976), p. 46.
105 Turner to DMS, 13 December 1939, KNA Health 1/292/27A; Goldthorpe, *African elite*, pp. 60, 62.
106 *Uganda Herald*, 18 January 1951.
107 Address to Makerere University Medical Students' Association, 23 June 1989, in Syed A.H. Abidi (ed.), *Challenges to leadership in the developing world: speeches of Dr Samson Kisekka* ([?Kampala, 1992]), p. 176.
108 David E. Reiser and David H. Rosen, *Medicine as a human experience* (Rockville, 1985), p. 75.
109 Senkubuge, 'The work', p. 100.
110 *Matalisi*, 25 July 1928; memorandum on Mulago quoted in Grossmith, minute, 19 May 1939, CO 536/204/40251; E.G. Holmes, 'Makerere College Medical School and Mulago Hospital: an appreciation of the present situation', 24 November 1947, BW 90/16.
111 *Uganda Herald*, 24 July 1947.
112 Owen, 'Medical education', p. 661.
113 *Makerere College Magazine*, December 1940, p. 18.
114 Ian McAdam, 'Medical Faculty – the next step', *Makerere Medical Journal*, 11 (November 1967); 8; A.B. Karugaba, 'Undergraduate training at Makerere University Kampala, Uganda in maternal and child health – the changing curriculum', *Uganda Medical Journal*, 7, 1 (April 1990), 13.
115 See, e.g., Renée C. Fox, *Essays in medical sociology* (New York, 1979), pp. 51–77; Howard S. Becker and others, *Boys in white: student culture in medical school* (Chicago, 1961), ch. 6; Joseph W. Lella and Dorothy Pawluch, 'Medical students and the cadaver in social and cultural context', in Margaret Lock and Deborah Gordon (eds.), *Biomedicine examined* (Dordrecht, 1988), pp. 125–53; Frederic W. Hafferty, *Into the valley: death and the socialization of medical students* (New Haven, 1991); Byron J. Good, *Medicine, rationality, and experience* (Cambridge, 1994), ch. 3.
116 Peter H. Sebuwufu, 'Foreword', *Makerere Medical Journal*, 17 (September 1972), 5; A.W. Williams, 'Some Mulago buildings', *Medmak*, 1 (1958), 6–7; J.N.P. Davies, Memoirs, Davies papers, RH.
117 Makerere College, *Faculty of Medicine handbook 1952* (in KNA Health 3/579/73).
118 Owen, 'Medical education', p. 665.
119 Mwankemwa, 'Transcript', p. 2, is revealing on this.
120 *Medicus*, May 1983, p. 1.
121 J.P. Mitchell, 'The Uganda Medical School: its origin and objectives', *Uganda Teacher's Journal*, 1 (1939), 90.
122 Odonga, *First fifty years*, p. 87.
123 A.W. Williams, 'East African notes', typescript, n.d., Williams papers, RH.
124 Odonga, *First fifty years*, p. 79; de Boer to CS, 14 February 1945, UNA 4313/1.
125 J.N.P. Davies, Memoirs, Davies papers, RH.
126 Aloni Lubwama, quoted in Odonga, *First fifty years*, p. 86.
127 B.J. M[ukasa], 'Some aspects of education in the United States', *Makerere College Magazine*, December 1937, pp. 119–22; Kenneth James King, *Pan-*

Africanism and education (Oxford, 1971), pp. 71–2, 228–31, 240–5; *Matalisi*, 20 December 1937.

128 *Uganda Herald*, 27 April 1938. See also Akiki K. Nyabongo, *Africa answers back* (London, 1936) and 'Religious practices and beliefs of Uganda', DPhil thesis, University of Oxford, 1939.

129 *Makerere College Magazine*, December 1938, p. 207, and August 1937, p. 97; *Uganda Church Review*, 1948, p. 24.

130 J.F. Gitau in *Makerere College Magazine*, July 1936, p. 8.

131 Sam K. Mukasa, 'Our neighbours', *ibid.*, April 1938, pp. 169–70.

132 *Ibid.*, November 1936, pp. 36, 49.

133 A.K. Kibaya, 'Native medicines', *ibid.*, April 1937, pp. 82–3.

134 See Mwankemwa, 'Transcript', p. 6.

135 Baker, *From exile*, p. 51.

136 *Matalisi*, 23 January 1942.

137 Baker, *From exile*, pp. 50–1; *Makerere College Newsletter*, 40 (March 1967); 'Makerere register (confidential)', vol. I, s.v. E.S. Lubulwa; *Uganda Argus*, 13 January 1960.

138 C.W. Davies, Comments on aide-mémoire, Davies papers, RH.

139 *Matalisi* substituted *Omusawo* for *Omwami* around 1945.

140 Undated statement by E.F. Mwaisela, FCB papers 121/1/48, RH.

141 Uganda, *AMR* 1927 p. 8; Semple to Paterson, 20 February 1942, KNA Health 1/292/185; D.N. Kiremerwa, pension record 1933–57, UNA 4055/19; Paterson to CS, 7 May 1940, TNA SMP 28540/4b.

142 Motani, 'Growth', p. 244.

143 Uganda Medical Board minutes, 5 April 1963, appendix F, UMOH GCM.4/108; *Makerere College Newsletter*, 49 (December 1974).

144 Uganda Medical Board minutes, 5 April 1963, appendix Cl, UMOH GCM.4/108; Semambo to CMO, 16 October 1962, UMOH GCM.4/88; *Voice of Uganda*, 7 July 1978.

145 *EAMJ*, 41 (1964), 31–2; P.E. Mitchell, diary, 27 April 1939, Mitchell papers, RH.

146 J.C. Likimani, 'Annual medical report 1950 – Narok', KNA Health BY/9/578/13.

147 *Makerere register*, s.v. N.O.P. Edyegu.

148 A.G. Farr, 'Service in Africa', Farr papers, RH.

149 *Kwetu*, 5 November 1940.

150 Minute, 5 August 1944, on Young to CS, 12 July 1944, TNA SMP 29043/32; J.K. Shija, *Surgery in Tanzania* (reprinted, Dar es Salaam, 1990), p. 5.

151 A.G. Farr, 'Service in Africa', Farr papers, RH; *Kwetu*, 5 November 1940.

152 *Kwetu*, 11 June 1941.

153 N. Chilton, 'Medical Department, Lake Province: annual report, 1947', TNA 450/1423/18.

154 J.B. Mtahangarwa, 'Shanwa Hospital annual report 1943', TNA 87/119/I/104A.

155 *Ibid.*

156 A.G. Farr, 'Sukumaland Rural Medical Service: report for 1945', TNA 215/850/II/300.

157 J.B. Mtahangarwa, 'Shanwa Hospital annual report 1944', TNA 87/119/I/113.

158 W.A. Young, 'Annual medical report, Lake Province, 1945', TNA 450/1266/11/1.
159 J.B. Mtahangarwa, 'Shanwa Hospital annual report 1943', TNA 87/119/I/104A.
160 J.B. Mtahangarwa, 'Shanwa Hospital annual report 1944', TNA 87/119/I/113.
161 J.M. [sic] Mutahangarwa, 'Superstition', *Makerere College Magazine*, August 1937, pp. 107–8.
162 A.G. Farr, 'Service in Africa', Farr papers, RH.
163 J.B. Mtahangarwa, 'Shanwa Hospital annual report 1944', TNA 87/119/I/113.
164 R.J. Kafamba, 'Shanwa Hospital – Maswa District: annual medical report 1946', TNA 87/119/I/117.
165 Mutahangarwa to DMS, 25 June 1944, TNA SMP 29043/32A.
166 E.F. Mwaisela, undated statement, FCB papers 121/1/48, RH.
167 A. Mackenzie, 'Annual report of the Western Province, 1944', TNA 63/24/91; 'Annual report Western Province, 1945', TNA 450/1266/27.
168 *Mambo Leo*, July 1947.
169 *Ibid.*, October 1945, April 1946, November 1946, July 1947, August 1944; Thom papers, RH.
170 E.H. Risley, 'Annual report, 1951 – Nzega District', TNA library; Macpherson, *They built*, p. 95.
171 M. Webster, 'Nursing in Uganda – colonial service 1937–1941', Webster papers, RH.
172 *Makerere College Newsletter*, 30 (March 1962).
173 Mitchell, diary, 20 November 1938, Mitchell papers, RH.
174 A.M. Odonga, 'Makerere medical graduates' "good old days"', *Makerere Medical Journal*, 7 (November 1964), 8.
175 Goldthorpe, *African elite*, p. 79. The best description of this world is Erasto A.M. Mang'enya, *Discipline and tears: reminiscences of an African civil servant on colonial Tanganyika* (Dar es Salaam, 1984).
176 Hassan S. Mayala in *Mambo Leo*, October 1945; *Matalisi*, 1 April 1949 and 16 April 1943.
177 Uganda, *Parliamentary debates*, 11 July 1967, col. 764.
178 Minute VI/45 of a meeting of Masai Local Native Councils, n.d. [1945] KNA DC Kajiado 3/4/1/1.
179 *Matalisi*, 1 October 1948, 26 May 1950, 18 August 1950.
180 Uganda, *AMR* 1938 pp. 8, 14; *Uganda Herald*, 3 October 1945.
181 Kiremerwa to DMS, 27 May 1946, UMOH C.740/8.
182 Kiremerwa to DMS, 28 July 1946, UMOH C.740/10.
183 *Matalisi*, 29 December 1950; Muganwa to Lumu, 16 November 1965, UMOH C.379/88; 'Makerere register (confidential)', vol. I, s.v. E.S. Lubulwa; 'Report on deployment of Ugandan MOs since 1980' [?June 1986] UMOH ECM.3/8/III/151.
184 Paterson to Macpherson, 15 August 1947, MUL UZ.35.
185 *Makerere*, May 1947, p. 84; P.W. Hutton, 'Some reflections on medecine [sic] in Uganda 1937–61', Hutton papers, RH.
186 A.W. Williams, 'East African notes', n.d., Williams papers, RH.
187 Medical report on D.N. Kiremerwa, 27 October 1972, UMOH C.740/37.
188 'Meeting held at Government House at 2.30 p.m. on 11 September 1957',

UMOH GCM.6/2/11; 'List of prominent personalities in Uganda', Goldthorpe papers, RH; Uganda Medical Board minutes, 19 November 1959, UMOH GCM.4/22.

189 Uganda Medical Board minutes, 5 April 1963, appendix G, UMOH GCM.4/108; Howell to Dean of Medicine, 24 February 1954, UMOH GCM.6/I/98.

190 Abidi, *Challenges*, p. 325.

191 Mitchell, diary, 30 August 1939, Mitchell papers, RH.

192 Baker, *From exile*, p. 56.

193 Gardner Thompson, 'Colonialism in crisis: the Uganda disturbances of 1945', *African Affairs*, 91 (1992), 615.

194 H.C. Trowell, J.N.P. Davies, and R.F.A. Dean, *Kwashiorkor* (reprinted, New York, 1982), p. xxiv.

195 Trowell, transcribed interview, p.62, Trowell papers, RH.

196 See above, pp. 142–3.

197 Uganda, *AMR* 1936 p. 66; Odonga, *First fifty years*, p. 56.

198 Trowell, transcribed interview, p. 35, Trowell papers, RH.

199 E.M.K. Muwazi, H.C. Trowell, and R.S.F. Hennessey, 'Liver diseases and jaundice in natives of Uganda', *EAMJ*, 19 (1942), 40–66 (quotation on p. 41).

200 E.M.K.Muwazi and H.C. Trowell, 'Neurological disease among African natives of Uganda: a review of 269 cases', *EAMJ*, 21 (1944), 2–19.

201 H.C. Trowell and E.M.K. Muwazi, 'Severe and prolonged underfeeding in African children (the kwashiorkor syndrome of malignant malnutrition)', *Archives of Disease in Childhood*, 20 (1945), 110–16.

202 E.M.K. Muwazi, 'Penicillin in treatment of relapsing fever', *EAMJ*, 23 (1946), 55–64.

203 E.M.K.Muwazi, H.C. Trowell, and J.N.P. Davies, 'Congenital syphilis in Uganda', *EAMJ*, 24 (1947), 152–70 (quotation on p. 152).

204 Holmes to Adams, 28 October 1947, BW 90/16; A.W. Williams, 'East African notes', Williams papers, RH.

205 J.N.P. Davies, I.S. Kadama, and T. D'Souza, 'Pemphigoid eruption following burns', *EAMJ*, 23 (1946), 115–17; A.K. Kibaya, 'Possible case of Crohn's disease in a Rwanda native', *ibid.*, 317–20; J.N.P. Davies, Memoirs, Davies papers, RH.

206 W.H. Kirkaldy-Willis and A.S. Mbuthia, 'Treatment of tuberculosis of bone and joint', *EAMJ*, 23 (1946), 326–44, A.S. Mbuthia and W.H. Kirkaldy-Willis, 'Recent advances in orthopaedics', *EAMJ*, 31 (1954), 235–7.

207 W.A.K. Aruwa, 'A case of relapsing fever in a child of nine days old', *EAMJ*, 27 (1950), 176–7.

208 See David E. Apter, *The political kingdom in Uganda* (2nd edn, Princeton, 1967), chs. 11 and 12.

209 Report of Medical Commission, 30 October 1944, Anti-Slavery Society file G.552, RH. For Mukiibi's affinities, see de Boer to Director of Intelligence and Security, 4 October 1945, UMOH 1/A; Apter, *Political kingdom*, p. 214; Uganda, *Report of the Commission of Inquiry into the Disturbances in Uganda during April 1949* (Entebbe, 1950), p. 109.

210 Mukibi Mwanjale to Trowell, 9 November 1944, Anti-Slavery Society file G.552, RH; Odonga, *First fifty years*, p. 74.

211 See Uganda, *Report of the Commission of Inquiry into the Disturbances which occurred in Uganda during January 1945* (Entebbe, 1945); Thompson, 'Colonialism', pp. 605–24.
212 H.S. de Boer, 'Strike of African employees at Kampala and Mulago Hospitals', 16 January 1945, and Boase, 'Strike – Mulago', 16 February 1945, both in UMOH 1/A.
213 E. Wilson, Memoirs, Wilson papers, RH.
214 Bamundaga to DMS, 19 January 1945, UMOH 1/A.
215 Apter, *Political kingdom*, p. 230.
216 Thompson, 'Colonialism', p. 624.
217 Wiltshire to DMS, n.d., UMOH 1/A.
218 de Boer to Director of Intelligence and Security, 4 October 1945, UMOH 1/A.
219 Odonga, *First fifty years*, p. 74.
220 Director of Security Intelligence to DMS, 14 February 1946, and Robinson to Director of Security Intelligence, 20 February 1946, UMOH 1/A.
221 *Matalisi*, 27 July 1945; Bell to DMS, 16 February 1946, Curtis to Lester, 18 December 1946, Hall to CS, 25 December 1946, and information recorded by C.V. Curtis, 29 December 1946, all in UMOH 1/A.
222 Curtis to Lester, 18 December 1946, UMOH 1/A.
223 Commissioner of Police (Special Branch) to Lester, 11 December 1946, UMOH 1/A.
224 Hall to CS, 25 December 1946, UMOH 1/A.
225 Information recorded by Curtis, 30 December 1946, and Commissioner of Police (Special Branch) to DMS, 21 January 1949, UMOH 1/A.
226 Black to DMS, 16 May 1949, UMOH 1/A.
227 Ladkin to Hennessey, 16 May 1949, UMOH 1/A.
228 See Luise White, '"They could make their victims dull": genders and genres, fantasies and cures in colonial southern Uganda', *American Historical Review*, 100 (1995), 1379–402.
229 Uganda, *Report into Disturbances during 1945*, p. 7; *Uganda Herald*, 19 September 1945.
230 Ladkin to Hennessey, 16 May 1949, UMOH 1/A; *Matalisi*, 26 May 1950.
231 Ladkin to Hennessey, 16 May 1949, and Ladkin to DMS, 16 May 1949, UMOH 1/A; Uganda, *Report into Disturbances during 1949*, p. 32.

5 THE PURSUIT OF PROFESSIONAL STATUS

1 Murray Last, 'The professionalisation of African medicine', in Last and Chavunduka, *Professionalisation*, p. 10.
2 *Uganda Herald*, 16 June 1949.
3 Odonga, *First fifty years*, p. 62; Odonga, 'Makerere graduates', p. 7.
4 'Meeting of the Joint East African Examining Board in Medicine', 25–28 October 1943, CO 822/112/11/1.
5 *Uganda Herald*, 16 June 1949; Kununka to GMC, 15 May 1950, BW 90/1191; Odonga, 'Makerere graduates', p. 8.
6 Kununka to GMC, 15 May 1950, BW 90/1191.
7 'Meeting of the Joint East African Examining Board in Medicine', 25–28

October 1943, CO 822/112/11/1; *Uganda Herald*, 21 February and 9 May 1945; correspondence in FCB papers 125/1B, RH.,

8 Odonga, *First fifty years*, p. 87; Creech Jones to Hinden, 17 December 1946, FCB papers 25/1/287, RH.

9 Odonga, 'Makerere graduates', p. 7.

10 Pridie, minute, 16 October 1950, CO 822/144/3/10; Uganda, *AMR* 1931 p. 12.

11 Kauntze, circular memorandum no. 1426, 6 July 1938, KNA Health 1/292/185A.

12 Minutes of DMS conference, 25–26 September 1946, KNA Health BY/19/45/40; P.A.T. Sneath, 'Case for the Asian and African professional staff based upon 1946 conditions', 27 March 1947, Sneath papers, RH.

13 Kununka to GMC, 15 May 1950, BW 90/1191.

14 S. of S. to Governor of Kenya, 1 July 1946, and minutes of DMS conference, 25–26 September 1946, KNA Health BY/19/45/27 and 40.

15 P. Wyn Harris to Minister of Health and Local Government, 21 April 1948, KNA Health BY/19/45/91.

16 Odonga, *First fifty years*, pp. 97–8; Uganda Medical Practitioners and Dentists Ordinance No. 36 of 1949 (in BW 90/1193).

17 D.N. Kiremerwa, pension record 1933–57, UNA 4055/19.

18 Odonga, *First fifty years*, p. 93; P. Rogers and E.L. Scott, 'Differential salaries in East Africa', November 1952, CO 822/284/12.

19 Great Britain, *Report on Higher Education*, p. 58.

20 'Minutes of the 409th meeting of the Colonial Advisory Medical Committee', 16 April 1940, CO 859/31/4/9.

21 Henry Tidy, 'Report to the General Medical Council on a visitation of Makerere College Medical School', January 1950, CO 822/144/3/7. On Tidy's visit, see also the correspondence in BW 90/1191.

22 Holmes to Adams, 9 January 1950, BW 90/1191.

23 Tidy to Pridie, 25 September 1950, CO 822/144/3/7. This was confirmed by *Minutes of the General Medical Council*, 1957, p. 6.

24 'GMC: Executive Committee, May, 1950', memorandum by W.J. Dilling: BW 90/1191.

25 Tidy to de Bunsen, 31 January 1950, BW 90/1191/3.

26 Adams to de Bunsen, 8 August 1950, BW 90/1192/34.

27 Kununka to GMC, 27 April and 15 May 1950, and Kadama to GMC, 25 May 1950, BW 90/1191

28 I infer this from its failure to refute several of Tidy's criticisms, e.g. regarding the predominance of tropical diseases.

29 Kununka to GMC, 15 May 1950, BW 90/1191.

30 Kafero and Onyango to S. of S., 1 May 1951, BW 90/1195.

31 Odonga, *First fifty years*, p. 62; Zeller, 'Establishment', p. 244.

32 Adams to de Bunsen, 6 November 1950, BW 90/1193.

33 Hall to Cohen, 19 March 1951, CO 822/144/4/4.

34 T.H. Davey, 'Registration of the Makerere Medical Diploma in East Africa', 24 September 1951, BW 90/1195.

35 Davey to Vowles, 14 August 1951, BW 90/1195.

36 Campbell to Carr-Saunders, 22 August 1951, de Bunsen to Campbell, 5

September 1951, Trim to de Bunsen, 11 October 1951, and Howell to de Bunsen, 27 October 1951, BW 90/1195.

37 E.R. Boland, J.M. Graham, and A.J. McNair, 'General Medical Council: Visitation of Makerere College Medical School, 1951', CO 822/532/44.

38 Cohen to Rogers, 8 July 1952, CO 822/532/43.

39 Hennessey, 'Notes on the recommendations of the Faculty of Medicine on the report of the GMC visitors', 6 November 1952, UMOH GCM.6/I/1.

40 *Ibid.*; Hicks to DMS, 8 March 1954, KNA Health 3/579/167; Anderson to Likimani and others, 19 February 1953, KNA Health 3/579/99.

41 *Uganda Argus*, 8 June 1956; J.K. Hunter, safari note, 10 December 1953, UMOH GCM.6/I/79; Kyalwazi and Semambo to IUC, 21 October 1953, BW 90/1196; note for Mr Gayward [May 1956] UMOH GCM.6/I/134(I).

42 Board of Assessors to DMS, 14 April and 25 November 1954, UMOH GCM.6/I/114 and 130; Galloway to DMS, 25 June 1955, KNA Health BY/36/7/108.

43 Frazer Committee minutes, 2 November 1955, C.D. Williams papers 19/E/3/2, Wellcome Institute for the History of Medicine.

44 Uganda, *Proceedings of the Legislative Council*, 17 December 1956, col. 37.

45 *Ibid.*, 18 December 1956, col. 77.

46 *Ibid.*, col. 86.

47 Sembeguya, 'Presidential address', p. 40; Goldthorpe, *African elite*, p. 13.

48 Uganda, *AMR* 1959–60 p. 3; *New Vision*, 16 September 1996.

49 Holden, *Doctors*, p. 168; Anderson to Bozman, 5 July 1954, KNA Health BY/36/7/28.

50 Flood to O'Brien, 27 December 1939, and Kauntze to O'Brien, 9 March 1940, CO 536/207/40267/16 and 8; *Munno*, 13 August 1964.

51 *Uganda Argus*, 19 April 1963.

52 Turner to Perham, 12 June 1945, Turner papers, RH; Williams to Adams, 15 July 1946, BW 90/2.

53 Sheldon to Adams, 2 February 1949, BW 90/222/33. See also A.W. Williams, 'Report on facilities for postgraduate training in Great Britain for African Medical Officers', March 1947, BW 90/2.

54 Extract from DMS conference [1947] BW 90/2.

55 *Makerere*, December 1947, p. 57.

56 *Matalisi*, 21 October 1949; Uganda, *AMR* 1950 p. 45; 'Makerere register (confidential)', vol. I, s.v. J.C. Likimani.

57 DMS to Director of Education, 11 June 1956, UMOH C.740/20.

58 Ouko to DMS, 13 May 1952, KNA Health BY/19/45/157/1; *Who's who*, s.v. William Ouko.

59 Odonga, *First fifty years*, pp. 132, 144; I.W.J. McAdam, 'Presidential address', *EAMJ*, 35 (1958), 207.

60 Odonga, *First fifty years*, p. 104; Uganda, *AMR* 1951 p. 77; *Uganda Herald*, 5 January 1952.

61 Clyde, *History*, p. 147; Uganda Medical Board minutes, 5 August 1960, UMOH GCM.4/42.

62 Uganda, *AMR* 1952 p. 60, 1953 p. 60; Uganda, *Medical and health services in Uganda* (Entebbe, 1956), p. 53,

63 'Record of interview granted by H.E. to representatives of the Makerere Medical Graduates Association', 19 March 1953, UMOH GCM.6/2/5.
64 *Uganda Herald*, 21 February 1953 and 8 July 1954; D.N. Kiremerwa, pension record 1933–57, UNA 4055/19.
65 Uganda, *Medical and health services*, p. 97; 'Brief for H.E. the Governor', 11 September 1957, UMOH GCM.6/2/7.
66 'The KAMSA Newsletter', August 1957, KNA Health BY/3/37/34; J.E. Goldthorpe, note on visit to Nairobi, 2 January 1960, Goldthorpe papers, RH.
67 Clyde, *History*, p. 159.
68 Uganda, *Medical and health services*, pp. ii, 90–1, 94–5, 98, 107, 177.
69 MMGA evidence to Frazer Committee, Kampala, 4 November 1955, C.D. Williams papers 19/E/3/2, Wellcome Institute for the History of Medicine.
70 Uganda, *Medical and health services*, p. 79.
71 Uganda, *Proceedings of the Legislative Council*, 7 June 1956, col. 95.
72 Uganda, *Statement by the Protectorate Government on the Report of the Committee on Medical and Health Services in Uganda*, Sessional Paper No. 1 of 1956/57 (Entebbe, 1956), pp. 28–9; Uganda, *AMR* 1959–60 p. 2.
73 Bernard de Bunsen, *Adventures in education* (Kendal, 1995), p. 131.
74 President's address to the General Council, 28 May 1957, *Minutes of the GMC*, 1957, pp. 6–7.
75 Paul ? to Maxwell, 10 June 1957, BW 90/190.
76 *Minutes of the GMC*, 1958, pp. 111–12; *East African Standard*, 18 March 1964.
77 J.C. Likimani, 'Annual medical report 1950 – Narok', KNA Health BY/9/578/13.
78 J.C. Likimani, 'Annual medical report 1954 – Kajiado', KNA Health BY/9/450/5.
79 See esp. J.C. Likimani, 'Annual report, 1957' on Kajiado, KNA Health BY/9/464/3.
80 Uganda, *Parliamentary debates*, 29 March 1963, col. 369.
81 W, Kahugu, 'Presidential address', *EAMJ*, 51 (1974), 2.
82 M.R. Migue, 'Annual report: Kajiado District Hospital – 1960', KNA Health BY/9/484/6.
83 T.K. Evelia, 'Annual medical report, Kilifi District, 1962', KNA Health BY/9/488/14.
84 D.B. Byaruhanga, 'Treatment and control of leprosy in Uganda with special reference to the Kingdom of Toro', DPH thesis, University of St Andrews (Dundee), 1962–3, pp. 100c, 133.
85 Eria M. Bahumba, 'An African patient', *EAMJ*, 31 (1954), 373–6.
86 W. Ouko, 'Discussions on approaches to the African mind in effecting health education and hygiene matters (health education and the African)', *EAMJ*, 37 (1960), 167–70.
87 N. Chilton, 'Medical Department, Lake Province: annual report, 1947', TNA 450/1423/18.
88 See Priscilla Copeland Reining, 'The Haya: the agrarian system of a sedentary people', PhD thesis, University of Chicago, 1967, pp. iv, 85–92, 304.
89 C.V. Mtawali, 'A health campaign in Tanganyika Territory', *Community Development Bulletin*, 2 (1951), 54–6.

90 This account is based on B.H. Omondi, 'Annual report, District Hospital Kerugoya, 1959', KNA Health BY/9/479/1.
91 W.S. Haynes, 'Port Reitz Chest Hospital and Infectious Diseases Hospital annual report for 1960', KNA Health BY/9/483/16.
92 G.S. Nelson and Y.B. Semambo, 'The treatment of tropical ulcers in the West Nile District of Uganda', *EAMJ*, 33 (1956), 189–202.
93 Frazer Committee, minutes of evidence, Soroti, 4 September 1955, C.D. Williams papers 19/E/3/2, Wellcome Institute for the History of Medicine.
94 E.S. Atieno-Odhiambo, 'The formative years, 1945–55', in B.A. Ogot and W.R. Ochieng' (eds.), *Decolonization and independence in Kenya 1940–93* (London, 1995), p. 33; J.E. Goldthorpe, Notes on tour, Mbale, 14 March 1954, Goldthorpe papers, RH.
95 R.J. Southall, *Parties and politics in Bunyoro* (Kampala, 1972), p. 8; Cohen to Rogers, 23 May 1952, CO 822/285/1.
96 Odonga, *First fifty years*, p. 111; Muganwa to Lumu, 16 November 1965, UMOH C.379/38.
97 Sembeguya to Prime Minister, 4 October 1965, UMOH C.379/37; DDMS to Governor, 10 September 1957, UMOH GCM. 6/2/9.
98 *Makerere College Newsletter*, 45 (December 1970).
99 *Ibid.*, 24 (March 1959).
100 C.L. Ssali, 'A country practitioner's difficulties', *Medmak*, 1 (1958), 35.
101 J.E. Goldthorpe, Diary of tour, Toro, 1 February 1954, Goldthorpe papers, RH.
102 Goldthorpe, *African elite*, p. 58.
103 T.H. Davey, 'Registration of the Makerere Medical Diploma in East Africa', draft, 24 September 1951, BW 90/1195; 'Note of discussion at Government House on 18 March 1953', UMOH GCM.6/2/5.
104 For Katwe, see *Uganda Empya*, 4 June 1953; Gutkind, *Royal capital*, pp. 240–1; Apter, *Political kingdom*, pp. 239–42.
105 *Uganda Herald*, 15 September 1954; *Uganda Argus*, 8 August 1964.
106 J.E. Goldthorpe, Diary of tour, Masaka, 26 May 1952, Goldthorpe papers, RH.
107 *Uganda Argus*, 1 June 1956.
108 J.C. Deans, 'Report and valuation – Dr Babumba's Nursing Home', 30 June 1966, and N. Kanyarutoke, 'Dr Babumba's Nursing Home', 14 June 1966, UMOH GCD.11/22 and 27; *Munno*, 22 August 1964.
109 *Uganda Argus*, 5 January 1962.
110 J.E. Goldthorpe, Notes on tours, Nairobi, 2 January 1960, Goldthorpe papers, RH.
111 *East African Standard*, 1 April 1960; *Weekly Review*, 17 January 1977.
112 *EAMJ*, 37 (1960), 297–8.
113 Ssali, 'Country practitioner's difficulties', p. 37.
114 *EAMJ*, 37 (1960), 297.
115 See Uganda Medical Board minutes in UMOH GCM.4.
116 *Uganda Argus*, 12 December 1962; *Uganda Empya*, 6 May 1953; *EAMJ*, 37 (1960), 298.
117 Sembeguya to Prime Minister, 29 January 1966, UMOH GCD.11/13.

118 Sembeguya to MOH, 31 May 1966, UMOH GCD.11/14; Abidi, *Challenges*, p. xxiv.

119 Buganda, 'Annual report: medical and health services, 1961', Albert Cook Library, Mulago.

120 Buganda, 'Annual report: medical and health services 1962', MP.

121 Judith Listowel, *The making of Tanganyika* (London, 1965), ch. 18; Pease to her parents, 13 January 1951, Pease papers, RH.

122 *Daily News*, 19 January 1979; Mwanjisi to Chairman, TANU, 1955, TANU 107 (see Iliffe, *Modern history*, p. 578); *Daily News*, 11 March 1988.

123 Muthoni Likimani, *Passbook number F.47927: women and Mau Mau in Kenya* (Basingstoke, 1985), p. 161.

124 B.H. Omondi, 'Annual report – 1954', KNA Health BY/9/448/12; E.P. Rigby, 'Annual report of King George VI Hospital 1953', KNA Health BY/9/442/7; Kenya, *AMR* 1954, p. 8.

125 'Monthly report on progress and policies: Medical Department – October, 1954', KNA Health BY/9/574/13; Kenya, *AMR* 1954 p. 38; E.P. Rigby, 'Annual report of King George VI Hospital 1953', KNA Health BY/9/442/7.

126 Kenya, *AMR* 1952 p. 2; E. de M. Connett, 'Medical annual report Narok 1953', KNA Health BY/9/445/9.

127 *Weekly Review*, 21 April 1975 and 17 January 1977; Michael Chege, 'A tale of two slums: electoral politics in Mathare and Dagoretti', *Review of African Political Economy*, 20 (January 1981), 84–5.

128 *East African Standard*, 20 January and 28 February 1961, 28 and 31 May 1963; Chege, 'Tale', p. 78.

129 Cherry Gertzel, *Party and locality in northern Uganda, 1945–1962* (London, 1974), pp. 35, 61.

130 Southall, *Parties*, pp. 8, 25, 28.

131 *Makerere College Newsletter*, 17 (September 1955); Apter, *Political kingdom*, pp. 315–16.

132 *Uganda Argus*, 6 September 1955.

133 Uganda, *Proceedings of the Legislative Council*, 22 September 1955, col. 39.

134 *Ibid.*, 24 September 1955, col. 124.

135 *Ibid.*, 11 January 1956, col. 53.

136 Kenneth Ingham, *Obote: a political biography* (London, 1994), p. 37.

137 Uganda, *Proceedings*, 24 April 1956, col. 2.

138 *Ibid.*, 6 June 1956, cols. 48–9.

139 *Ibid.*, 19 October 1956, cols. 170–3.

140 See above, pp. 118–19.

141 *Uganda Argus*, 23 November 1957, 7 December 1957, 2 December 1958, 2 and 17 March 1959.

142 *Ibid.*, 24 September and 8 October 1960.

143 *Ibid.*, 11 November and 5 and 28 December 1961.

144 *Ibid.*, 3 March 1962, 26 February 1962, 26 April 1962, 1 May 1962.

145 *Ibid.*, 28 December 1961.

146 *Ibid.*, 25 March 1961, 18 December 1961, 27 April 1962.

147 Correspondence in W.K. Hancock papers (Buganda file 24), Institute of

Commonwealth Studies, London; *Uganda Argus*, 11 and 28 July 1962; Southall, *Parties*, pp. 38–9.

148 *Uganda Argus*, 10 May 1962.

149 *New Vision*, 28 July 1987.

6 THE TRANSFER OF POWER

1 General Notice 1062 of 16 October 1952, CO 822/2690/1/appendix 3.

2 DDMS, 'Meeting held at Government House at 2.30 p.m. on 11 September 1957', UMOH GCM.6/2/11; *Uganda Argus*, 13 January 1960.

3 Uganda, *Future developments in the public service of Uganda*, Sessional Paper No. 2 of 1961 (Entebbe, 1961), p. 8; Cartland to Minister of Finance, 21 December 1961, UMOH GCI.2/49.

4 *Who's who*, s.v. I.S. Kadama; C.W. Davies, comments on aide-mémoire, Davies papers, RH.

5 'Ministry of Health progress report since independence' [April 1964] UMOH GCR.16/13.

6 Richard M. Titmuss and others, *The health services of Tanganyika* (London, 1964), p. 71.

7 Cranford Pratt, *The critical phase in Tanzania 1945–1968* (Cambridge, 1976), pp. 91–2, 105–8, 121–5.

8 *Daily News*, 10 April 1976 and 25 March 1989.

9 Craig to Director of Establishments, 6 April 1960, KNA Health BY/19/21/93; Kenya, *Report on the working of the Civil Service Commission for the year 1961* (Nairobi, 1962), pp. 1, 8.

10 *East African Standard*, 12 December 1963.

11 *Ibid.*, 4 September 1962; Extract from minutes of the Kenya Council of Ministers, 19 September 1962, CO 822/2693/49; above, p. 171.

12 Kenya, *The National Assembly: House of Representatives: official report*, 13 October 1965, col. 937.

13 Clyde, *History*, p. 169; *Who's who*, s.v. S.B. Asea.

14 Zanzibar, *AMR* 1955 p. 14; J. de Zulueta, G.W. Kafuko, A.W.R. McCrae, J.R. Cullen, C.K. Pedersen, and D.F.B. Wasswa, 'A malaria eradication experiment in the highlands of Kigezi (Uganda)', *EAMJ*, 41 (1964), 102–20; report on smallpox eradication in East Africa [1985] UMOH GCP.16; below, ch. 10.

15 Raphael Owor, 'Foreword', *Makerere Medical Journal*, 24 (October 1978), 1.

16 T. Farnworth Anderson, 'Presidential address to the Kenya branch of the British Medical Association', *EAMJ*, 38 (1961), 364; Kenya, *AMR* 1957 p. 2; K.V. Adalja, 'The development of the medical services in Kenya', *EAMJ*, 39 (1962), 114; *EAMJ*, 36 (1959), 443.

17 Oscar Gish, *Planning the health sector: the Tanzanian experience* (London, 1975), pp. 71, 186; Meredeth Turshen, *The political ecology of disease in Tanzania* (New Brunswick, 1984), p. 164.

18 Uganda, *Medical and health services*, pp. 53, 86.

19 John A. Carman, *A medical history of the Colony and Protectorate of Kenya: a personal memoir* (London, 1976), p. 13; 'Distribution of private medical practitioners in comparison with the non-native population' [1947] Sneath papers, RH.

20 Correspondence in KNA Health BY/11/100 and BY/1/261.
21 Kenya, *AMR* 1959 p. 2; *Makerere College Newsletter*, 38 (March 1966); *EAMJ*, 56 (1979), 461–2, 467–8.
22 *EAMJ*, 31 (1954), 294, 350, 570; 'Brief for H.E. the Governor', 11 September 1957, UMOH GCM.6/2/7; Uganda Medical Board minutes in UMOH GCM.4.
23 Uganda Medical Board minutes, 19 October 1962, UMOH GCM.4/95.
24 Uganda, *Parliamentary debates*, 18 February 1963, col. 415; Uganda Medical Board minutes, 30 January 1964, UMOH GCM.4/113.
25 Muganwa to Lumu, 16 November 1965, Lumu to Muganwa, 7 October 1965, and Pincombe to MOH, 14 May 1966, UMOH C.379/38 and 40.
26 *Uganda Argus*, 17 July 1968; *Uganda Practitioner*, 2 (1969), 3–6.
27 N.P.H. Milner, 'Safari Masaka and Western Region', 28 March 1963, UMOH RPB.5/9.2.
28 See Harry Eckstein, *Pressure group politics: the case of the British Medical Association* (London, 1960); Terence J. Johnson and Marjorie Caygill, 'The British Medical Association and its overseas branches: a short history', *Journal of Imperial and Commonwealth History*, 1 (1972–3), 303–29.
29 J.N.P. Davies, 'The history of the Uganda branch of the British Medical Association, 1913 to 1932', *EAMJ*, 31 (1954), 93–5; BMA (Uganda Division) minutes, 23 December 1914 [?1913] MP 7; Johnson and Caygill, 'BMA', p. 309.
30 Bottomley to Craig, 7 May 1919, T1/12472/4756/42927. For the negotiations, see *British Medical Journal*, 1920–1.
31 *British Medical Journal*, 1926/1, supplement, pp. 9–10, 27–8, 175.
32 Maclennan to Minister for Health and Local Government, 7 June 1949, and Drury to Maclennan, 16 June 1949, KNA Health BY/38/38/173 and 178.
33 E.g. Crawford to DMS, 28 September 1957, UMOH GCA.3/1.
34 Andrew Hicks, 'Forty years of the British Medical Association (Kenya Branch)', *EAMJ*, 38 (1961), 46.
35 Microfilm in RH seen by the kindness of Dr M.G. Redley.
36 BMA (Kenya Branch) Council minutes, 18 April 1934, 8 February 1939, 21 June 1939, 5 June 1940, RH; Hicks, 'Forty years', p. 46.
37 BMA (Kenya Branch) Council minutes, 3 April 1940, RH; *EAMJ*, 36 (1959), 186.
38 *EAMJ*, 29 (1952), 79.
39 Davies, 'History', p. 98; *EAMJ*, 18 (1941–2), 318; *ibid.*, 20 (1943), 128; *ibid.*, 29 (1952), 492; Kununka to GMC, 15 May 1950, BW 90/1191.
40 Roy Billington, 'The story of the Uganda Medical Association', *Makerere Medical Journal*, 8 (May 1965), 22–4; *Uganda Argus*, 22 December 1961; A.M. Odonga, 'Presidential address', *EAMJ*, 42 (1965), 171; *Uganda Practitioner*, 1 (1968), 1–4, 35–6, and 2 (1969), 7; *East African Standard*, 10 March 1970
41 *East African Standard*, 10 August 1960, 7–8 July 1961; A. Hicks, 'Notice of the inaugural meeting of the Medical Association of Kenya to be held on Friday May 10th, 1963', KNA Health BY/3/20/6; *EAMJ*, 41 (1964), 302.
42 Ramniklal Devshi Shah, 'The Kenya Medical Association', *EAMJ*, 53 (1976), 725–6; above, pp. 194–5.
43 *EAMJ*, 40 (1963), 587–8; above, p. 209.
44 Amos O. Odenyo, 'Professionalisation and change: the emergent Kenyan

lawyer', duplicated, City University of New York, n.d., pp. 12–14 (KNA library); *Nairobi Law Monthly*, 61 (February 1996), 31.

45 Odonga, *First fifty years*, p. 159.

46 'Minutes of a Council meeting of the BMA (Kenya Branch)', 12 September 1961, KNA Health BY/3/19/26; Terence J. Johnson and Marjorie Caygill, *Community in the making: aspects of Britain's role in the development of professional education in the Commonwealth* (London, 1972), pp. 250–2.

47 See esp. Nsekela and Nhonoli, *Development*, pp. 36, 55.

48 *Uganda Argus*, 1 October 1960; Uganda, *AMR* 1960–1 p. 48; *Tanganyika Standard*, 20 October 1960.

49 Craig to Establishments Division, 9 December 1960, KNA Health BY/19/89; 'Medical education with particular reference to the needs of Kenya' [?1962] A.W. Williams papers, RH.

50 Makerere Medical Faculty Board, 'Statement on the quinquennial estimates of Makerere College Medical School', 20 July 1960, MUL UZ.35.

51 Paterson, in Mitchell, diary, 21 August 1936, Mitchell papers, RH.

52 Kenya, *AMR* 1957 p. 3; T.F. Anderson, 'Memorandum on the establishment of a Medical Training School in Nairobi' [10 July 1956] KNA Health BY/19/51/70/1; Aird to de Bunsen, January 1961, and Aird to McAdam, 27 February 1961, BW 90/139/12 and 15.

53 A.W. Williams, 'Chief Medical Officers' Conference, Nairobi, 13 September 1962', Williams papers, RH; de Bunsen to Maxwell, 20 March 1961, BW 90/139.

54 One of the earliest is H.G. Kayamba to African Association, Dodoma, 21 April 1944, Hassan Suleiman papers 54, TNA.

55 *Uganda Argus*, 29 November 1955.

56 Roger Southall, *Federalism and higher education in East Africa* (Nairobi, 1974), pp. 36–7.

57 *Ibid.*, pp. 53–71.

58 Fendall to Cambournac, 12 July 1963, KNA Health BY/12/36/2.

59 Southall, *Federalism*, p. 74; Kenya, *AMR* 1966 p. 1.

60 Southall, *Federalism*, pp. 75–8.

61 Roger J. Southall, 'The politics of medical higher education in East Africa', *SSM*, 6 (1972), 422.

62 *Tanganyika Standard*, 30 December 1961; A.M. Rankin, 'Dar es Salaam School of Medicine – the first five years', *Dar es Salaam Medical Journal*, 1, 1 (September 1968), 3–4.

63 'Minutes of the DMSs' conference,' 13–14 September 1962, UMOH GCC.5/3/1.

64 Sembeguya, 'Presidential address', p. 44.

65 Fendall, diary, 28 August 1965, Fendall papers, RH; Hilary P. Ojiambo, 'Presidential address: new perspectives in medical education in Middle Africa', *EAMJ*, 45 (1968), 84.

66 A.W. Williams notebook, 30–31 August 1962, Williams papers, RH. See also Nsekela and Nhonoli, *Development*, pp. 89–93, who blame it on expatriates.

67 Rankin, 'Dar es Salaam School of Medicine', pp. 3–4; Tanzania, *AMR* 1966, part 1, pp. 2, 43; *Sunday News*, 4 March 1984.

68 Hobokela Mbelile, *Storm in a teacup* (Dar es Salaam, 1990).

69 Nsekela and Nhonoli, *Development*, p. 81; 'Medical education with particular reference to the needs of Tanganyika', June 1962, A.W. Williams papers, RH.
70 Nsekela and Nhonoli, *Development*, pp. 77–8; *Daily News*, 21 November 1989; Clyde, *History*, p. 201.
71 M.P. Mandara, 'Health services in Tanzania: a historical overview', in G.M.P. Mwaluko, W.L. Kilama, P.M. Mandara, M. Murru, and C.N.L. Macpherson (eds.), *Health and disease in Tanzania* (London, 1991), p. 5; W.K. Chagula and E. Tarimo, 'Meeting basic needs in Tanzania', in Kenneth W. Newell (ed.), *Health by the people* (Geneva, 1975), p. 160.
72 Kenya, *AMR* 1960 p. 35, 1966 p. 94. 'Parchment curtain' comes from de Craemer and Fox, *Emerging physician*, p. 6.
73 Kenya, *National Assembly*, 1 August 1963, col. 1662.
74 'Medical education in relation to the needs of Uganda' [1962] A.W. Williams papers, RH.
75 Quoted in E.B. Turya, 'Practical therapeutics: lessons for primary health care from experience with medical assistants in Uganda', *EAMJ*, 62 (1985), 525.
76 *Uganda Argus*, 22 May 1963.
77 Turya, 'Which way?' pp. 147, 152, 180.
78 Kenya, *The economic development of Kenya* (Nairobi, 1963), pp. 174–5; N.R.E. Fendall, 'Planning health services in developing countries', *Public Health Reports*, 78 (1963), 978–9.
79 World Bank, *The economic development of Uganda, October 1961* (Entebbe, n.d.), p. 312.
80 Titmuss and others, *Health services*, pp. 28, 88; *Tanganyika Standard*, 20 May 1961.
81 E.M. Nordberg, 'The true disease pattern in East Africa: part 2', *EAMJ*, 60 (1983), 533; W.J.M. Evans in Clyde, *History*, p. 206; J.N.P. Davies, Memoirs, Davies papers, RH.
82 Latimer K, Musoke, 'An analysis of admissions to the paediatric division, Mulago Hospital in 1959', *Archives of Disease in Childhood*, 36 (1961), 314; Tanganyika, *AMR* 1959, part 2; Tanzania, *AMR* 1964, part 2, p. 14.
83 'Dar es Salaam Hospitals Group: annual report 1957', TNA 450/1614/12A; Kenya, *AMR* 1959 p. 23.
84 *East African Standard*, 19 April 1963 and 16 March 1964; Uganda, *AMR* 1959–60 p. 2.
85 See Pridie to Anderson, 10 December 1952, KNA Health BY/18/14/97.
86 *East African Standard*, 22 May 1963; *Uganda Argus*, 18 March 1963.
87 Uganda, *AMR* 1934 pp. 61–4; C.W. Davies, comments on aide-mémoire, Davies papers, RH; Kenya, *AMR* 1946 p. 1.
88 J.A. Ouya, 'Annual medical report: Elgon Nyanza, Bungoma, 1962', KNA Health BY/9/496/8.
89 N.R.E. Fendall, 'Health centres in Kenya', *EAMJ*, 37 (1960), 179.
90 Fendall, 'Planning', p. 980.
91 Maurice King (ed.), *Medical care in developing countries* (Nairobi, 1966), ch. 2, p. 14; Kenya, *Economic development*, p. 170.
92 *Tanganyika Standard*, 1 June 1961; Uganda, *AMR* 1959–60 pp. 2, 35; Fendall, diary, 11 September 1965, Fendall papers, RH.
93 Tanganyika/Tanzania, *Annual medical reports*, 1954–67.

94 *New Vision*, 14 October 1996.
95 M.F. Natkanski, 'Poliomyelitis in Tanganyika: some epidemiological aspects', DPH thesis, Usher Institute, Edinburgh, 1959, p. 48; B. Kaur and D. Metselaar, 'Poliomyelitis in Kenya: the 1965–1966 epidemic', *EAMJ*, 44 (1967), 74–82.
96 Charles C. Hughes and John M. Hunter, 'Disease and "development" in Africa,' *SSM*, 3 (1970), 458.
97 Clyde, *Malaria*, pp. 58, 103.
98 World Bank, *World development report 1993: investing in health* (New York, 1993), p. 29.
99 *Kikuyu News*, 192 (June 1950), 1093.
100 Frazer Committee minutes, 3 November 1955, C.D. Williams papers 19/E/3/2, Wellcome Institute for the History of Medicine.
101 L.P. Gerlach, 'Some basic Digo conceptions of health and disease', in East African Institute of Social Research, *One-day symposium*, p. 25.
102 Susan Reynolds Whyte, 'The power of medicines in East Africa', in van der Geest and Whyte, *Context*, p. 220.
103 *Uganda Argus*, 9 December 1961; R. Dreschfield, 'Legal report on an ordinance entitled "The Medical Practitioners (Amendment) Ordinance, 1953"', 10 October 1953, UNA G.697/13; above, p. 122.
104 Whyte in van der Geest and Whyte, *Context*, pp. 217–33.
105 Lloyd William Swantz, 'The role of the medicine man among the Zaramo of Dar es Salaam', PhD thesis, University of Dar es Salaam, 1974, pp. iii–iv, 72, 319–21, 340–62.
106 Walter D. Abilla, 'Are nurses ready to take some control away from doctors in medical profession?' *Medicus*, August 1990, pp. 17–19.

7 UGANDA: DOCTORS AND A DISINTEGRATING STATE

1 'Medical education in relation to the needs of Uganda' [1962] A.W. Williams papers, RH; Richard Baraza, 'News and statistics', *Makerere Medical Journal*, 16 (September 1971), 46.
2 Uganda Cabinet Memorandum CT (1965) 215: 'Progress report on smallpox outbreak in Uganda and measures of control' [c. 7 September 1965] UMOH GCP.16/118; R.L. Huckstep, 'The cripple in Africa', *Makerere Medical Journal*, 14 (January 1970), 15; City Council of Kampala, *Annual report of the Medical Officer of Health for 1967 and 1968* (printed, UMOH library).
3 Uganda, *Parliamentary debates*, 13 November 1962, cols. 275–8, and 11 July 1963, col. 1001; Stanley Scheyer and David Dunlop, 'Health services and development in Uganda', in Cole P. Dodge and Paul D. Wiebe (eds.), *Crisis in Uganda: the breakdown of health services* (Oxford, 1985), p. 33.
4 Uganda, *Parliamentary debates*, 19 June 1963, col. 318, and 20 March 1969, col. 1047; 'A report by the working committee on the review of Mulago Hospital and related medical services in the Kampala Metropolitan Area', n.d. (UMOH library).
5 King, *Medical care*, ch. 12, pp. 3, 9; Colin Leys, *Politicians and policies: an essay on politics in Acholi, Uganda, 1962–65* (Nairobi, 1967), pp. 66–7.
6 Uganda, *Parliamentary debates*, 29 March 1963, cols. 353–4.
7 Leys, *Politicians*, pp. 4, 11–12; Grace Stuart Ibingira, *African upheavals since*

independence (Westview, 1980), p. 76; Uganda Cabinet Minute 8, 7 January 1964, UMOH GCR.2/22.

8 The figure was chosen because the colonial government had built twenty-two hospitals. See Uganda, *Parliamentary debates*, 30 November 1964, col. 8, and 4 December 1964, cols. 139–40; 'Health services – building the new hospitals', August 1969, UMOH GCR.16/37; Leys, *Politicians*, pp. 69–70.

9 E.A. Brett, 'Adjustment policy and institutional reform', in P. Langseth, J. Katorobo, E. Brett, and J. Munene (eds.), *Uganda: landmarks in rebuilding a nation* (Kampala, 1995), p. 32; Scheyer and Dunlop in Dodge and Wiebe, *Crisis*, p. 33; 'Record of a meeting . . . to discuss financial matters concerning the Ministry', 7 September 1966, UMOH *10/23. (For references marked with an asterisk, see below, p. 313.)

10 Uringi to MOH, 26 September 1968, UMOH *10/150; Uganda, *Parliamentary debates*, 5 October 1970, col. 160; Scheyer and Dunlop in Dodge and Wiebe, *Crisis*, p. 27.

11 Uganda Medical Association, 'Private clinics owned by government employed doctors: memorandum submitted to H.E. the President of Uganda', 14 February 1989 (UMOH library).

12 Southall, *Parties*, pp. 10–46; *Munno*, 14 September 1963 and 23 November 1964; J.W.P. Okwirri, 'Machakos Provincial General Hospital: annual report 1974', KNA Health BY/9/610/19.

13 *Uganda Argus*, 18 June 1963.

14 Uganda, *Parliamentary debates*, 4 February 1966, col. 1027.

15 For rival accounts of this crisis, see Leys, *Politicians*, pp. 7–9; Ibingira, *Upheavals*, pp. 113–46; Ingham, *Obote*, pp. 100–6.

16 Uganda, *Parliamentary debates*, 29 June 1966, cols. 502–6.

17 Sembeguya to MOH, 31 May 1966, UMOH GCD.11/14.

18 *Uganda Argus*, 21 February and 5 September 1967, 12 January 1970.

19 *Ibid.*, 22 May 1967.

20 Uganda, *Parliamentary debates*, 1 October 1970, col. 126; Zeller, 'Establishment', p. 253.

21 *Uganda Argus*, 18 June 1963, 21 October 1964, 2 May 1966.

22 Uganda, *Parliamentary debates*, 29 June 1966, col. 508.

23 *Ibid.*, 13 October 1967, col. 37; Expedit Ddungu, 'Popular forms and the question of democracy', in Mahmood Mamdani and Joe Oloka Onyango (eds.), *Uganda: studies in living conditions, popular movements, and constitutionalism* (Vienna, 1994), pp. 398–9.

24 *Uganda Argus*, 18 December 1969; Redshaw to FCO, 20 July 1970, BW 90/1376/79.

25 Uganda Cabinet Minute 362, 10 August 1965, UMOH GCD.11/12; 'Mulago/Makerere Joint Advisory Committee: minutes', 26 September 1968, UMOH GCC.31/1/32; *Uganda Argus*, 8 February 1969.

26 J.S.W. Lutwama, 'East Africa', in Elizabeth Purcell (ed.), *World trends in medical education* (Baltimore, 1971), pp. 110–12; University of East Africa, 'External examiners' reports for the 1968/69 academic year', duplicated, MUL LD; *Makerere Medical Journal*, 8 (May 1965), 25; *Uganda Argus*, 19 March 1969.

27 J.S.W. Lutwama and M.S.R. Hutt, 'Makerere University Faculty of Medicine, Kampala', Hutt papers, RH.

28 *Makerere College Newsletter*, 45 (December 1970).
29 Joel D. Barkan, *An African dilemma: university students, development and politics in Ghana, Tanzania and Uganda* (Nairobi, 1975), pp. 187, 57, 113.
30 Mahmood Mamdani, *And fire does not always beget ash: critical reflections on the NRM* (Kampala, 1995), p. 4.
31 Odonga, *First fifty years*, pp. 216–18.
32 N.O. Bwibo, 'Medical education in a developing country', *EAMJ*, 64 (1987), 707–8; Baraza, 'News', p. 47.
33 M.S.R. Hutt, Answers to aide-mémoire, Hutt papers, RH; Alex B. Nganwa-Bagumah, 'From the President's desk', *Makerere Medical Journal*, 14 (January 1970), 49.
34 H.G.K. Rwabugahya, 'Experience in an up-country hospital', *Makerere Medical Journal*, 9 (November 1965), 21.
35 Musoke, 'Analysis', pp. 309–14, 305.
36 Aaron E. John Masawe, 'Syphilis in Uganda (the history, clinical features and cellular immunity)', MMed thesis, Makerere University, 1971, pp. 2, 5, 60.
37 J.W. Kibukamusoke, 'Nephrotic syndrome of quartan malaria', in A.G. Shaper, J.W. Kibukamusoke, and M.S.R. Hutt (eds.), *Medicine in a tropical environment* (London, 1972), p. 424.
38 J.N.P. Davies, 'Pathology of Central African natives: cardio-vascular diseases', *EAMJ*, 25 (1948), 464.
39 J.W. Kibukamusoke, M.S.R. Hutt, and N.E. Wilks, 'The nephrotic syndrome in Uganda and its association with quartan malaria', *Quarterly Journal of Medicine*, NS, 36 (1967), 393.
40 John W. Kibukamusoke, *Nephrotic syndrome of quartan malaria* (London, 1973).
41 John W. Kibukamusoke (ed.), *Tropical nephrology* (Canberra, 1984).
42 John W. Kibukamusoke, 'The nephrotic syndrome of quartan malaria', *Medical Journal of Australia*, 1971/1, p. 191.
43 *Uganda Argus*, 14 April 1972.
44 Raphael Owor, 'The pathology of chronic pancreatic disease in Uganda', MD thesis, University of East Africa, 1970; S.K. Kajubi, 'Clinical and functional aspects of chronic pancreatic disease in Uganda', MD thesis, Makerere University, 1971.
45 J.N.P. Davies, J. Knowelden, and Barbara A. Wilson, 'Incidence rates of cancer in Kyadondo County, Uganda, 1954–1960', *Journal of the National Cancer Institute*, 35 (1965), 790.
46 J.N.P. Davies, Sally Elmes, M.S.R. Hutt, L.A.M. Mtimavalye, R. Owor, and Lorna Shaper, 'Cancer in an African community 1897–1956', *British Medical Journal*, 1964, 1, pp. 259, 261 (and editorial comments, pp. 321–2).
47 *Ibid.*, p. 340; Davies, Knowelden, and Wilson, 'Incidence rates', pp. 813, 817–18; J.K.G. Mati and S. Auma, 'Cancer of the stomach', *Makerere Medical Journal*, 8 (May 1965), 38–40; M.S.R. Hutt, D.P. Burkitt, J.J. Shepherd, B. Wright, J.K.G. Mati, and S. Auma, 'Malignant tumours of the gastrointestinal tract in Ugandans', *National Cancer Institute Monograph*, 25 (1967), 41–7.
48 C.L.M. Olweny and F.K. Nkrumah, 'Treatment of Burkitt's lymphoma: the African experience', in G.M. Lenoir, G.T. O'Conor, and C.L.M. Olweny (eds.), *Burkitt's lymphoma* (Lyon, 1985), p. 376.

49 Denis Burkitt, 'A sarcoma involving the jaws in African children', *British Journal of Surgery*, 46 (1958–9), 218–23.
50 Davies to Robinson, 24 January 1975, J.N.P. Davies papers, RH.
51 John L. Ziegler, 'Cancer and HIV infection', *Makerere Medical Journal*, 32 (December 1995), 7–8.
52 S.K. Kyalwazi, 'Kaposi's sarcoma', *Tropical Doctor*, 2 (1972), 68–72; Charles L. Vogel and Sebastian K. Kyalwazi, 'Recent advances in hepatocellular carcinoma research', *Makerere Medical Journal*, 16 (September 1971), 13–14; S.K. Kyalwazi, 'Carcinoma of the penis', *EAMJ*, 43 (1966), 415–25.
53 S.K. Kyalwazi, 'Treatment of Kaposi's sarcoma', *EAMJ*, 46 (1969), 450–8; S.K. Kyalwazi, 'Problems of cancer treatment in Africa', *Uganda Medical Journal*, 3 (1974), 9–14.
54 C.L.M. Olweny, 'Cancer', in E.H.O. Parry (ed.), *Principles of medicine in Africa* (2nd edn, Oxford, 1984), pp. 983–5.
55 Kyalwazi, 'Problems', p. 11.
56 *New Vision*, 5 February 1992.
57 Charles L.M. Olweny, 'Hepatocellular carcinoma in Uganda', MD thesis, Makerere University, 1976; Charles L.M. Olweny, Edward Katongole-Mbidde, David Otim, Stephen K. Lwanga, Ian T. Magrath, and John L. Ziegler, 'Long-term experience with Burkitt's lymphoma in Uganda', *International Journal of Cancer*, 26 (1980), 261–6; Charles L.M. Olweny, John L. Ziegler, Costan W. Berard, and A.C. Templeton, 'Adult Hodgkin's disease in Uganda', *Cancer*, 27 (1971), 1295–301.
58 J.N.P. Davies, 'Endocardial fibrosis in Africans', *EAMJ*, 25 (1948), 10.
59 J. Freers, H. Mayanja-Kizza, J.L. Ziegler, and M. Rutakingirwa, 'Echocardiographic diagnosis of heart disease in Uganda', *Tropical Doctor*, 26 (1996), 125; M.S. Valiathan, Krishna Somers, and C. Chandrasekharan Kartha (eds.), *Endomyocardial fibrosis* (Delhi, 1993); above, p. 159.
60 P.G. D'Arbela, 'The epidemiology and consequences of degenerative heart diseases in the African environment', in F.J. Bennett, A.M. Nhonoli, and H. Nsanzumuhire (eds.), *Degenerative disorders in the African environment* (Nairobi, 1976), pp. 308–9; J.O.M. Pobee, 'Cardiovascular research: a luxury in tropical Africa?' *EAMJ*, 64 (1987), 399–400; *Makerere Medical Journal*, 12 (February 1969), 15.
61 E.g. Muhangi, *Psychiatry*, pp. 3–5.
62 Odonga, *First fifty years*, p. 189.
63 *Uganda Argus*, 4 February and 30 January 1971.
64 *Ibid.*, 12 February 1971.
65 *Ibid.*, 24 February 1971.
66 *Ibid.*, 7 July 1971, 25 February 1971, 17 February 1972.
67 David Martin, *General Amin* (London, 1974), pp. 139–40; Henry Kyemba, *A state of blood: the inside story of Idi Amin* (New York, 1977), p. 40.
68 Kyemba, *State*, pp. 55, 164; Odonga, *First fifty years*, p. 193.
69 *Uganda Argus*, 10–31 August 1972.
70 E.g. Monica Byrne, 'Nursing in Uganda', Byrne papers, RH; Kyemba, *State*, pp. 122, 125; *Voice of Uganda*, 5 July 1974.
71 Kyemba, *State*, pp. 149, 156; Odonga, *First fifty years*, p. 193.
72 Martin, *Amin*, p. 227; *Voice of Uganda*, 12 and 15 March 1973.

73 J.M. Theakstone, 'Visit to IUC by Professor J. Kibuuka-Musoke', 23 March 1973, BW 90/1386/116.

74 Musisi to PS, 28 June 1977, UMOH ECS.9/8/7; 'Minutes of the meeting between H.E. the Life President and members of the Uganda Medical Association', 2 September 1977, UMOH ECT.28; 'Ministry of Health draft policy proposal, September, 1979', UMOH *1; Senteza Kajubi, 'Integration and national development from the viewpoint of education in Uganda', in Dodge and Wiebe, *Crisis*, p. 22.

75 *Voice of Uganda*, 11 October 1973; Kyemba, *State*, pp. 132–3; *Daily News*, 28 May 1977.

76 Kyemba, *State*, p. 42.

77 *Voice of Uganda*, 22 April 1978.

78 *Ibid.*, 15 February 1974.

79 Sam Agatre Okuonzi and Joanna Macrae, 'Whose policy is it anyway? International and national influences on health policy development in Uganda', *Health Policy and Planning*, 10 (1995), 123; World Bank, *Uganda population, health and nutrition sector review* (Washington, 1985), p. 30; Cole P. Dodge, 'Uganda – rehabilitation, or redefinition of health services?' *SSM*, 22 (1986), 756.

80 'Ministry of Health draft policy proposal, September, 1979', UMOH *1; F.K. Banegura, G.M.R. Munube, A.G. Senyakazana, and E. Nzaro, 'An epidemic of typhus in Ankole, Uganda, 1975–1976', *EAMJ*, 60 (1983), 55–9; F.S. Matovu, 'Rhodesian sleeping sickness in south-eastern Uganda', *EAMJ*, 59 (1982), 390–3; above, p. 152.

81 'Meeting of the Senior Staff with the Minister held on 19 December 1980', UMOH GCM.15/V/19; *Voice of Uganda*, 20 January 1976; 'Report on inspections at Mulago Hospital', 24 July 1978, UMOH GCH.3/4/II/97; Kirya to MS, Mulago, 2 March 1978, UMOH GCH.3/4/II/91; *Uganda Times*, 6 October 1983.

82 Department of Medicine, 'Quinquennial development 1976/77–1980/1', UMOH GCU.5/19; Pobee, 'Cardiovascular research', p. 399; above, p. 177.

83 R.D. Mugerwa, 'Heart diseases in Uganda and their control', *Medicom*, 8 (1986), 133.

84 Correspondence in BW 90/1377 and 90/1389; Bryan Langlands, 'Students and politics in Uganda', *African Affairs*, 76 (1977), 3–20.

85 Makerere University, 'University examinations: external examiners' reports', 1974, 1974–1976/77, 1979, duplicated, MUL UC.64, UH.4, UH.3.

86 *Minutes of the General Medical Council*, 1975 p. 198, 1976 pp. 309 and 15; Jeffery, 'Allopathic medicine', p. 565.

87 Babumba to MOH, 12 March 1973, UMOH GCD.11/95; Musa Dawha, 'A review of the activities of voluntary health organizations in the Central Province of Uganda', DPH thesis, Makerere University, 1978, pp. 12, 67; Nyangabyaki Bazaara, 'Land policy and the evolving forms of land tenure in Masindi District', in Mamdani and Oloka-Onyango, *Uganda*, pp. 35–6; *Voice of Uganda*, 21 March 1973.

88 'Minutes of the meeting between H.E. the Life President and members of the Uganda Medical Association', 2 September 1977, UMOH ECT.28.

89 Uganda, 'Report and recommendations of the Health Policy Review Commission under the chairmanship of Professor Raphael Owor', Entebbe, 1987, p. 82 (UMOH library).
90 *Voice of Uganda*, 8 December 1974; Kyemba, *State*, pp. 130–1; Kanyerezi to Amin [1976] UMOH ECT.28; *Voice of Uganda*, 30 January 1976 and 31 July 1978.
91 H.P. Dinwiddy, 'Return to Northcote, 1980', Dinwiddy papers, RH; R. Schram, 'Kampala: memoirs', Schram papers, RH; William Parson, 'Medical education in Uganda today', in Dodge and Wiebe, *Crisis*, pp. 247–8.
92 S.K. Kyalwazi, 'Foreword', *Makerere Medical Journal*, 23 (July 1977), 1.
93 *New Vision*, 7 December 1995.
94 Tony Avirgan and Martha Honey, *War in Uganda* (Westport, 1982), pp. 108–9, 202; *Uganda Times*, 1 August 1979.
95 Ingham, *Obote*, p. 164; *Uganda Times*, 20 November 1979.
96 Francis A.W. Bwengye, *The agony of Uganda* (London, 1985), pp. 44, 93, 95, 233–6; Baker, *From exile*, p. 78; *New Vision*, 22 January 1995.
97 Pat Holden, 'Colonial sisters: nurses in Uganda', in Pat Holden and Jenny Littlewood (eds.), *Anthropology and nursing* (London, 1991), p.78; 'First Senior Staff meeting held under the new Government', 23 April 1979, UMOH *1.
98 J.M. Jagwe, 'A retrospective study of causes of death among Ugandan African doctors', *Health Information Quarterly*, 3, 3 (September 1987), 12.
99 *Uganda Times*, 28 July 1979. Generally, see Avirgan and Honey, *War*, pp. 206–7.
100 *Uganda Times*, 23 July 1979.
101 *Ibid.*, 1 August 1979.
102 Cutting enclosed in A.W. Williams, 'East African notes', Williams papers, RH; Baker, *From exile*, pp. 82–6; *New Vision*, 5 September 1996 and 9 August 1994.
103 'Senior Staff Conference', 12 October 1979, and 'Extra-ordinary Senior Staff meeting', 20 March 1980, UMOH *1.
104 Recovery Programme Task Force, '1982–84 Recovery Programme review: health sector', 18 August 1983, p. 11, UMOH GCR.37/I.
105 Yoweri Kaguta Museveni, *What is Africa's problem?* (Kampala, 1992), p. 44.
106 C. Michaud and C.J.L. Murray, 'External assistance to the health sector in developing countries: a detailed analysis, 1972–90', *Bulletin of the WHO*, 72 (1994), 643; World Bank, *Uganda population*, p. 45.
107 *Uganda Times*, 9 August and 13 September 1979; Recovery Programme Task Force, '1982–84 Recovery Programme review: health sector', 18 August 1983, UMOH GCR.37/I; Ruberantwari to DMS, 9 September 1980, UMOH GCH.3/4/II/131.
108 P.J. Shipp, 'The current situation of health manpower in Uganda', duplicated, Nairobi, 1986, pp. 14–15 (UMOH library); Uganda, 'Health Policy Review Commission', p. 21.
109 Jagwe to DMS, 9 September 1980, UMOH GCH.3/4/II/129; Bryan Pearson, 'Uganda: picking up the pieces', *Africa Health*, 6, 3 (February 1984), 27; Okiria to MS, Mulago, 16 August 1984, UMOH GCH.3/4/II/212; *Uganda Times*, 2 July 1984.

110 Badru Buwembo-Kakande, 'Post operative wound infection in Mulago Hospital', *Uganda Medical Journal*, 8 , 1 (April 1991), 55–61; Jagwe to PS, MOH, 20 February 1985, UMOH GCH.3/4/III/1.
111 World Bank, *Uganda population*, p. 33; Dodge, 'Uganda', pp. 757–8; 'Minutes of the Senior Staff meeting', 2 December 1982, UMOH GCM.15/V/38.
112 Uganda, 'Health Policy Review Commission', p. 91; 'First AGM of Uganda Community Based Health Care Association', October 1986 (UMOH library).
113 World Bank, *Uganda population*, p. 14; 'Minutes of the meeting between Ministry of Health and the Ministry of Planning and Economic Development', 3 September 1980, UMOH GCM.15/V/14.
114 'Minutes of the Ministry of Health Headquarters Senior Staff meeting for working out a common stand on the future of EPI' [c. April 1980] UMOH *1; Dodge, 'Uganda', p. 758; World Bank, *Uganda population*, p. 20; E.M. Kaijuka, 'Uganda without polio by year 2000', *Mbarara University Medical Journal*, 2, 1 (January 1996), 38; F.M. Kaharuza, 'Measles in Nyakibale Hospital', *Health Information Quarterly*, 5, 1 (June 1989), 7.
115 'Extra-ordinary Senior Staff meeting', 20 March 1980, UMOH *1; G.R. Nzarubara, 'The Ugandan losses', *Proceedings of the Association of Surgeons in East Africa*, 8 (1986), supplement, p. 40; *Uganda Times*, 8 April 1981, 2 April 1982, 20 June 1983; DMS to MOH, 25 June 1984, UMOH ECM.3/8/III/89; Parson in Dodge and Wiebe, *Crisis*, pp. 249–50; C.E. Cory, 'Report of the Nuffield Foundation visitors concerning Makerere University Medical School', October 1982, UMOH GCM.5/II/56.
116 Uganda: Ministry of Health, 'Report on the first meeting of District Medical Officers', 2–7 June 1986, duplicated, pp. 31, 101 (UMOH library).
117 World Bank, *Uganda population*, p. 27; *Uganda Times*, 14 July 1979 and 6 September 1980.
118 'Minutes of the Senior Staff meeting', 6 November 1980 and 8 January 1981, UMOH GCM.15/V/18 and 21.
119 'Minutes of the Senior Staff meeting', 5 February 1981, UMOH GCM.15/V/24; *Uganda Times*, 29 September 1980.
120 *Uganda Times*, 9 February 1982 and 31 August 1983.
121 Uganda: Ministry of Local Government, 'Report of the annual conference of DMOs, M/Ss and NGOs', June 1988, p. 117 (UMOH library); *New Vision*, 5 April 1989, 7 April 1993, 3–6 April 1995.
122 *Weekly Topic*, 3 February 1986. See also Abidi, *Challenges*, pp. 207–8.
123 *New Vision*, 28 July 1987.
124 *Ibid.*, 18 November 1988 and 5 November 1991.
125 Uganda, 'Health Policy Review Commission', *passim*; Z.K.R. Kaheru, 'Statement in the National Resistance Council on the 1989/90 budget', p. 6 (UMOH library); Uganda: Ministry of Health, 'Approach and guidelines for health planning 1996/97 and 1997/98', June 1995, p. 1 (UMOH library).
126 Joanna Macrae, Anthony B. Zwi, and Lucy Gilson, 'A triple burden for health sector reform: "post"-conflict rehabilitation in Uganda', *SSM*, 42 (1996), 1098–102.
127 Museveni, *Africa's problem*, p. 44; *New Vision*, 26 September 1996.
128 Emmanuel Tumusiime-Mutebile, 'Management of the economic reform programme', in Langseth and others, *Uganda*, pp. 3, 9.

129 Uganda Medical Association, ‘Private clinics’; *New Vision*, 1 April 1995.
130 Uganda, ‘Health Policy Review Commission’, p. 68; *New Vision*, 26 May 1988, 15 February 1996.
131 Uganda: Ministry of Health, ‘The three year health plan frame 1993/94–1995/96’, p. iv (UMOH library).
132 *New Vision*, 24 May 1989.
133 E.g. Uganda: Ministry of Local Government, ‘Report’, p. 9; Holden in Holden and Littlewood, *Anthropology*, p. 79; Tim Allen, ‘The quest for therapy in Moyo district’, in Holger Bernt Hansen and Michael Twaddle (eds.), *Changing Uganda* (London, 1991), pp. 150–2.
134 Charles Onyango-Obbo in *EastAfrican*, 30 December 1996.
135 *New Vision*, 18 June and 2 August 1996; Jane Shaw, ‘Recurrent costs of Mulago Hospital’, 1 September 1990, UMOH PHC/HP/1/I/41.
136 *New Vision*, 12 December 1986 and 2 August 1995.
137 Kaheru, ‘Statement on 1989/90 budget’, p. 21; Uganda, ‘Mulago Hospital: annual report 1990’ (UMOH library); *EastAfrican*, 17 March 1997.
138 Yoweri Kaguta Museveni, *Tackling the tasks ahead* (n.p., 1996), p. 40.
139 Jane Shaw, ‘Recurrent costs of Mulago Hospital’, 1 September 1990, UMOH PHC/HP/1/I/41; Uganda: Ministry of Health, ‘National health personnel study’ (Entebbe, 1991), p. 11.
140 *New Vision*, 15 August 1995 and 11 November 1994.
141 J.C. Munene, ‘Organisational pathology and accountability in health and education in rural Uganda’, in Langseth and others, *Uganda*, p. 140.
142 Quoted in *ibid.*
143 *New Vision*, 2 August 1993; Uganda, ‘Health Policy Review Commission’, p. 33; *New Vision*, 19 August 1994.
144 *New Vision*, 18 December 1989 and 10 May 1991.
145 Lawrence Ojom, ‘District Medical Office, Kitgum District, annual report 1993’ (UMOH library).
146 Damian Ndagij’Imana and others, ‘St Francis Hospital, Mutolere, 1989–1991’ (UMOH library); *New Vision*, 30 April 1994.
147 J.G.S. Makumbi, ‘The 1993/94 budget statement to the National Resistance Council’, p. 1 (UMOH library); Uganda: Ministry of Health, ‘Approach and guidelines’, p. 2.
148 Uganda: Ministry of Health, ‘Approach and guidelines’, pp. 8–9.
149 ‘Proceedings of the seventh annual general meeting of the Uganda Community Based Health Care Association’, 5–6 November 1992 (UMOH library).
150 *New Vision*, 9 September 1996.
151 *Ibid.*, 16 July 1993; J.G.S. Makumbi, ‘Ministry of Health budget policy statement to the National Resistance Council for 1994/95 fiscal year’, p. 7 (UMOH library).
152 *New Vision*, 18 September 1996.
153 *Daily News*, 6 May 1989; *New Vision*, 15 February 1994; *Daily Nation*, 20 April 1996.
154 *New Vision*, 11 November 1989; Uganda, ‘Mulago Hospital: annual report 1990’ (UMOH library); *EastAfrican*, 28 October 1996.
155 Uganda: Ministry of Health, ‘National health personnel study’, p. 97; *New Vision*, 19 October and 16 November 1990.

156 *Makerere Medical Journal*, 30 (February 1994), i–iv, 28; *ibid.*, 32 (December 1995), 17–18, 21–3, 30; *Med.Info.* (Makerere), 1 (May 1993), 1; A.B. Nganwa-Bagumah, 'Community based medical education', *Mbarara University Medical Journal*, 2, 1 (January 1996), 5–7.

157 *New Vision*, 11 January 1994; Anne Merriman, 'The medical profession in Uganda and palliative care', *Makerere Medical Journal*, 31 (October 1994), 5–7; *New Vision*, 31 August and 12 September 1996.

158 C.L. Sezi, 'New findings: EMF a disease of growing children and child bearing women', *Uganda Medical Journal*, 8, 3 (September 1991), 2–4; C.L. Sezi, 'The role of mechanical factors in the pathogenesis of endomycardial fibrosis', *ibid.*, 5–6; C.L. Sezi, 'The interaction of various factors in the pathogenesis of endomyocardial fibrosis', *ibid.*, 7–9; C.L. Sezi, 'Theory: the cause of endomyocardial fibrosis', *ibid.*, 10–16. These should be compared with Freers and others, 'Echocardiographic diagnosis'; Valiathan and others, *Endomyocardial fibrosis*.

159 Uganda: Ministry of Health, 'National health personnel study', pp. ii, iv; *New Vision*, 8 February 1992 and 16 July 1993; Peter Langseth, 'Civil service reform in Uganda', in Langseth and others, *Uganda*, pp. 111, 113.

160 Z.K.R. Kaheru, 'Statement in the National Resistance Council on the 1990/91 budget', p. 6 (UMOH library).

161 *New Vision*, 27 January, 2 June, and 18 August 1995; Uganda: Ministry of Health, 'Three year plan frame', p. ii; Uganda: Ministry of Health, 'Approach and guidelines', p. 2.

162 World Bank, *Uganda population*, pp. 32, 46; Samwiri Etyono, 'Cost-sharing for health in my view', *Health Information Quarterly*, 8, 1 (June 1991), 16–17; Uganda, 'Health Policy Review Commission', pp. 16–17; Uganda: Ministry of Local Government, 'Report', pp. 168, 176; *New Vision*, 8 July 1989.

163 Munene in Langseth and others, *Uganda*, pp. 146–7; *New Vision*, 10 August 1990; Uganda, 'Terminal report of the health cost sharing co-ordination unit', October 1990, appendix 6 (UMOH library).

164 Z.K.R. Kaheru, 'Health cost-sharing policy', 25 March 1990 (UMOH library); Kaheru, 'Statement on 1989/90 budget', p. 20; Okuonzi and Macrae, 'Whose policy?' pp. 127–8; *New Vision*, 27 September 1990.

165 Sandra Wallman and others, *Kampala women getting by* (London, 1996), p. 7; *New Vision*, 13 July 1992 and 11 December 1993.

166 *New Vision*, 22 February 1994 and 9 March 1995; R. Francis Mwesigye, 'Health care financing', *Uganda Health Bulletin*, 1, 3 (May 1994), 40–1.

167 *New Vision*, 13 September 1995 and 11 October 1996.

168 Uganda: Ministry of Health, 'National health personnel study', p. 8. There were many other, often contradictory, figures.

169 Langseth in Langseth and others, *Uganda*, p. 113.

170 Uganda Medical Association, 'Private clinics'.

171 Uganda: Ministry of Health, 'National health personnel study', p. 8; *New Vision*, 12 November 1995 and 13 September 1988.

172 *New Vision*, 30 September 1989; Uganda: Ministry of Health, 'White paper on health policy up-date and review (1993)', pp. 46–7 (UMOH library).

173 *New Vision*, 29 September 1987 and 23 August 1988; Medical Officer of

Health, Masaka, to Pharmacy Board, 19 August 1992, UMOH PHC.D/3/7; Uganda: Ministry of Health, 'National health personnel study', p. vii.

174 *New Vision*, 21 September and 25 August 1995.

175 *Ibid.*, 16 June 1994.

176 *Ibid.*, 3 April 1992 and 19 October 1993; *Weekly Topic*, 12 April 1991.

177 Susan Reynolds Whyte, 'Medicines and self-help: the privatization of health care in eastern Uganda', in Hansen and Twaddle, *Changing Uganda*, pp. 134–5; Wallman and others, *Kampala women*, p. 124.

178 Harriet Kashagire, 'The problems associated with health facilities in Ibanda County Mbarara District since 1900', BA thesis, Makerere University, 1993, p. 13.

179 Robert J. Mwesigwa, 'Rural private clinics and health, a case study of Rwampara County Mbarara District', BA thesis, Makerere University, 1995, pp. 45, 50, 53–4, 65.

180 Jack G.M. Jagwe, 'Drug use in Uganda: a growing concern for the professionals', *Medical Review (Uganda Edition)*, 1, 5 (September 1995), 19; Whyte in Hansen and Twaddle, *Changing Uganda*, p. 146.

181 *New Vision*, 19 June 1994.

182 Joachim Buwembo in *EastAfrican*, 19 August 1996. For an admirable survey of medical provision, see Christine Obbo, 'Healing: cultural fundamentalism and syncretism in Buganda', *Africa*, 66 (1996), 183–201.

183 Wallman and others, *Kampala women*, pp. 122–5, 146; *New Vision*, 11 October 1988; Whyte in Hansen and Twaddle, *Changing Uganda*, p. 137; Assistant Inspector of Drugs, Kampala, to Pharmacy Board, 1 April 1992, UMOH PHC.D/3/19.

184 Uganda, 'Health Policy Review Commission', pp. 86, 108; Jagwe, 'Drug use', p. 19; Wallman and others, *Kampala women*, p. 147.

185 *New Vision*, 12 April 1988 and 2 June 1992; Okuonzi and Macrae, 'Whose policy?' pp. 128–9; *EastAfrican*, 22 December 1997.

186 Whyte in Hansen and Twaddle, *Changing Uganda*, p. 142.

187 *Ibid.*, pp. 144–5.

188 *East African Standard*, 12 April 1972; 'Report on the visit of Hon. Minister of Health to the Natural Chemotherapeutic Research Laboratory, Wandegeya, 31 December 1986', UMOH *8; N.K. Mubiru and others, *Ethnomedicine in Uganda* (17 vols., Kampala, 1992–).

189 Uganda: Ministry of Health, 'Review of health facilities in Rakai District' [1993] p. 14 (UMOH library); Oona Lynch and Marc Derveeuw, 'The impact of training and supervision of traditional birth attendants', *Tropical Doctor*, 24 (1994), 103–7; *Makerere Medical Journal*, 30 (February 1994), ii.

190 Above, p. 242; *New Vision*, 23 June 1996; Allen in Hansen and Twaddle, *Changing Uganda*, p. 153; Obbo, 'Healing', pp. 188–90.

191 Mwesigwa, 'Rural private clinics', p. 52.

192 *New Vision*, 20 September 1993 and 1 March 1996.

193 Uganda, 'Health Policy Review Commision', p. 90.

194 Obbo, 'Healing', p. 190; *New Vision*, 10 August 1991.

195 *Ibid.*, 15 July 1996.

196 *Ibid.*, 7 August 1992 and 29 September 1993; *Uganda Medical Journal*, 8, 1

(April 1991), 62; A. Karugaba, 'Speech of the President of Uganda Medical Association', *ibid.*, 3.
197 *EastAfrican*, 12 August 1996.
198 Munene in Langseth and others, *Uganda*, p. 150.
199 *New Vision*, 19 July 1995.
200 Uganda Medical Association, 'Private clinics'.
201 *New Vision*, 1 December 1995, 10 February 1996, 20 March 1996.
202 Uganda Medical Association, 'Private clinics'.
203 Erich Ogoso Opolot in *New Vision*, 24 July 1995.
204 *New Vision*, 18 May 1996.
205 *Ibid.*, 8 February 1994.
206 Diana Dyason, 'The medical profession in colonial Victoria, 1834–1901', in Roy MacLeod and Milton Lewis (eds.), *Disease, medicine, and empire* (London, 1988), p. 200; McClelland, *German experience*, pp. 131–2, 140–2, 181.
207 See esp. S. Ogoh Alubo, 'The political economy of doctors' strikes in Nigeria', *SSM*, 22 (1986), 467–77.
208 Langseth in Langseth and others, *Uganda*, p. 114; *New Vision*, 27 September 1995.
209 *New Vision*, 15 March and 21 July 1996.
210 *Monitor*, 18 September 1995.
211 *New Vision*, 22 September 1995.
212 *Ibid.*, 16 July 1996.
213 *Ibid.*, 20, 23, 25 September 1995.
214 *Ibid.*, 21 October 1995.
215 *Monitor*, 25 September 1995.
216 *New Vision*, 28–29 September 1995.
217 *Ibid.*, 16 October and 23 November 1995.
218 *Ibid.*, 21 and 24 July 1996; *Sunday Vision*, 4 August 1996; *EastAfrican*, 28 October 1996.

8 KENYA: DOCTORS AND A CAPITALIST TRANSITION

1 D.K. Fieldhouse, *Black Africa 1945–1980* (London, 1986), p. 74; Paul Collier and Deepak Lal, *Labour and poverty in Kenya 1900–1980* (Oxford, 1986), pp. 78–85.
2 Beck, *Medicine*, pp. 52–3.
3 World Bank, *World development report*, 1990, p. 228.
4 Nordberg, 'True disease pattern', p. 533; Kenya, *AMR* 1955 p. 1; Anthony E. Thomas, 'Adaptation to modern medicine in lowland Machakos, Kenya', PhD thesis, Stanford University, 1970, p. 182; A.M. Salyani, 'Nandi District – annual report on medical and health services, 1965', KNA Health BY/9/518.
5 Kenya, *AMR* 1965 p. 1; J.J. Thuku, 'Annual report: Provincial Medical Officer, Rift Valley Province, 1965', KNA Health BY/9/518.
6 Kenya, *National Assembly*, 4 October 1966, col. 355; Kenya, *AMR* 1965 p. 47, 1967 p. 78; D.V. Bhatt, 'Annual report for the year 1965 on medical and health services: Meru and Isiolo Districts', and J.K. Kamau, 'Annual report 1965: District Hospital Kitui', KNA Health BY/9/522.
7 J.J. Thuku, 'Annual report: Provincial Medical Officer, Rift Valley Province,

1965', KNA Health BY/9/518; Kenya, *National Assembly*, 5 December 1967, col. 2898.

8 *East African Standard*, 28 November 1963; Robert M. Maxon, 'Social and cultural changes', in Ogot and Ochieng', *Decolonization*, p. 134.

9 *Sunday Nation*, 7 July 1996; 'Minutes of the Senior Medical Staff Conference – 1966', KNA Health BY/2/19/118.

10 Kenya, *AMR* 1967 p. 60; Kenya, *National Assembly*, 4 October 1966, col. 351.

11 Kenya, *AMR* 1967, p. 60; J.K. Kamau, 'Medical Department, Eastern Province, annual report 1967', KNA Health BY/9/530; Anthony E. Thomas, 'Health care in *Ukambani* Kenya', in Stanley R. Ingman and Anthony E. Thomas (eds.), *Topias and utopias in health* (The Hague, 1975), pp. 273–4.

12 Kenya, *National Assembly*, 13 July 1967, col. 2194.

13 *Ibid.*, 4 October 1966, col. 359, and 4 October 1973, col. 779.

14 *Ibid.*, 7 August 1969, col. 3002, and 29 September 1966, cols. 198–9.

15 S.N. Ngure, 'Annual report of 1964', KNA Health BY/9/514.

16 Kenya, *National Assembly*, 4 October 1973, col. 770.

17 K. Koinange, 'Some reflections on development of health services in Kenya', *EAMJ*, 60 (1983), 601; J.A. Ouya, 'Ministry of Health: Western Province: annual report 1970' (KNA library).

18 Kenya, *A report by the Director of the Medical Services on status of health in Kenya 1979* (Nairobi, 1982), pp. 61–2; *Daily Nation*, 13 October 1971; Kenya, *National Assembly*, 28 October 1970, col. 1444.

19 Kenya, *National Assembly*, 14 February 1969, cols. 5036–9.

20 A.M. Baker, 'Visit to Kenya: January/February 1976', BW 90/1341/101.

21 Gerlinde Katerina Janovsky, 'Planning as organizational transaction and bargaining: the case of health in Kenya', EdD thesis, Harvard University, 1979, pp. 48–55; 'Visit by Dr P.W. Dill-Russell to Kenya from January 31–February 15 1973', BW 90/2370.

22 Kenya, *National Assembly*, 15 October 1969, cols. 723–4.

23 'Kangundo Sub-District Hospital: annual report for 1975', KNA Health BY/9/614/3.

24 Kenya, *National Assembly*, 9 October 1973, col. 896, and 14 February 1969, cols., 5034 et seq.

25 See the excellent account in Elizabeth Maina-Githinji, 'The outpatient and the staff satisfaction with the treatment provided in a district hospital Kiambu', MA thesis, University of Dar es Salaam, 1977.

26 Walter Dan Abilla, 'Life in the ward: a sociological study of the inpatient in a general hospital in Kenya (Kisumu)', duplicated, University of Nairobi, 1977, p. 10; Thomas, 'Adaptation', pp. 93–5; Maxon in Ogot and Ochieng', *Decolonization*, p. 134.

27 *Medicus*, June 1984, p. 32.

28 T. Ogada, 'Tana River District – annual medical report, 1964', KNA Health BY/9/509.

29 J.N. Obare, 'Annual report for the year 1976', KNA Health BY/9/604/22.

30 A.T.T. Forrester, 'Address of the President of the Association of Physicians of East Africa', *EAMJ*, 47 (1970), 594–5.

31 T.K. Evelia, 'Republic of Kenya: Ministry of Health: Nyanza Province: annual report 1975', KNA Health BY/9/668.

32 *East African Standard*, 28 November 1963; Kenya, *National Assembly*, 26 May 1966, col. 78; *Daily Nation*, 11 March 1995; *Weekly Review*, 8 July 1994.
33 Joseph M. Mungai, 'Medical sciences in Africa', *Nairobi Journal of Medicine*, 4, 2 (September 1971), 67–8; Joseph M. Mungai, 'Medical practice in East Africa', *ibid.*, 1 (1968–9), 24–6.
34 *Medicus*, May 1984, pp. 3–4.
35 Correspondence in KNA Health BY/12/36; *East African Standard*, 2 August and 12 December 1968; *Weekly Review*, 19 October 1984; Paul Starr, *The social transformation of American medicine* (New York, 1982), p. 433.
36 Kenya, *AMR* 1968 p. 61; Charles Walekhwa, 'Out-patient services of Kenyatta National Hospital: annual report for the year 1980', duplicated, p. 13 (UNMS library); *Weekly Review*, 17 May 1985.
37 *Weekly Review*, 25 January 1980; Kenya, *Report by DMS 1979*, p. 37.
38 Kenya: Ministry of Health, *Kenyatta National Hospital annual report 1976*, pp. 4–7; Kenya: Ministry of Health, *Kenyatta National Hospital annual report 1979*, pp. 3–10, 56; P.W. Dill-Russell, 'Visit to Kenya: 22–28 January and 2–5 February 1972', BW 90/2370.
39 Kenya: Ministry of Health, *Kenyatta National Hospital annual report 1976*, pp. 10, 22; *Weekly Review*, 18 May 1979.
40 *Medicus*, July 1984, p. 1.
41 E.g. *Standard*, 7 March 1974; *The Student Doctor*, 1, 1 [?1991], 1.
42 *Weekly Review*, 6 May 1988; P.M. Nyarango, 'Medical education for doctors in Kenya: an overview of its organisation and conduct', duplicated, 1987, p. 12 (UMNS library); *The Student Doctor*, 1, 1 [?1991], 24; Tiyambe Zeleza, 'The labour system in independent Kenya', in W.R. Ochieng' and R.M. Maxon (eds.), *An economic history of Kenya* (Nairobi, 1992), p. 351.
43 *Medicus*, December 1986, p. 27; N.O. Bwibo, 'Medical and paediatric clerkship', *Medicom*, 3 (1981), 48.
44 P. Masajjage and D. Sgarabotto, letter in *EAMJ*, 59 (1982), 4; N. Anjicki, letter in *Medicus*, November 1983, p. 2.
45 Letter in *Medicus*, September 1987, p. 2.
46 *Ibid.*, p. 7; *Weekly Review*, 12 June 1992.
47 Germano Mwabu, 'Health care reform in Kenya: a review of the process', *Health Policy*, 32 (1995), 251; *Daily Nation*, 18 April 1996; *Weekly Review*, 12–26 June 1992; *Medicus*, October 1992, p. 1.
48 *Daily Nation*, 30 March 1996.
49 William Lore, 'Undergraduate medical curriculum in a developing country: the case for community orientation', *Nairobi Journal of Medicine*, 16, 1 (February 1990), 9.
50 William Lore, 'Community-oriented medical education in developing countries', *Medicus*, December 1989, pp. 4, 7.
51 *Daily Nation*, 4 June 1994, 11 March 1995.
52 W. Lore, 'Authorship in the *East African Medical Journal*', *EAMJ*, 71 (1994), 762–5; Davy K. Koech, 'Challenges to health scientists in Africa', *African Journal of Health Sciences*, 1 (1994), 4.
53 Scheyer and Dunlop in Dodge and Wiebe, *Crisis*, p. 35.
54 Edward George Kasili, 'Leukaemia in Kenya', MD thesis, University of Nairobi, 1979, pp. x, 86, 110.
55 Edward George Kasili, 'Childhood leukaemia: is it a problem in tropical

Africa?' *Leukemia and Lymphoma*, 1 (1989–90), 187; *Daily Nation*, 3 January 1995.

56 E.G. Kasili, 'Children's cancer ward at the KNH', *Medicus*, August 1986, p. 3; Edward G. Kasili, 'Coping with cancer in sub-Saharan Africa', *World Health Forum*, 4 (1983), 149.

57 Edward G. Kasili, 'Palliative care of the terminally ill cancer patient in the Kenyan context', *Nairobi Journal of Medicine*, 16, 1 (February 1990), 7.

58 E.G. Kasili, *A synopsis of the management of some cancers in Kenya* (Nairobi, 1991).

59 *Daily Nation*, 3 January 1995.

60 J.M. Mukiibi and J. Kyobe, 'Pattern of multiple myeloma in Kenyans', *Tropical and Geographical Medicine*, 40 (1988), 20–5; W.M. Macharia, 'Highlight on childhood lymphomas', *EAMJ*, 73 (1996), 341–2.

61 *Weekly Review*, 15 December 1978; *Medicus*, July 1985, pp. 3–4, and December 1986, p. 28.

62 P.A. Odhiambo, 'Organ transplant', *Medicom*, 6 (1984), 121–3; G.M. Anabwani, 'Heart disease in Africa: what is known?' *EAMJ*, 73 (1996), 213.

63 H.P. Ojiambo, J. Okanga, and A.H.T. Parker, 'The pattern of heart disease', in L.C. Vogel, A.S. Muller, R.S. Odingo, Z. Onyango, and A. de Geus (eds.), *Health and disease in Kenya* (Nairobi, 1974), p. 474; *Daily Nation*, 1 June 1981; Hilary Ojiambo, *You and your health* (Nairobi, 1986), p. 9.

64 H.P. Ojiambo, inaugural lecture in *Weekly Review*, 20 March 1978; East African Medical Research Council, *Report of the Consultative Committee on Cardiology Research in East Africa* (Arusha, 1976), p. 23; Ojiambo, *You and your health*, pp. 19–20, 54.

65 Hillary P. Ojiambo, 'Postgraduate medical training in Kenya', *The Lancet*, 30 December 1967, p. 1416; Hillary P. Ojiambo, 'Medical education and research – an agenda for change and action', *Medicus*, November 1993, pp. 315–20.

66 E.g. M.S. Abdullah, 'Hypertension – the Kenyan experience', *Medicom*, 1 (1979), 9–13.

67 P.A. Odhiambo, 'The first ten years of heart surgery in Kenya – aspirations, dilemmas and possibilities', *EAMJ*, 69 (1992), 520–4.

68 A. Wasunna, 'The diagnosis and conservative management of peptic ulcer', *Kenya Nursing Journal*, 2, 2 (December 1973), 22; E.N. Mngola and J.W. Odeny, 'Retrospective study of cases of gouty arthritis', *ibid.*, 2, 1 (June 1973), 11; E.N. Mngola, 'Current management of diabetes mellitus: part 1', *Medical Review (Uganda Edition)*, 1, 5 (September 1995), 2; D.M. Ndetei, 'Psychiatry in Kenya: yesterday, today and tomorrow', *Acta Psychiatrica Scandinavia*, 62 (1980), 201.

69 Kihumbu Thairu, *The African civilization* (Kampala, 1975), pp. 9, 201–2. The review was in *Weekly Review*, 15 September 1975.

70 Kihumbu Thairu, 'The direction of medical research in Africa', in J.B.O. Were, M.W. Mutugi, and J.I. Githure (eds.), *Recent advances in medical research with a symposium on the rational use of drugs* (Nairobi, 1992), pp. 5–8.

71 Nyarango, 'Medical education', p. 18; *Medicus*, July 1984, pp. 10, 25; S.N. Kinoti, P.G. Waiyaki, and J.B.O. Were (eds.), *Recent advances in medical research with a symposium on appropriate technology in disease control* (Nairobi, 1988); *Weekly Review*, 15 December 1989.

72 Davy K. Koech, 'Editorial', *African Journal of Health Sciences*, 1 (1994), 1.

73 Others included *Medicus*, *Medicom*, *African Journal of Sexually Transmitted Diseases*, *Medical Review*, and *African Medical News*.
74 *East African Standard*, 2 July 1970.
75 *Daily Nation*, 5 and 6 October 1971; Kenya, *National Assembly*, 5 October 1971, col. 860.
76 *Daily Nation*, 22–23 October 1971.
77 Kenya, *National Assembly*, 22 October 1971, cols. 1566, 1568; *Sunday Nation*, 24 October 1971; *Daily Nation*, 26 October 1971.
78 *Daily Nation*, 5–6 November 1971; *East African Standard*, 8 November 1971.
79 *Daily Nation*, 9 November 1971; *East African Standard*, 9–10 November 1971.
80 Growth rates in *Sunday Nation*, 24 March 1996; Maxon in Ogot and Ochieng', *Decolonization*, p. 136.
81 Kenya, *Report by DMS 1979*, pp. 10, 59; Kenya: Ministry of Health, 'Annual report 1981', duplicated, ch. 9 (UNMS library); V.A. Orinda, Peter Bjerregaard, and Dominic Mutie, 'Immunisation services in Kenya', *Medicus*, January 1987, pp. 9–12; Dan C. Owino Kaseje and Esther K.N. Sempebwa, 'An integrated rural health project in Saradidi, Kenya', *SSM*, 28 (1989), 1063; Karin E. Johnson, Wilson K. Kisubi, J. Karanja Mbugua, Douglas Lackey, Paget Stanfield, and Ben Osuga, 'Community-based health care in Kibwezi, Kenya', *SSM*, 28 (1989), 1039.
82 Kenya: Ministry of Health, *Medical Practitioners and Dentists Board: annual report 1978*, pp. 25–6.
83 *Weekly Review*, 8 August 1977.
84 *Ibid.*
85 *Ibid.*, 4 January 1980.
86 *Ibid.*, 4 January and 1 February 1980, 13 February 1981; Kenya: Ministry of Health, *KNH annual report 1979*, p. 37; *EAMJ*, 56 (1979), 467.
87 *Weekly Review*, 30 January and 6 and 13 February 1981.
88 *Daily Nation*, 7–9 May 1981.
89 *Weekly Review*, 15 May 1981.
90 *Ibid.*; *Daily Nation*, 9 and 11 May 1981; *Sunday Nation*, 10 and 24 May 1981.
91 *Daily Nation*, 16 May–3 June 1981.
92 *Weekly Review*, 9 October 1981 and 17 May 1985; above, pp. 194–5; *Medicus*, February 1987.
93 The figures are confusing and contradictory, but see Kenya, *Economic survey*, 1995, p. 187; *Weekly Review*, 8 July 1994; *EastAfrican*, 25 November 1996.
94 Kenya, *National development plan for the period 1989 to 1993* (Nairobi, n.d.), p. 240.
95 *Medicus*, May 1984, p. 1.
96 Kenya, *National Assembly*, 4 October 1966, col. 338.
97 Somba Kivungu, letter in *Medicus*, September 1989, p. 2.
98 Nyarango, 'Medical education', p. 18; *Medicus*, May 1986, p. 2, June 1983, p. 8, and May 1984, p. 2; *Weekly Review*, 31 May 1985.
99 *Weekly Review*, 15 July 1994; S.K. Masara (ed.), *Nairobi medical directory 93/94* (Nairobi, n.d.)
100 *Daily Nation*, 9 December 1994.
101 There is a lively fictional account of such a practice in Wamugunda Geteria, *Nice people* (Nairobi, 1992).

102 Wetungu to DMS, 15 July 1968, KNA Health BY/9/326/175.
103 'The code of professional conduct and discipline', in *Medicus*, July 1985, pp. 30–4.
104 H.K. Colebatch, 'Government services at the district level in Kenya: roads, schools and health services', University of Nairobi Institute of Development Studies discussion paper no. 38, May 1974, p. 43.
105 'The code', *Medicus*, July 1985, p. 32.
106 'Annual report 1976 – Inspector of Drugs, Western Kenya', KNA Health BY/9/604/42; Colebatch, 'Government services', p. 49; *Makerere College Newsletter*, 47 (December 1972); *Weekly Review*, 9 August 1976.
107 E.g. 'Minutes of Medical Practitioners and Dentists Board', 21 March 1967, KNA Health BY/9/326/12; C.J. Wanguku, 'Inspector of Drugs 1975 annual report Coast and North Eastern Provinces', KNA Health BY/9/608/60.
108 *Daily Nation*, 2, 20, and 30 December 1976.
109 Fendall, diary, 17 September 1965, Fendall papers, RH; 'Inspector of Drugs report – quarter ending 31st March '70', KNA Health BY/14/4/48; *Medicus*, December 1986, p. 4, and September 1989, p. 20; M.N. Kikindas, 'Ministry of Health: Kiambu District: 1983 annual report', KNA library.
110 Kenya, *National Assembly*, 9 October 1973, cols. 887–91; above, p. 182.
111 Masara, *Directory*, *passim*.
112 *Weekly Review*, 1 July 1988.
113 Masara, *Directory*, p. 6; *Medical Review (Uganda Edition)*, 2, 3 (May 1996), 37–9.
114 *Medical Review (Uganda Edition)*, 2, 2 (April 1996), 38–44.
115 *Weekly Review*, 21 May 1993, 9 June 1995, 4 August 1995; P.A. Odhiambo, 'How practical is free health care system in a developing country?' *Medicom*, 5 (1983), 164; Kenya, *Economic survey*, 1995, p. 188; Kenya, *National Assembly*, 9 October 1973, col. 898.
116 Odenyo, 'Professionalisation', pp. 29–30.
117 P.A. Odhiambo, 'Consultations – dilemmas and dare-devilry', *Medicom*, 8 (1986), 3; William Lore, 'Some ethical issues in the medical profession in Kenya', *Medicus*, 12, 11 (November 1993), 322; David M. Ndetei, 'Family/marital problems in Kenya and the practising doctor', *Medicom*, 4 (1982), 105.
118 Above, p. 185; *Weekly Review*, 13 October 1975.
119 Felix Lado Swaka, 'Practice of drug peddlers and health workers in relation to sexually transmitted diseases in Kenya', MPH thesis, University of Nairobi, 1992, pp. 25, 40; Karuga Wandai, 'Dr Stephen Nicholas Ngure Muthu', in his *Thika leaders* (Thika, 1989), p. 62; Ojiambo, 'Medical education', p. 322; Kenya: Ministry of Health, *Medical Practitioners and Dentists Board: annual report 1978*, p. 20.
120 *Medicus*, November 1981, p. 9, and September 1992, pp. 5–6.
121 There are two versions with slightly different figures: C. Sekadde-Kigondu and others, 'Knowledge, attitudes, practice and provision of family planning services by Kenyan medical doctors', duplicated, 1992, p. 22 (UNMS library); C. Sekadde-Kigondu and others, 'A survey of knowledge of family planning methods among Kenyan medical doctors: secondary data analysis', *Journal of Obstetrics and Gynaecology in Eastern and Central Africa*, 11, 1 (1995), 33. I have recalculated the figures from the second version.

122 *Daily Nation*, 1 August 1994; *East African Standard*, 23 June 1967, 13 January 1969, 8 December 1969.
123 Wandai, 'Dr James Flavian Chege Munene', in his *Thika leaders*, pp. 40–1.
124 Chege, 'Tale', pp. 84–8; David Throup, 'Elections and political legitimacy in Kenya', *Africa*, 63 (1993), 378–81; *Weekly Review*, 8 November 1996.
125 Chege, 'Tale', pp. 78–83; *Weekly Review*, 6 April 1979 and 7 March 1997.
126 Wetungu to DMS, 22 October 1968, KNA Health BY/9/326/187.
127 *Weekly Review*, 11 April 1986 and 29 July 1988; *Medicus*, December 1985, p. 6; *Daily Nation*, 17 April 1996; *EastAfrican*, 19 May 1997.
128 Thomas in Ingman and Thomas, *Topias*, pp. 274–5.
129 Violet N. Kimani and David Nyamwaya, 'Potential contribution of indigenous health personnel to primary health care', KEMRI conference paper, 1981, p. 23.
130 *EastAfrican*, 5 May 1997.
131 See above, p. 258 n103.
132 A.E.O. Wasunna and M. Wasunna, 'Drugs in wrong hands', in A.F. Bagshawe, G. Maina, and E.N. Mngola (eds.), *The use and abuse of drugs and chemicals in tropical Africa* (Nairobi, 1974), pp. 161–2.
133 Swaka, 'Practice', p. 7.
134 David Nyamwaya, 'A case study of the interaction between indigenous and Western medicine among the Pokot of Kenya', *SSM*, 25 (1987), 1277–8; Violet N. Kimani, 'The role of traditional medical practice', *Medicus*, 2, 2 (January 1983), 12.
135 C.M. Good and V.N. Kimani, 'Urban traditional medicine: a Nairobi case-study', *EAMJ*, 57 (1980), 306–9; Charles M. Good, *Ethnomedical systems in Africa: patterns of traditional medicine in rural and urban Kenya* (New York, 1987), p. 170.
136 See, e.g., Isaac Sindiga, Chacha Nyaigotti-Chacha, and Mary Peter Kanunah (eds.), *Traditional medicine in Africa* (Nairobi, 1995).
137 Kenya, *National Assembly*, 19 February 1969, cols. 5296 et seq.; *East African Standard*, 18 January 1969 and 4 February 1970; Ouma to Provincial Police Officer, Nyeri, 7 April 1970, KNA Health BY/14/4/28.
138 Sindiga and others, *Traditional medicine*, pp. 177, 31; Charles B.K. Nzioka, 'The social construction and management of HIV and AIDS among low-income patients in Nairobi', PhD thesis, University of London, 1994, p. 104.
139 Thairu, *African civilization*, ch. 8.
140 *Medicus*, May 1985, p. 22.
141 *New Vision*, 27 February 1989; David C. Nyamwaya, 'The management of illness in an East African society: a study of choice and constraint in health care among the Pokot', PhD thesis, University of Cambridge, 1982, p. 185.
142 J.O. Kokwaro, *Medicinal plants of East Africa* (Nairobi, 1976).
143 *Daily News*, 21 August 1991; Zysk, *Asceticism*, p. 78.
144 Kenya: Ministry of Health, *National guidelines for the implementation of primary health care in Kenya* (Nairobi, 1986), p. 106; Sindiga and others, *Traditional medicine*, p. 178; Kenya: Ministry of Health, 'Report of the proceedings of the first AIDS awareness seminar for traditional healers and herbalists', 14 March 1989 (UNMS library).

145 Good, *Ethnomedical systems*, pp. 193, 212–13, 302, 306; Mary Kigasia Amuyunzu, 'The management of illness in a plural health care setting: a case study of the Duruma of coastal Kenya', PhD thesis, University of Cambridge, 1994, p. 127.

146 Jack K. Githae, 'Ethnomedical practice in Kenya: the case of the Karati Rural Service Centre', in Sindiga and others, *Traditional medicine*, p. 63. See also *New Vision*, 20 March 1989.

147 Maxon in Ogot and Ochieng', *Decolonization*, p. 134; Kenya, *Economic survey*, 1995, p. 186; *Medicus*, October 1984, p. 1.

148 Kenya, *Economic survey*, 1995, p. 187; *Medicus*, December 1984, p. 25.

149 World Bank, *World development report*, 1995, p. 162; *Sunday Nation*, 7 July 1996; *New Vision*, 26 September 1996; Kenya: National Council for Population and Development, *Kenya demographic and health survey 1989: summary report* (Nairobi, n.d.), p. 2.

150 *Daily Nation*, 10 July 1996; *EastAfrican*, 5 August 1996; *Weekly Review*, 30 August 1996.

151 G.D. Moore, 'Essential drugs for Kenya's rural population', *World Health Forum*, 3 (1982), 196–9; 'Essential drug kits for rural Kenya: an interview with Dr Wilfred Koinange', *WHO Chronicle*, 40 (1986), 57–60; German Mwabu, James Mwanzia, and Wilson Liambila, 'User charges in government health facilities in Kenya', *Health Policy and Planning*, 10 (1995), 168.

152 Kenya: Ministry of Health, *Health information system: 1989 annual report* (Nairobi, 1991), p. 34.

153 *EAMJ*, 47 (1970), 301, and 54 (1977), 166; *Medicus*, November 1981, pp. 8–9.

154 *Medicus*, June 1985, p. 46, January 1983, p. 3, November 1981, p. 9, and June 1984, p. 24.

155 Vincent Akoko Orinda, 'The mother of a sick child in a paediatric ward – her role in ward management', MMed thesis, University of Nairobi, 1982.

156 James Wambura Nyikal, 'Socio-economic background of children admitted to Kenyatta National Hospital with kwashiorkor', MMed thesis, University of Nairobi, 1984, p. ii.

157 *Medicus*, September 1983, p. 25; *Weekly Review*, 15 December 1978.

158 Yusuf Ali Eraj, 'The organization of doctors and the crisis in medicine', paper to the Commonwealth Medical Association Annual Conference, Nairobi, 1980 (UNMS library).,

159 *Medicus*, November 1981, p. 8, and April 1982, pp. 4–5.

160 *Ibid.*, November 1981, pp. 3 4, and December 1981, p. 5.

161 *Ibid.*, December 1981, p. 10, January 1982, pp. 10–11, 17, April 1982, pp. 5–6, 19–21.

162 *Ibid.*, June 1984, pp. 1, 20–6.

163 *Ibid.*, September 1984, pp. 1–2, 7–15, 19, 23; *Weekly Review*, 19 October 1984.

164 *Daily Nation*, 27 May 1994.

165 *Ibid.*, 9 July 1994.

166 *Ibid.*, 29 June 1994.

167 *Weekly Review*, 8 July 1994.

168 *Ibid.*

169 See Ogot and Ochieng', *Decolonization*, ch. 9.

170 *Medicus*, January 1993, p. 7; F.G. Njenga, 'Doctors must stand up for human rights', *Nairobi Law Monthly*, 32 (April 1991), 34–5; *ibid.*, 42 (April 1992), p. 28, and 62 (March 1996), p. 25; *Daily Nation*, 1 July and 22 November 1993.
171 *Weekly Review*, 27 May 1994; *Daily Nation*, 27–28 May 1994.
172 *Daily Nation*, 17 June 1994.
173 *Weekly Review*, 24 June 1994.
174 *Daily Nation*, 22 June and 5 July 1994.
175 *Ibid.*, 23 June 1994; *Weekly Review*, 24 June 1994.
176 *Daily Nation*, 2 July 1994.
177 *Weekly Review*, 8 July 1994.
178 *Daily Nation*, 12–13 July 1994.
179 *Ibid.*, 7 July–2 August 1994.
180 *Ibid.*, 5 August 1994.
181 *Ibid.*, 20 August 1994.
182 *Ibid.*, 3–19 September 1994.
183 *Ibid.*, 23 September 1994.
184 *Ibid.*, 30 September 1994.
185 *Ibid.*, 23 September 1994.
186 Mwabu, 'Health care reform', pp. 245–55; D. Collins, J.D. Quick, S.N. Murau, D. Kraushaar, and I.M. Hussein, 'The fall and rise of cost sharing in Kenya', *Health Policy and Planning*, 11 (1996), 52–63; J. Karanja Mbugua, Gerald H. Bloom, and Malcolm M. Segall, 'Impact of user charges on vulnerable groups: the case of Kibwezi in rural Kenya', *SSM*, 41 (1995), 829–35.
187 Kenya, *National development plan 1989–93*, pp. 236–43.
188 *Sunday Nation*, 7 July 1996.
189 Obeid Mumamari in *Medicus*, January 1984, p. 4.
190 *Sunday Nation*, 7 July 1996.

9 TANZANIA: DOCTORS AND A SOCIALIST EXPERIMENT

1 *EastAfrican*, 27 January 1997.
2 Tallack, 'Aspects', p. 40.
3 Pratt, *Critical phase*, p. 138; *East African Standard*, 18 August 1964; *Daily News*, 12 January 1974, 14 June 1980, 23 May 1987.
4 Pratt, *Critical phase*, p. 131.
5 Gish, *Planning*, p. 52; Pratt, *Critical phase*, p. 175.
6 Titmuss and others, *Health services*, p. 84.
7 Tanzania, *Five-year plan for economic and social development, 1st July, 1964–30th June, 1969* (2 vols., Dar es Salaam, 1964), vol. I, p. 70; Gish, *Planning*, pp. 21–2.
8 Gish, *Planning*, pp. 23, 123–4; Kris Heggenhougen, Patrick Vaughan, Eustace P.Y. Muhondwa, and J. Rutabanzibwa-Ngaiza, *Community health workers: the Tanzanian experience* (Oxford, 1987), p. 26; Chagula and Tarimo in Newell, *Health*, p. 156.
9 Gish, *Planning*, pp. 71, 145; Tanganyika, *AMR* 1961 vol. II; Tanzania, *AMR* 1967 vol. I, p. 1.
10 See Pratt, *Critical phase*, chs. 7–8.
11 P.S. Mganga, 'Visit to China', *Afya*, 2, 2 (February 1968), 4–7.

12 *Sunday News*, 4 October 1981; L. Nangwanda Sijaona, 'Medical practice in the context of the socialistic pattern of society', *Dar es Salaam Medical Journal*, 2, 1 (March 1970), 11–14.
13 Tanzania, *Second five-year plan for economic and social development, 1st July, 1969–30th June, 1974* (2 vols., Dar es Salaam, 1969), vol. I, ch. 11.
14 Gish, *Planning*, pp. 25–31, 189.
15 *Daily News*, 13 September 1978.
16 P. Stambuli, 'Rural health', *Afya*, 4, 7 (July 1970), 3–6.
17 A.M. Nhonoli, 'Problems of promoting healthy living in East African rural areas with particular reference to Tanzania', in P. Correa and others, *Biomedical lectures: 1970–1973 series*, Afro Technical Papers No. 11 (Brazzaville, 1975), pp. 39–47.
18 Gish, *Planning*, *passim*.
19 E.g. *Sunday News*, 27 May 1973.
20 Gish, *Planning*, pp. 46–51, 72–3.
21 *Daily News*, 13 April 1973.
22 *Ibid.*, 22 May 1972.
23 *Ibid.*, 29 May 1973.
24 Nsekela and Nhonoli, *Development*, p. 103; *Daily News*, 15 May 1973; *Sunday News*, 8 December 1974.
25 *Daily News*, 2 July 1973.
26 *Sunday News*, 11 November 1973.
27 Tanzania, *Evaluation of the health sector 1979*, p. 31; Gish, *Planning*, p. 51n.
28 Knud Erik Svendsen, 'The creation of macroeconomic imbalances and a structural crisis', in Jannik Boesen, Kjell J. Havnevik, Juhani Koponen, and Rie Odgaard (eds.), *Tanzania: crisis and struggle for survival* (Uppsala, 1986), p. 67; Mandara in Mwaluko and others, *Health*, p. 6; Albert E. Henn, *Tanzania: health sector strategy* (Dar es Salaam, 1980), annex II, pp. 25–6.
29 Chagula and Tarimo in Newell, *Health*, p. 165; *Daily News*, 20 July 1989.
30 Heggenhougen and others, *Community health workers*, pp. 27–8; Gish, *Planning*, p. 56; Urban Johnson, 'Ideological framework and health development in Tanzania 1961–2000', *SSM*, 22 (1986), 748; Henn, *Tanzania*, annex II, p. 25.
31 G. van Etten, 'Towards research on health development in Tanzania', *SSM*, 6 (1972), 346.
32 *Daily News*, 20 May 1983; Oscar Gish, 'Some observations about health development in three African socialist countries: Ethiopia, Mozambique and Tanzania', *SSM*, 17 (1983), 1966; Brian Abel-Smith and Pankaj Rawal, 'Can the poor afford "free" health services? A case study of Tanzania', *Health Policy and Planning*, 7 (1992), 330.
33 G.M. van Etten, *Rural health development in Tanzania* (Assen, 1976), p. 49; *Daily News*, 4 December 1982.
34 *Daily News*, 21 January 1981.
35 See the excellent account in Heggenhougen and others, *Community health workers*.
36 *Daily News*, 19 March 1991, 21 May 1992;Tanzania, *Health profile 1991* (Dar es Salaam, 1991), p. 7.
37 Marilynn M. Rosenthal, *Health care in the People's Republic of China* (Boulder,

1987), pp. 2, 21, 23, 183; Naisu Zhu, Zhihua Ling, Jie Shen, J.M. Lane, and Shanlien Hu, 'Factors associated with the decline of the Cooperative Medical System and barefoot doctors in rural China', *Bulletin of the WHO*, 67 (1989), 431–41.

38 Tanzania: Bureau of Statistics, *Tanzanian demographic and health survey 1991/92: summary report* (Dar es Salaam, 1993), p. 12; *Daily News*, 18 March 1986, 10 January 1990, 11 November 1991.

39 WHO, *Annual report 1990–1*, p. 100; Tanzania: Bureau of Statistics, *Demographic and health survey*, p. 11.

40 Motomora Matomora, Angwana Kiwara, and Brian Cooksey, *The provision and acceptability of child immunization services in Tanzania* (Dar es Salaam, 1992), p. 3.

41 Elias H.O. Ayiemba and John O. Oucho, *The state of population in eastern and southern Africa* (Nairobi, 1994), p. 25; E. Renganathan and others, 'Evolution of operational research studies and development of a national control strategy against intestinal helminths in Pemba Island, 1988–92', *Bulletin of the WHO*, 73 (1995), 183; Mandara in Mwaluko and others, *Health*, p. 5; *New Vision*, 26 March 1994; *Daily News*, 3 November 1977; World Bank, *World development report*, 1995, p. 162.

42 Lucy Gilson, 'Management and health care reform in sub-Saharan Africa', *SSM*, 40 (1995), 707.

43 K.S. Mnyika and J.Z.J. Killewo, 'Irrational drug use in Tanzania', *Health Policy and Planning*, 6 (1991), 180; *Daily News*, 26 May 1988 and 13 December 1983; Ronald J. Vogel and Betsy Stephens, 'Availability of pharmaceuticals in sub-Saharan Africa', *SSM*, 29 (1989), 482–4.

44 Johnson, 'Ideological framework', p. 749.

45 *Daily News*, 3 August 1987.

46 *Ibid.*, 30 December 1982; *Sunday News*, 17 March 1991.

47 *Daily News*, 19 November 1985.

48 A.M. Kilonzo, 'Obstetric and gynaecologic cases and commentaries', MMed thesis, University of Dar es Salaam, 1987, p. 320.

49 World Bank, *World development report*, 1994, p. 222.

50 Tanzania, *Recorded population changes 1948–1967* (Dar es Salaam, 1968), p. 13; *Pears' cyclopaedia* (1996–7), p. K.43; Akim J. Mturi and Sian L. Curtis, 'The determinants of infant and child mortality in Tanzania', *Health Policy and Planning*, 10 (1995), 386.

51 E. Tarimo, 'Primary health care in Tanzania', *Tanzania Medical Journal*, special issue, September 1985, p. 22; Hamza J. Chum, Richard J. O'Brien, T. Martin Chonde, Petra Graf, and Hans L. Rieder, 'An epidemiological study of tuberculosis and HIV infection in Tanzania, 1991–1993', *AIDS*, 10 (1996), 308; *Daily News*, 2 June 1990.

52 *Daily News*, 29 June 1992. See also W.L. Kilama, *The war against mosquitoes and mosquito-borne diseases in Tanzania: some lost battles* (Dar es Salaam, 1994).

53 Henn, *Tanzania*, annex II, pp. 12–15; *Sunday News*, 13 June 1982, 28 December 1985, 19 June 1990.

54 *Daily News*, 21 May 1981, 16 June 1984.

55 *Ibid.*, 26 September 1973.

56 *Sunday News*, 17 May 1987; *Daily News*, 28 July 1988.
57 *Daily News*, 17 June 1983, 26 June 1986, 11 April 1987; E.M.A. Ombaka and E.S.T. Mosha, 'Some aspects of drug use in Dar es Salaam', *Tanzania Medical Journal*, 3, 1 (December 1986), 15.
58 Harald Kristian Heggenhougen, 'Health services: official and unofficial', in Boesen and others, *Tanzania*, p. 310; Tanzania, *Evaluation*, pp. 20–1; *Daily News*, 28 February 1984.
59 Tanzania, *Evaluation*, pp. 119–20.
60 *Daily News*, 12 February 1986.
61 *East African Standard*, 30 September 1968.
62 Nyerere in Stirling, *Tanzanian doctor*, p. xv.
63 *Sunday News*, 9 August 1981; *Daily News*, 29 May 1973; Dean E. McHenry Jr, *Tanzania's ujamaa villages* (Berkeley, 1979), p. 56; Reginald Herbold Green and Hans Singer, 'Sub-Saharan Africa in depression', *World Development*, 12 (1984), 292; *Daily News*, 22 November 1982; *Sunday News*, 8 February 1981.
64 *Tanganyika Standard*, 2, 6, 19, 20 December 1961.
65 *Ibid.*, 22 December 1961; Titmuss and others, *Health services*, pp. 70–1; Nsekela and Nhonoli, *Development*, pp. 99–100.
66 Chagula and Tarimo in Newell, *Health*, p. 162; *Daily News*, 10 April 1976.
67 *Daily News*, 18 June 1975, 10 November 1975.
68 *Sunday News*, 13 June 1976.
69 *Ibid.*, 4 July 1976 and 13 February 1977; *Daily News*, 28 April 1977.
70 Joseph T. Karashani, 'Welcome address', *Tanzania Medical Journal*, special issue, September 1985, pp. 2–3; *Daily News*, 1 January 1977.
71 *Daily News*, 18 January 1977.
72 *Weekly Review*, 28 April 1978; *Daily News*, 2 July 1980 and 1 January 1992.
73 *Daily News*, 19 December 1979, 24 July 1987; *Sunday News*, 4 March 1984.
74 Stirling, *Tanzanian doctor*, p. 141.
75 *Daily News*, 3 September 1982; *Sunday News*, 17 April 1983.
76 *Daily News*, 19 March 1985, 18 September 1986, 4 August 1987.
77 *Sunday News*, 1 October 1978. Chama Cha Mapinduzi (CCM) was TANU's successor.
78 *Daily News*, 24 September 1981.
79 *Ibid.*, 16 March 1990.
80 Ralph C. Croizier, *Traditional medicine in modern China* (Cambridge, Mass., 1968), pp. 183–5; Nathan Sivin, *Traditional medicine in contemporary China* (Michigan, 1987), p. 19.
81 Above, p. 202; *Daily News*, 31 October 1973.
82 Sijaona, 'Medical practice', p. 14; I.A.J. Semali, 'Associations and healers: attitudes towards collaboration in Tanzania', in Last and Chavunduka, *Professionalisation*, pp. 87–8; Tanzania, *Health profile*, p. 6.
83 Inga Hedberg, Olov Hedberg, Posanyi J. Madati, Keto E. Mshigeni, E.N. Mshiu, and Gunnar Samuelsson, 'Inventory of plants used in traditional medicine in Tanzania', *Journal of Ethnopharmacology*, 6 (1982), 29–60, and 9 (1983), 105–28 and 237–60; S.C. Chhabra, R.L.A. Mahunnah, and E.N. Mshiu, 'Plants used in traditional medicine in eastern Tanzania', *ibid.*, vols. 21–33 (1987–91); Mshigeni and others, *Proceedings*; Siegfried J. Nkinda, 'Traditional herbs for bronchial asthma in Tanga Region', MMed thesis,

University of Dar es Salaam, 1976; I.A.J. Semali and A.E. Masawe, 'Bronchial asthma as known by traditional healers', *EAMJ*, 62 (1985), 533–9.

84 *Daily News*, 26 July 1995.

85 Innocent Antony John Semali, 'The opinions of allopathic health workers on traditional medicine/healers and degree of contact between the two in Tanzania', DPH thesis, University of Dar es Salaam, 1982.

86 Tanzania, *Health profile*, p. 7; *Daily News*, 11 September 1990, 24 December 1991.

87 *Daily News*, 18 January 1973; Semali in Last and Chavunduka, *Professionalisation*, pp. 87–92.

88 Semali, 'Opinions', p. 47.

89 Rosenthal, *Health care*, ch. 5; Judith Farquhar, 'Re-writing traditional medicine in post-Maoist China', in Don Bates (ed.), *Knowledge and the scholarly medical traditions* (Cambridge, 1995), pp. 262–76.

90 *Daily News*, 28 February 1991, 4 August 1991.

91 World Bank, *World development report*, 1990, p. 178.

92 Tarimo, 'Primary health care', p. 20; Lucy Gilson, Martin Alilio, and Kris Heggenhougen, 'Community satisfaction with primary health care services: an evaluation undertaken in the Morogoro Region of Tanzania', *SSM*, 39 (1994), 771–8.

93 Quoted in *ibid.*, p. 779.

94 Information from Dr S.A. Mwankemwa; *Daily News*, 23 October 1976.

95 *Daily News*, 5 December 1976, 30 November 1984; Kihumuro-Apuuli to Undersecretary, 16 February 1989, UMOH PHC/HP/1/I/33; *Daily News*, 29 March 1991.

96 C.H. Wood, 'The Michael Ngirwamungu memorial lecture', *Dar es Salaam Medical Journal*, 3, 2 (March 1971), 113–14; Nhonoli in Correa and others, *Biomedical lectures*, p. 44.

97 Nhonoli, 'Analysis', p. 99.

98 *Ibid.*

99 Jesse Kagimba, 'The Mafia campaign, June 1970', *Dar es Salaam Medical Journal*, 4, 1 (December 1971), 136–7.

100 Alanagh Raikes, 'Medical education in a developing country: a survey of Tanzanian medical students', MA thesis, University of Dar es Salaam, 1978. See also A.M. Raikes, 'Medical education in transition: Tanzania', in Ingman and Thomas, *Topias*, pp. 159–73.

101 *Daily News*, 27 November 1974.

102 F.D.E. Mtango and M.T. Leshabari, 'Medical students performance: pre- and post-Musoma Resolution', *TNR*, 92 (1985), 89–94.

103 *Daily News*, 16 July 1983; *Sunday News*, 4 March 1984; *Daily News*, 9 October 1991.

104 *Daily News*, 4 August 1987, 29 November 1988, 9 October 1991.

105 *Ibid.*, 21 September 1991, 9 October 1991, 1 January 1992.

106 Editorial in *East African Journal of Medical Research*, 3, 4 (October 1976), 171.

107 A.M.M. Nhonoli, 'An enquiry into the infant mortality rate in rural areas of Unyamwezi', *EAMJ*, 31 (1954), 1–12.

108 A.M. Nhonoli, 'Cutaneous anthrax in Moshi District', *EAMJ*, 37 (1960), 37–32; A.M. Nhonoli, 'The differential diagnosis of malnutrition in children',

ibid., 336–42; J.S. Meredith and A.M. Nhonoli, 'Intraperitoneal blood transfusion in infantile anaemia', *ibid.*, 39 (1962), 274–87; A.M. Nhonoli, 'Some aspects of duodenal ulcer in Dar es Salaam', *ibid.*, 46 (1969), 64–6.

109 Aloysius Mwessa Nhonoli, 'Hookworm disease and its cardio-vascular manifestations', MD thesis, University of East Africa, 1969, p. 56.

110 A.M. Nhonoli, F.E. Kihama, and B.D. Ramji, 'Infection rates of Tanzanian rural communities by the common parasites and some of their haematological effects', *EAMJ*, 51 (1974), 829–36; A.M. Nhonoli and F.E. Kihama, 'The health status of a rural population in mid-eastern Tanzania', *ibid.*, 122–30; A.M. Nhonoli, B.D. Ramji, and J.Y. Shemaghoda, 'The effect of malaria infection in the placenta and foetal growth, and the concept of congenital malaria', *East African Journal of Medical Research*, 2, 2 (April 1975), 149–61; A.M. Nhonoli and others, 'Haemoglobin quantitation and the distribution of sickle haemoglobin gene among Tanzanians', *ibid.*, 4, 1 (January 1977), 17–24; A.M. Nhonoli, B.D. Ramji, and J. Kujwalile, 'The white blood cell counts in Africans and the probable causes of neutropenia', *ibid.*, 2, 4 (October 1975), 293–303.

111 H.M. Kitange, A.B.M. Swai, P.M. Kilima, G. Masuki, K.G.M.M. Alberti, and D.G. McLarty, 'Anaemia as a major public health problem in Tanzania', *Health Policy and Planning*, 8 (1993), 413–18.

112 W.B.P. Matuja and W.J. Makene, 'Neurological disease pattern in adults admitted to the medical wards at Muhimbili Medical Centre', *Tanzania Medical Journal*, 4, 1 (June 1989), 18–21; *Daily News*, 1 October 1990; Kilama, *War against mosquitoes*.

113 *Daily News*, 23 July 1982.

114 V.P. Kimati and B. Lyaruu, 'Measles complications as seen at Mwanza Regional Consultant and Teaching Hospital in 1973', *EAMJ*, 53 (1976), 322–40; V.P. Kimati and N.S. Scrimshaw, 'The nutritional status of Tanzanian children', *EAMJ*, 62 (1985), 105–17; V.P. Kimati, 'Review of sickle cell haemoglobinopathy in Tanzania', in R. Owor, V.L. Ongom, and B.G. Kirya (eds.), *The child in the African environment* (Nairobi, 1975), pp. 171–80; V.P. Kimati, *The world's best medicine and a new health prescription* (Dar es Salaam, 1983); *Sunday News*, 1 May 1977.

115 Joseph K. Shija, *Paediatric surgical care in developing countries* (Nairobi, 1989).

116 B.S. Kilonzo, 'Observations on the epidemiology of plague in Tanzania during the period 1974–1988', *EAMJ*, 69 (1992), 494–9; F.S. Mhalu, F.D.E. Mtango, and A.E. Msengi, 'Hospital outbreaks of cholera transmitted through close person-to-person contact', *The Lancet*, 1984/2, pp. 82–4; F.S. Mhalu, D.S.M. Mwakagile, and R. Linje, 'End of the penicillin era in the management of gonorrhoea at first level health care in Dar es Salaam', *Tanzania Medical Journal*, 2, 1 (September 1985), 47–52.

117 A.M. Nhonoli, 'Heart disease in Dar es Salaam', *EAMJ*, 45 (1968), 118–21; A.M. Nhonoli, 'The incidence of hypertensive heart disease in Dar es Salaam', *ibid.*, 46 (1969), 55–7.

118 W.J. Makene and J. Maindi, 'The frequently of cardiomyopathies in Dar es Salaam', in Bennett and others, *Degenerative disorders*, pp. 325–30.

119 W.J. Makene, 'Presiding Chairman's address', *EAMJ*, 51 (1974), 823.

120 *Sunday News*, 2 August 1987; *Daily News*, 5 May 1988; C.A. Mkony, 'Kidney

transplantation in developing countries', *Tanzania Medical Journal*, 7, 1 (September 1992), 1–3; *Sunday News*, 6 January 1985.

121 Boesen and others, *Tanzania*, p. 25.
122 *EastAfrican*, 23 September 1996; *Daily News*, 15 November 1989 and 7 June 1986.
123 *EastAfrican*, 6 January 1997.
124 *Daily News*, 18 September 1986, 27 January 1987, 19 September 1991.
125 *Ibid.*, 28 July 1988 and 20 July 1989.
126 *Ibid.*, 10 November 1990, 10 January 1991; *Sunday News*, 24 March 1991.
127 *Daily News*, 18 June 1990, 11 February 1981, 13 September 1985, 27 November 1991.
128 *Ibid.*, 9 October 1991 and 24 January 1992.
129 *Ibid.*, 18 July 1988, 29 June 1990, 20 June 1991.
130 *Ibid.*, 23 January–2 February and 10–11 March 1992.
131 'Proceedings of the East Africa burden of disease, cost effectiveness of health care interventions and health policy regional workshop', Nairobi, August 1994, pp. 73–5, 98–9 (UMOH library); Gilson, 'Management', p. 697.
132 K. Wyss and others, 'Utilisation of government and private health services in Dar es Salaam', *EAMJ*, 73 (1996), 357–8; A.H. Ahmed, D.P. Urassa, F. Gherardi, and N.Y. Game, 'Patients' perception of public, voluntary and private dispensaries in rural areas of Tanzania', *ibid.*, 370.
133 'Proceedings of the . . . regional workshop', p. 16; *Daily News*, 7 March 1997.
134 *Daily News*, 1 January and 30 March 1992; Ahmed and others, 'Patients' perception', p. 370.
135 *Sunday News*, 12 January 1992; *Daily News*, 5 March 1997.
136 Gilson, 'Management', p. 697; Abel-Smith and Rawal, 'Can the poor?' pp. 329–41; *Daily News*, 7 July 1995; Gijs Walraven, 'Willingness to pay for district hospital services in rural Tanzania', *Health Policy and Planning*, 11 (1996), 434.
137 *Daily News*, 6 July and 24 October 1995.
138 *Ibid.*, 12 April 1986; *EastAfrican*, 16 September 1996; *New Vision*, 16 April 1994; *Daily News*, 22 February 1993.
139 *Daily News*, 1 January and 11 June 1992.

10 AIDS

1 A.M.T. Lwegaba, 'Preliminary report of "an unusual wasting disease" complex nicknamed "Slim" a slow epidemic of Rakai District, Uganda', November 1984, photocopy of typescript, UMOH library.
2 For the early history of AIDS in the region, see also Ed Hooper, *Slim: a reporter's own story of AIDS in East Africa* (London, 1990).
3 *New Vision*, 9 April 1991.
4 J.M. Jagwe, quoted in *New Vision*, 2 January 1990.
5 A.J. Nahmias and others, 'Evidence for human infection with an HTLV III/LAV-like virus in central Africa, 1959', *The Lancet*, 1986/1, pp. 1279–80; Manfred Eigen and Katja Nieselt-Struwe, 'How old is the immunodeficiency virus?' *AIDS*, 4 (1990), supplement, S90–S92.
6 Mirko D. Grmek, *History of AIDS* (trans. R.C. Maulitz and J. Duffin, Princeton, 1990), pp. x, 135.

7 Nelson Sewankambo and others, 'Enteropathic AIDS in Uganda', *AIDS*, 1 (1987), 9; James W. Curran and others, 'Epidemiologic aspects of the current outbreak of Kaposi's sarcoma and opportunistic infections', *New England Journal of Medicine*, 306 (1982), 248–52.
8 Olweny in Parry, *Principles*, p. 986.
9 Grmek, *History*, p. 32.
10 Hooper, *Slim*, p. 346.
11 D. Serwadda and others, 'Slim disease: a new disease in Uganda and its association with HTLV-III infection', *The Lancet*, 1985/2, pp. 849–52.
12 J. Wilson Carswell, Roy Mugerwa, Nelson Sewankambo, Fred Kigozi, and Rick Goodgame, 'AIDS in Uganda: a special report by the Clinical Committee on AIDS', *Health Information Quarterly*, 2, 1 (February 1986), 11–20.
13 *Weekly Topic*, 13 September 1985.
14 Minutes on Undersecretary to PS, 22 November 1985, UMOH GCH.3/4/III/20.
15 Hooper, *Slim*, p. 347; *Weekly Topic*, 20 March 1986.
16 'Minutes of the meeting between the Hon. Minister of Health and AIDS Surveillance Sub-Committee', 5 September 1986, UMOH *7; Hooper, *Slim*, pp. 347–8; *New Vision*, 12 July 1988.
17 The meeting was on 8 September 1986. Its outcome is inferred from *New Vision*, 9 September 1986, and 'Speech by the Deputy Minister of Health Dr I.J. Batwala at the launching of an "AIDS" seminar', 25 September 1986, *Health Information Quarterly*, 2, 4 (December 1986), 18–21.
18 Hooper, *Slim*, p. 153; Uganda: Ministry of Health, 'AIDS Control Programme: proposals for a five year action plan (1987–1991)', duplicated, 1987, p. 5 (UMOH library).
19 Quoted in *New Vision*, 4 September 1993.
20 *Daily News*, 28 September 1985 and 2 June 1989; F.S. Mhalu, A. Dahoma, E. Mbena, S. Maselle, V. Bredberg-Rådén, and G. Biberfeld, 'Some aspects of the epidemiology of AIDS and infections with the Human Immunodeficiency Virus in the United Republic of Tanzania', in G. Giraldo, E. Beth-Giraldo, N. Clumeck, M.R. Gharbi, S.K. Kyalwazi, and G. de Thé (eds.), *AIDS and associated cancers in Africa* (Basel, 1988), pp. 50–2.
21 Mhalu and others in Giraldo and others, *AIDS*, pp. 50, 52; *Sunday News*, 24 March 1985.
22 *Sunday News*, 2 June 1985 and 12 January 1986.
23 *Ibid.*, 11 May 1986; *Daily News*, 2 August 1986.
24 Kenya: Ministry of Health, 'First AIDS awareness seminar', p. 20; *Weekly Review*, 25 January 1985 and 9 February 1990.
25 *Weekly Review*, 13 September 1985 and 29 November 1985; Alfred J. Fortin, 'The politics of AIDS in Kenya', *Third World Quarterly*, 9 (1987), 914
26 Robert J. Biggar and others, 'Regional variation in prevalence of antibody against Human T-Lymphotropic Virus types I and III in Kenya', *International Journal of Cancer*, 35 (1985), 763–7; J.W. Carswell, N. Sewankambo, G. Lloyd, and R.G. Downing, 'How long has the AIDS virus been in Uganda?' *The Lancet*, 1986/1, p. 1217.
27 Okware, 'Brief report and policy considerations on AIDS Control Programme', 15 April 1989, UMOH *6; *New Vision*, 8 November 1988.

28 *New Vision*, 10 February 1987; *Daily News*, 29 July 1988.
29 *Medicus*, January 1987, p. 1.
30 *Weekly Review*, 11 October 1985; Fortin, 'Politics', pp. 908–13.
31 PS to MOH, 5 June 1989, UMOH GCD.2/1/5.
32 Okware to ACP staff, 7 December 1987, UMOH *5; Jagwe to National Committee for the Prevention and Control of AIDS, 23 February 1987, UMOH GCC.42/AIDS/IV/39; Okware, 'Brief report and policy considerations on AIDS Control Programme', 15 April 1989, UMOH *6.
33 R.D. Mugerwa, D. Serwadda, S.K. Kyalwazi, E. Beth-Giraldo, F.M. Buonaguro, and G. Giraldo, 'Some clinical aspects of AIDS in Uganda', in Giraldo and others, *AIDS*, pp. 134–7.
34 Nelson K. Sewankambo and others, 'HIV infection through normal heterosexual contact in Uganda', *AIDS*, 1 (1987), 113–16.
35 J. Wilson Carswell, 'HIV infection in healthy persons in Uganda', *ibid.*, 225.
36 Okware, quoted in *New Vision*, 11 November 1988.
37 David Serwadda, Maria J. Wawer, Stanley D. Musgrave, Nelson K. Sewankambo, Jonathan E. Kaplan, and Ronald H. Gray, 'HIV risk factors in three geographic strata of rural Rakai District', *AIDS*, 6 (1992), 983–9.
38 David Serwadda and others, 'The social dynamics of HIV transmission as reflected through discordant couples in rural Uganda', *AIDS*, 9 (1995), 745; Maria J. Wawer and others, 'Incidence of HIV-1 infection in a rural region of Uganda', *British Medical Journal*, 308 (1994), 172–3; Nelson K. Sewankambo and others, 'Demographic impact of HIV infection in rural Rakai District', *AIDS*, 8 (1994), 1707.
39 Andrew J. Nunn, Jane F. Kengeya-Kayondo, Sam S. Malamba, Janet A. Seeley, and Daan W. Mulder, 'Risk factors for HIV-1 infection in adults in a rural Uganda community', *AIDS*, 8 (1994), 81, 84, 86; Daan W. Mulder, Andrew J. Nunn, Hans-Ulrich Wagner, Anatoli Kamali, and Jane F. Kengeya-Kayondo, 'HIV-1 incidence and HIV-1 associated mortality in a rural Ugandan population cohort', *ibid.*, 92; H. Pickering, M. Okongo, B. Nnalusiba, K. Bwanika, and J. Whitworth, 'Sexual networks in Uganda', *AIDS Care*, 9 (1997), 206–7.
40 Y.K. Konde-Lule, 'Syphilis in pregnant mothers at Mulago Hospital', DPH thesis, Makerere University, 1977.
41 Joseph K. Konde-Lule, Seth F. Berkley, and Robert Downing, 'Knowledge, attitudes and practices concerning AIDS in Ugandans', *AIDS*, 3 (1989), 513–18; J.K. Konde-Lule and A.J.N. Sebina, 'The impact of AIDS in a rural Ugandan community', *EAMJ*, 70 (1993), 725–9. For subsequent findings, see *EastAfrican*, 15 September 1997.
42 Joseph K. Konde-Lule, M. Musagara, and S. Musgrave, 'Focus group interviews about AIDS in Rakai District of Uganda', *SSM*, 37 (1993), 679–84; Joseph K. Konde-Lule and others, 'Adolescents, sexual behaviour and HIV-1 in rural Rakai District, Uganda', *AIDS*, 11 (1997), 791–9.
43 Joseph K. Konde-Lule, 'The effects of urbanization on the spread of AIDS in Africa', *African Urban Quarterly*, 6 (1991), 13.
44 J. Seeley, E. Kajura, C. Bachengema, M. Okongo, U. Wagner, and D. Mulder, 'The extended family and support for people with AIDS in a rural population

in south west Uganda', *AIDS Care*, 5 (1993), 117–22; A. Kamali, J.A. Seeley, A.J. Nunn, J.F. Kengeya-Kayondo, A. Ruberantwari, and D.W. Mulder, 'The orphan problem', *AIDS Care*, 8 (1996), 509–15.

45 Hubert Nsanze, 'Sexually transmitted diseases', *Afya*, 18 (1984), 109–13.

46 F.A. Plummer, E.N. Ngugi, and S. Moses, 'The Pumwani experience: evolution of a partnership in disease control', in Network of AIDS Researchers of Eastern and Southern Africa, *Focusing interventions among vulnerable groups for HIV infection* (Nairobi, 1994), pp. 75–81.

47 Stephen Moses and others, 'Sexual behaviour in Kenya: implications for sexually transmitted disease transmission and control', *SSM*, 39 (1994), 1656.

48 Elizabeth N. Ngugi and Francis A. Plummer, 'Health outreach and control of HIV infection in Kenya', *Journal of AIDS*, 1 (1988), 566–70; F.A. Plummer and S. Moses, 'Transmission dynamics of STD and HIV', in Network, *Focusing interventions*, pp. 1–9.

49 S.Y. Maselle and D.S.M. Mwakagile, 'Genital ulcer disease in Dar es Salaam', *Tanzania Medical Journal*, special issue, September 1985, p. 31; W.K. Urassa, S. Moshi, A. Rutahindurwa, J. Mbwana, and F.S. Mhalu, 'Bacteriological findings among patients attending a referral clinic for sexually transmitted diseases in Dar es Salaam', *ibid.*, 5, 1 (March 1990), 15–17.

50 Fred Mhalu and others, 'Prevalence of HIV infection in healthy subjects and groups of patients in Tanzania', *AIDS*, 1 (1987), 217–21; Japhet Killewo and others, 'Prevalence of HIV-1 infection in the Kagera region of Tanzania', *AIDS*, 4 (1990), 1081–5.

51 Mhalu and others in Giraldo and others, *AIDS*, p. 53.

52 *Daily News*, 8 August 1986 and 9 July 1988.

53 Editorial in *Tanzania Medical Journal*, 6, 2 (September 1991), 33.

54 F.S. Mhalu, 'Inter-relationships between HIV infection and other sexually transmitted diseases', *EAMJ*, 67 (1990), 512.

55 Kagoma S. Mnyika, Knut-Inge Klepp, Gunnar Kvåle, Steinar Nilssen, Peter E. Kissila, and Naphthal Ole-King'ori, 'Prevalence of HIV-1 infection in urban, semi-urban and rural areas in Arusha Region', *AIDS*, 8 (1994), 1477–81; Longin R. Barongo and others, 'The epidemiology of HIV-1 infection in urban areas, roadside settlements and rural villages in Mwanza Region', *AIDS*, 6 (1992), 1521–8.

56 Heiner Grosskurth and others, 'Impact of improved treatment of sexually transmitted diseases on HIV infection in rural Tanzania: randomised controlled trial', *The Lancet*, 346 (1995), 534.

57 Daan Mulder, Andrew Nunn, Anatoli Kamali, and Jane Kengeya-Kayondo, 'Decreasing HIV-1 seroprevalence in young adults in a rural Ugandan cohort', *British Medical Journal*, 311 (1995), 833; *New Vision*, 29 July 1994.

58 Wallman and others, *Kampala women*, pp. 176, 180, 185.

59 Magdalene K. Ngaiza, 'Women's bargaining power in sexual relations', *Tanzania Medical Journal*, 6, 2 (September 1991), 59; G.G. Mbugua and others, 'Epidemiology of HIV infection among long distance truck drivers in Kenya', *EAMJ*, 72 (1995), 515, 517; *New Vision*, 24 June 1992.

60 See above, p. 234.

61 *New Vision*, 25 January 1988.

62 *Weekly Review*, 3 August 1990; Don Balmer, 'The impact of HIV/AIDS on the African community', in Craig Newnes (ed.), *Death, dying, and society* (Hove, 1991), p. 382.
63 *Weekly Review*, 15 December 1989.
64 Davy K. Koech, Arthur O. Obel, Jim Minowada, Val A. Hutchinson, and Joseph M. Cummins, 'Low dose oral alpha-interferon therapy for patients seropositive for human immunodeficiency virus type-1', *Molecular Biotherapy*, 2 (1990), 91–4.
65 *Weekly Review*, 9 February 1990 and 15 December 1989.
66 *Medicus*, February 1990, p. 1.
67 Joseph Oliech, 'The AIDS situation and its containment', *EAMJ*, 67 (1990), supplement, SS29–SS30.
68 *Weekly Review*, 8 March 1996.
69 *Daily News*, 11 May, 28 July, and 24 September 1990.
70 *Weekly Review*, 3 August 1990; *Daily News*, 20 September 1990; *Weekly Review*, 12 October and 21 December 1990.
71 *New Vision*, 6 October 1995 and 21 July 1993.
72 Koech, 'Challenges', p. 4.
73 *Weekly Review*, 18 January 1991.
74 *Economic Review*, 18 March 1996.
75 *Weekly Review*, 8 March 1996.
76 *African Medical News*, 15 February 1996.
77 *Economic Review*, 18 March 1996.
78 *Weekly Review*, 10 May 1996; *AIDS Analysis Africa*, June 1996; *AIDS Newsletter*, April 1997.
79 Uganda: Ministry of Health, 'AIDS Control Programme: proposals'; 'Meeting of interested participating parties', 21–22 May 1987, UMOH *5; Okware, 'Brief report', 15 April 1989, UMOH *6.
80 *Daily News*, 24 July 1987; *Sunday News*, 6 March 1988.
81 *Kenya AIDS Newsletter*, July 1989, p. 1.
82 'Proposals for plan of action for health information and education on AIDS in Uganda (1987–1991)', UMOH *5; D. Wilson, 'African contributions on AIDS/HIV', *AIDS Care*, 1 (1989), 196; *New Vision*, 3 January 1994.
83 *Sunday News*, 6 March 1988; *Medicus*, May 1994, p. 168; World Bank, *Tanzania: AIDS assessment and planning study* (Washington, 1992), p. xxxii.
84 Charles Nzioka, 'AIDS policies in Kenya', in Peter Aggleton, Peter Davies, and Graham Hart (eds.), *AIDS: foundations for the future* (London, 1994), pp. 160–5, 171–3.
85 *Daily News*, 4 December 1989, 24 December 1993; Nzioka in Aggleton and others, *AIDS*, p. 167; *AIDS Analysis Africa*, June 1995; Edward C. Green, *AIDS and STDs in Africa* (Boulder, 1994), p. 1; A.A. Opio, G. Asiimwe-Okiror, J. Musinguzi, D. Kaweesa-Kintu, and P. Nsubuga, 'Condom use in two rural districts of Lira and Soroti in Uganda', *AIDS*, 11 (1997), 547.
86 Naamara to MOH, 28 January 1988, UMOH *6; *Daily News*, 1 December 1988; World Bank, *Tanzania*, p. xxiv; *Kenya AIDS Newsletter*, July 1989, p. 5.
87 Uganda AIDS Commission, 'AIDS control in Uganda: the multi-sectoral strategy', revised draft, December 1992, p. 5 (UMOH library); R.O. Swai and

H. Van Asten, 'Epidemiology of HIV-1 infection in Tanzania', *Tanzania Medical Journal*, 6, 2 (September 1991), 36; Uganda: Ministry of Health, 'STD/AIDS Control Programme: annual report for the year 1993', p. 27 (UMOH library).

88 Uganda: Ministry of Health, 'AIDS Control Programme: proposals', p. 35; '15th NCPA meeting, 28 October 1987', UMOH *5; 'NCPA (extra-ordinary) meeting H.E. the President, 10 July 1987', UMOH *5; *New Vision*, 13 July 1988.

89 Uganda: AIDS Control Programme, 'AIDS surveillance report, June 1992', duplicated, p. 3; *Daily News*, 13 November 1987; M. Christian Mukoyogo and Glen Williams, *AIDS orphans: a community perspective from Tanzania* (London, 1991), p. 21; Nzioka, 'Social construction', p. 244; *New Vision*, 1 December 1996.

90 K. Nyamuryekung'e, 'Achievements, constraints and future perspectives of the Tanzania National AIDS Control Programme', *Tanzania Medical Journal*, 6, 2 (September 1991), 39.

91 World Bank, *Tanzania*, pp. xxxi–xxxii; *Daily News*, 29 March 1990.

92 *New Vision*, 21 January 1992; Kaheru, 'Statement on 1990/91 budget', p. 8.

93 *New Vision*, 19 March 1993; J. Chin and S.K. Lwanga, 'Estimation and projection of adult AIDS cases: a simple epidemiological model', *Bulletin of the WHO*, 69 (1991), 399–406.

94 PS to Okware, 5 January 1988, UMOH *5; *New Vision*, 1 December 1996; *Weekly Review*, 22 December 1995.

95 *New Vision*, 21 January 1992 and 2 March 1993; Uganda: Ministry of Health, 'The report of the joint evaluation of the Uganda AIDS Commission and Secretariat', typescript, 16 October 1992 (UMOH library).

96 Uganda AIDS Commission, 'Uganda national operational plan for HIV/AIDS/STD prevention, care and support 1994–1998' (UMOH library); Uganda: Ministry of Health, 'AIDS Control Programme 1993 plan and budget' (UMOH library).

97 *New Vision*, 1 December 1996.

98 *AIDS Analysis Africa*, January 1995; *EastAfrican*, 4 August 1997.

99 *AIDS Analysis Africa*, October 1996.

100 *Ibid.*, August 1995; *AIDS Newsletter*, August 1997.

101 *EastAfrican*, 2 September 1996 and 24 November 1997.

102 *New Vision*, 14 March and 8 July 1994; *Daily Nation*, 28 July 1994; *AIDS Newsletter*, February and August 1997.

103 R.D. Mugerwa, L.H. Marum, and D. Serwadda, 'Human Immunodeficiency Virus and AIDS in Uganda', *EAMJ*, 73 (1996), 20; Mulder and others, 'Decreasing HIV-1 seroprevalence', pp. 833, 835.

104 *New Vision*, 8 July 1994; *Daily Nation*, 18 July 1994.

105 *AIDS Analysis Africa*, February and August 1996; T.E. Mertens and D. Low-Beer, 'HIV and AIDS: where is the epidemic going?' *Bulletin of the WHO*, 74 (1996), 128; Maria J. Wawer and others, 'Trends in HIV-1 prevalence may not reflect trends in incidence in mature epidemics: data from the Rakai population-based cohort, Uganda', *AIDS*, 11 (1997), 1023–30.

106 Mulder and others, 'Decreasing HIV-1 seroprevalence', pp. 833, 835.

107 *New Vision*, 17 November 1995.
108 D. Schopper and J. Walley, 'Care for AIDS patients in developing countries: a review', *AIDS Care*, 4 (1992), 95.
109 Janie Hampton, *Living positively with AIDS: The AIDS Support Organization (TASO)* (London, 1990), p. 23; G. Lwihula, L. Dahlgren, J. Killewo, and A. Sandström, 'AIDS epidemic in Kagera region', *AIDS Care*, 5 (1993), 355; Jill Armstrong, *Uganda's AIDS crisis*, World Bank discussion paper no. 298 (Washington, 1995), p. 36.
110 *New Vision*, 2 December 1996.
111 Nzioka, 'Social construction', pp. 116–17; D.H. Balmer, *HIV/AIDS: group counselling theory and practice* (Nairobi, 1993), p. 32.
112 G.T. Lie and P.M. Biswalo, 'Perceptions of the appropriate HIV/AIDS counsellor in Arusha and Kilimanjaro Regions', *AIDS Care*, 6 (1994), 143–8.
113 *New Vision*, December 1996; Armstrong, *Uganda's AIDS crisis*, p. 30; *AIDS Analysis Africa*, October 1996 and January 1995; *EastAfrican*, 16 June 1997.
114 David A. Okello, 'The resource use patterns and the factors affecting the cost of care of patients with the Acquired Immunodeficiency Syndrome in Mulago Hospital', MMedSc thesis, University of Newcastle (NSW), 1993, p. 33; 'St Francis Hospital, Nsambya: annual report 1988' (UMOH library).
115 Okello, 'Resource use', pp. i, 46–7; *Daily News*, 8 August 1987.
116 *Daily Nation*, 27 March 1996; *Medicus*, November 1993, p. 356.
117 Uganda, *Mulago Hospital: annual report 1990* (UMOH library); Francis A. Mmiro and others, 'The effect of Human Immunodeficiency Virus infection on the outcome of pregnancy in Ugandan women', *Journal of Obstetrics and Gynaecology of Eastern and Central Africa*, 12, 1 (1996), 25; *Medicus*, November 1993, p. 333.
118 Hampton, *Living positively*, p. 7.
119 Bernard Joinet and Theodore Mugolola, *Survivre face au sida en Afrique* (Paris, 1994), p. 72.
120 Nzioka, 'Social construction', ch. 5, is especially interesting on doctors' experiences and attitudes.
121 E.T. Katabira, 'Looking after AIDS patients', *Health Information Quarterly*, 4, 4 (December 1988), 25.
122 *New Vision*, 13 July 1988.
123 Kenya: Ministry of Health, *National guidelines on counselling for HIV infection* (Nairobi, 1988); G.T. Lie and P.M. Biswalo, 'Action research to improve the quality of HIV/AIDS counselling', *Tanzania Medical Journal*, 6, 2 (September 1991), 71–2; Nzioka in Aggleton and others, *AIDS*, p. 168; Philip Wittman Sitel, 'Bo'n town life: youth, AIDS, and the changing character of adulthood in Kilimanjaro', PhD thesis, Boston University, 1995, p. 322.
124 Hampton, *Living positively*; N. Kaleeba and others, 'Participatory evaluation of counselling, medical and social services of The AIDS Support Organization (TASO) in Uganda', *AIDS Care*, 9 (1997), 13–26; Mukoyogo and Williams, *AIDS orphans*; Nzioka, 'Social construction', p. 117.
125 Christine Obbo, 'The language of AIDS in rural and urban Uganda', *African Urban Quarterly*, 6 (1991), 83–92; Seeley and others, 'Extended family', pp. 117–22.
126 Jacob T. Kaimenyi and Francis L. Ndungu, 'Knowledge, attitudes and prac-

tices towards HIV positive and AIDS patients among public service dentists in Nairobi', *African Journal of Health Sciences*, 1 (1994), 116–21; Jacob T. Kaimenyi and Francis L. Ndungu, 'Knowledge, practices and attitudes towards HIV positive and AIDS patients among dental auxiliaries', *EAMJ*, 71 (1994), 304–10; M.N. Katsivo and others, 'Relationship between nurses' opinion on nursing care for HIV infected/AIDS patients and socio-economic factors in Nyeri District', in Were and others, *Recent advances*, pp. 34–7; Thecla Wankuru Kohi, 'The knowledge, attitudes, and perceived support of Tanzanian nurses when caring for patients with AIDS', MNursing thesis, Dalhousie University, 1992; Thecla W. Kohi and Mona June Horrocks, 'The knowledge, attitudes and perceived support of Tanzanian nurses when caring for patients with AIDS', *International Journal of Nursing Studies*, 31 (1994), 77–86.

127 See Rosaline S. Barbour, 'The impact of working with people with HIV/AIDS: a review of the literature', *SSM*, 39 (1994), 221–32.

128 I have taken these from Gerald H. Friedland, 'Clinical care in the AIDS epidemic', *Daedalus*, 118, 2 (Spring 1989), 66–71.

129 Quoted by Lydia Bennett, 'AIDS health care: staff stress, loss and bereavement', in Lorraine Sherr (ed.), *Grief and AIDS* (Chichester, 1995), p. 96.

130 Jagwe, 'Retrospective study', p. 12.

131 Joinet and Mugolola, *Survivre*, p. 99; Byahuka to ACP, 26 October 1988, UMOH *6; *New Vision*, 11 January 1994.

132 One such report in Uganda was alleged to have been suppressed: *New Vision*, 27 January 1995.

133 Bosenge N'galy and others, 'Human Immunodeficiency Virus infection among employees in an African hospital', *New England Journal of Medicine*, 319 (1988), 1123–7.

134 *Daily News*, 30 August 1990; B. Gumodoka, I. Favot, Z.A. Berege, and W.M.V. Dolmans, 'Occupational exposure to the risk of HIV infection among health care workers in Mwanza Region, United Republic of Tanzania', *Bulletin of the WHO*, 75 (1997), 133–40; *Daily Nation*, 27 May 1994; Katsivo and others in Were and others, *Recent advances*, pp. 36–7.

135 G.T. Lie and P.M. Biswalo, 'HIV-positive patients' choice of a significant other to be informed about the HIV-test result', *AIDS Care*, 8 (1996), 286.

136 C. Nzioka, 'Lay perceptions of risk of HIV infection and the social construction of safer sex: some experiences from Kenya', *AIDS Care*, 8 (1996), 567.

137 Kohi and Horrocks, 'Knowledge', p. 82; Barbour, 'Impact', p. 222.

138 Lwihula and others, 'AIDS epidemic', p. 355; Fortin, 'Politics', p. 918.

139 Raymond Kasirye, 'Community response to AIDS affected households: a case study of Kamwokya,' BA thesis, Makerere University, 1992, p. 36.

140 E.g. *ibid.*; J.W. McGrath, E. Maxine Ankrah, D.A. Schumann, S. Nkumbi, and M. Lubega, 'AIDS and the urban family: its impact in Kampala', *AIDS Care*, 5 (1993), 55–70, Kohi, 'Knowledge', pp. 61–2, 70.

141 Abidi, *Challenges*, p. 217.

142 Konde-Lule and others, 'Focus group interviews', p. 679; Susan S. Hunter, 'Orphans as a window on the AIDS epidemic in sub-Saharan Africa', *SSM*, 31 (1990), 681; *New Vision*, 6 December 1988.

143 Cynthia Haq, 'Management of AIDS patients: case report from Uganda', in Norman Miller and Richard C. Rockwell (eds.), *AIDS in Africa* (Lewiston, 1988), p. 92.
144 *Daily News*, 21 June 1974.
145 Wallman and others, *Kampala women*, pp. 131–41; Richard W. Goodgame, 'AIDS in Uganda – clinical and social features', *New England Journal of Medicine*, 323 (1990), 387.
146 Hooper, *Slim*, p. 83; Samuel I. Okware, 'Perspectives in AIDS control in Africa', in Commonwealth Secretariat, 'Report of the first inter-regional workshop on surveillance and control of Acquired Immuno-Deficiency Syndrome', duplicated (London, 1988), p. 27; S.S. Faya, 'HIV/AIDS – the real emergency of our times', *Medicus*, 12, 11 (November 1993), 338–9.
147 N.K. Ndosi and M.C. Waziri, 'The nature of parasuicide in Dar es Salaam', *SSM*, 44 (1997), 57, 59; *Weekly Review*, 16 June 1989; Christian Medical Board of Tanzania and others, *Participatory action research on AIDS and the community as a source of care and healing* (Uganda, 1993), p. 18.
148 *Daily News*, 25 April 1988; Ian Clarke, *The man with the key has gone!* (Chichester, 1993), p. 267.
149 Spencer Birungi, 'Exploratory study of the effects of counselling services on AIDS clients in Uganda: study of Mulago TASO branch', BA thesis, Makerere University, 1992, p. 38; Azariah O. Ndonji, 'Living positively', *AIDS Watch*, 11 (1990), 5; AIDSCAP, *AIDS in Kenya: socioeconomic impact and policy implications* (Arlington, 1996), p. 48.
150 *EastAfrican*, 14 October 1996; 'Kitovu Complex: annual report – 1993' (UMOH library); *New Vision*, 3 May 1996.
151 Hooper, *Slim*, pp. 251–4; Elly Katabira and Richard Goodgame, *AIDS care: diagnostic and treatment strategies for health workers* (Entebbe, 1989), p. 23.
152 Kenya: Ministry of Health, *National guidelines*, p. 10; Lie and Biswalo, 'HIV-positive patients' choice', p. 286; *Daily News*, 29 September 1988; Hooper, *Slim*, p. 294.
153 Kenya: Ministry of Health, *National guidelines*, p. 11; Nzioka, 'Social construction', pp. 145–9; AIDSCAP, *AIDS in Kenya*, p. 96; *Daily Nation*, 12 May 1994.
154 Maulidi R. Fataki, 'Clinical presentation of HIV disease in children at Muhimbili Medical Centre', MMed thesis, University of Dar es Salaam, 1989, p. 31; Clarke, *The man*, p. 262.
155 Faya, 'HIV/AIDS', p. 340.
157 Lie and Biswalo, 'HIV-positive patients' choice', pp. 290–5; Clarke, *The man*, p. 274; McGrath and others, 'AIDS', pp. 55, 60; Gladys Baingana, Kyung-Lee Choi, Donald C. Barrett, Ronald Byansi, and Norman Hearst, 'Female partners of AIDS patients in Uganda: reported knowledge, perceptions and plans', *AIDS*, 9 (1995), supplement, S16–S18; Kaleeba and others, 'Participatory evaluation', p. 20.
157 Alexander M. Odonga, *Practical medical ethics* (Kisubi, n.d.), p. 56.
158 *New Vision*, 2 January 1990.
159 Kenya: Ministry of Health, *National guidelines*, p. 16.
160 Michael W. Ross and Val Seeger, 'Determinants of reported burnout in health professionals associated with the care of patients with AIDS', *AIDS*, 2 (1988),

395–7; L. Bennett, P. Michie, and S. Kippax, 'Quantitative analysis of burnout and its associated factors in AIDS nursing', *AIDS Care*, 3 (1991), 181–92.

161 Joan M. Eakin and Kathryn M. Taylor, 'The psychosocial impact of AIDS on health workers', *AIDS*, 4 (1990), supplement, S261; Nelson K. Sewankambo, 'Care of HIV-infected people in the developing world', *AIDS*, 3 (1989), supplement, S198; Okello, 'Resource use patterns', p. 18.

162 Quoted by Glenn W. Geelhoed, 'Migration of African AIDS from town to country', *African Urban Quarterly*, 6 (1991), 45.

163 Hampton, *Living positively*, p. 10.

164 Katabira and Goodgame, *AIDS care*, pp. 6, 9, 14, 16, 18, 22.

165 *New Vision*, 19 October 1993; S. Kalibala and N. Kaleeba, 'AIDS and community-based care in Uganda: the AIDS support organization, TASO', *AIDS Care*, 1 (1989), 173–5; Sewankambo, 'Care,' pp. S195–S199; F.S. Mhalu, 'AIDS and infections with the human immunodeficiency virus in Tanzania', *Tanzania Medical Journal*, 4, 1 (June 1989), 1–6.

166 Fr Peter Le Jacq, quoted in *Maryknoll*, March 1989, p. 9; Janet M. Horsman and Paschal Sheeran, 'Health care workers and HIV/AIDS', *SSM*, 41 (1995), 1560.

167 Sitel, 'Bo'n town life', p. 323.

168 *New Vision*, 22 January 1995.

169 Goodgame, 'AIDS in Uganda', p. 386; Kenya: Ministry of Health, 'Report of the proceedings', pp. 7, 14; *Daily News*, 31 May 1990.

170 Okware in Commonwealth Secretariat, 'Report', p. 27; *New Vision*, 4 February 1994; *Weekly Review*, 24 March 1989; *Daily News*, 21 August 1991.

171 Museveni, *Africa's problem*, pp. 277–8.

172 *AIDS Analysis Africa*, September 1993; *New Vision*, 9 August 1994.

173 *New Vision*, 23 February 1995, 4, 5, 10, and 13 October 1996, 5 February 1997; *EastAfrican*, 4 August 1997.

174 *Daily News*, 2 January 1997.

175 Okware to DMS, 19 December 1988, UMOH *6.

176 *AIDS Analysis Africa*, February 1997.

177 *New Vision*, 21 June 1996.

178 Omwony Ojok and John Rwamushana, 'Uganda's response to the challenge of HIV/AIDS', *Uganda Journal*, 42 (December 1995), 6.

179 *Monitor*, 21 August 1996; *AIDS Analysis Africa*, February 1997; *New Vision*, 6 and 12 September 1996, 11 November 1996.

180 *New Vision*, 12 March 1994, 25 April 1994, 13 August 1996, 6 October 1996; *AIDS Analysis Africa*, February 1997.

181 *New Vision*, 2 August 1996; *AIDS Analysis Africa*, February 1997.

11 CONCLUSION

1 For a contrary view, see Obbo, 'Healing', p. 200.

2 The closest parallels were in South-East Asia. See T.H. Silcock (ed.), *Professional structure in South-East Asia* (Canberra, 1977).

Bibliography

I. DOCUMENTARY SOURCES

KENYA: KENYA NATIONAL ARCHIVES, NAIROBI (KNA)

I used chiefly the records of the Medical Department and its successor ministries. They were generally open to the mid-1960s, plus more recent annual reports. Records earlier than the 1920s are listed so inadequately as to be almost useless. Those for the 1920s and 1930s appear to have only partially survived. From about 1940 the records are full, well listed, and valuable. I also consulted a small number of education and other files and the records of the Church Missionary Society stations in Kenya.

TANZANIA: TANZANIA NATIONAL ARCHIVES, DAR ES SALAAM (TNA)

Only a handful of relevant German files survive. The Medical Department records of the British period have been deposited (TNA 450) but not unpacked. The archivists kindly found a few files which I especially wished to see, but there were limits. I supplemented these by Secretariat files, although a good many had been misplaced, and by some records collected from provincial and district medical offices. The fullest surviving copy of *Kwetu* is in SMP 23754.

UGANDA: UGANDA NATIONAL ARCHIVES, ENTEBBE (UNA)

The archives were in poor condition. A number of medical records prior to about 1940 were listed, but many of the most important could not be found.

UGANDA: MINISTRY OF HEALTH, ENTEBBE (UMOH)

Most records of the British Medical Department were apparently never transferred to the archives and cannot now be traced. In June 1986 the then Permanent Secretary said that the Ministry's archive 'was broken into and all files stolen about four months ago' ('Minutes of the meeting on expansion of the Ministry and personnel problems', 10 June 1986, UMOH *3). The current Permanent Secretary kindly allowed me to consult what remained. Some were in the Ministry Headquarters, others at a Records Repository, but I have listed them all as

UMOH because access to them was possible only through the Ministry. Ten files had no numbers and are cited here with an asterisk (UMOH *1–*10). The Ministry's library contains a valuable collection of unpublished reports and other documents.

UGANDA: ALBERT COOK LIBRARY, MULAGO (MP)

The Medical School Library houses the records of the CMS Mengo Mission. I used the mission registers and correspondence (cited by box number). The collection of case notes, dating continuously from 1897, was not relevant to this study but is a magnificent source for strictly medical history.

UGANDA: MAKERERE UNIVERSITY LIBRARY, KAMPALA (MUL)

There was only a scattering of relevant documents, mainly concerning the history of the University, but the library has a unique collection of Luganda newspapers.

GREAT BRITAIN: PUBLIC RECORD OFFICE, LONDON (PRO)

I made selective use of the original correspondence with Kenya (CO 533), Tanganyika (CO 691), Uganda (CO 536), and East Africa (CO 822), plus the papers of the Social Service Department (CO 859). An unexpectedly valuable source was the records of the Inter-University Council (BW 90).

GREAT BRITAIN: WELLCOME INSTITUTE FOR THE HISTORY OF MEDICINE, LONDON

The Contemporary Medical Archives Centre holds the (disappointing) diaries and some papers of Sir Albert Cook. I also used the papers of Cicely D. Williams, including notes and minutes of the Frazer Committee with which she visited Uganda in 1955.

GREAT BRITAIN: RHODES HOUSE LIBRARY, OXFORD (RH)

As part of the Oxford Development Records Project, the library has collected an extremely valuable body of papers from former colonial medical officers (and some missionary doctors) working chiefly in Nigeria, Tanganyika, and Uganda, but with a scattering from Kenya, Zanzibar, and elsewhere. There is a parallel collection of higher-education records. Relevant papers are scattered in other collections, notably those of the Anti-Slavery Society and Fabian Colonial Bureau.

GREAT BRITAIN: BIRMINGHAM UNIVERSITY LIBRARY (CMS)

The library houses the records of the Church Missionary Society. I used the papers of the Mombasa and Uganda missions before the First World War and the connected unofficial papers of individual missionaries. The records of the CMS Medical Department were not available for study during my period of research.

GREAT BRITAIN: EDINBURGH UNIVERSITY LIBRARY (EUL)

The library contains the papers of J.W. Arthur, although more valuable is its almost complete collection of *Kikuyu News*. The few missing numbers are available nearby at the National Library of Scotland.

II. NEWSPAPERS AND JOURNALS

African Medical News (Nairobi)
AIDS Analysis Africa (London)
AIDS Newsletter (London)
Central Africa (London)
Church Missionary Intelligencer (London)
CMS Monthly Reporter (London)
Daily Nation (Nairobi)
Daily News (Dar es Salaam)
EastAfrican (Nairobi)
East African Medical Journal (Nairobi)
East African Standard (Nairobi)
Ebifa mu Buganda (Mengo, Budo, Namirembe)
Economic Review (Nairobi)
Gambuze (Nairobi, Kampala)
Habari (Nairobi)
Inland Africa (Brooklyn)
Kenya AIDS Newsletter (Nairobi)
Kikuyu News (Edinburgh)
Kwetu (Dar es Salaam)
Makerere (Kampala)
Makerere College Magazine (Kampala)
Makerere College Newsletter (Kampala)
Mambo Leo (Dar es Salaam)
Maryknoll (Maryknoll)
Matalisi (Kampala)
Medicus (Nairobi)
Mercy and Truth (London)
The Mission Hospital (London)
Monitor (Kampala)
Muigwithania (Nairobi)
Munno (Kampala)
New Vision (Kampala)
Rafiki Yangu (Dar es Salaam)
Standard (Nairobi)
Sunday Nation (Nairobi)
Sunday News (Dar es Salaam)
Sunday Vision (Kampala)
Tanganyika Opinion (Dar es Salaam)
Tanganyika Standard (Dar es Salaam)
Target (Nairobi)

Uganda Argus (Kampala)
Uganda Church Review (Namirembe)
Uganda Empya (Kampala)
Uganda Herald (Kampala)
Uganda Notes (Namirembe)
Uganda Times (Kampala)
Voice of Uganda (Kampala)
Weekly Review (Nairobi)
Weekly Topic (Kampala)

III. OTHER WORKS

Abdullah, M.A. 'Hypertension – the Kenyan experience', *Medicom*, 1 (1979), 9–13.

Abel-Smith, Brian, and Pankaj Rawal. 'Can the poor afford "free" health services? A case study of Tanzania', *Health Policy and Planning*, 7 (1992), 329–41.

Abidi, Syed A.H. (ed.) *Challenges to leadership in the developing world: speeches of Dr Samson Kisekka*. [?Kampala, 199?.]

Abilla, Walter Dan. 'Life in the ward: a sociological study of the inpatient in a general hospital in Kenya (Kisumu)', duplicated, University of Nairobi, 1977.

Adeloye, Adelola. *African pioneers of modern medicine: Nigerian doctors of the nineteenth century*. Ibadan, 1985.

Ademuwagun, A.Z., John A.A. Ayoade, Ira E. Harrison, and Dennis M. Warren (eds.) *African therapeutic systems*. Waltham, 1979.

Aggleton, Peter, Peter Davies, and Graham Hart (eds.) *AIDS: foundations for the future*. London, 1994.

Ahmed, A.H., D.P. Urassa, F. Gherardi, and N.Y. Game. 'Patients' perception of public, voluntary and private dispensaries in rural areas of Tanzania', *EAMJ*, 73 (1996), 370–4.

AIDSCAP. *AIDS in Kenya: socioeconomic impact and policy implications*. Arlington, 1996.

Alubo, S. Ogoh. 'The political economy of doctors' strikes in Nigeria: a Marxist interpretation', *SSM*, 22 (1986), 467–77.

Amuyunzu, Mary Kigasia. 'The management of illness in a plural health care setting: a case study of the Duruma of coastal Kenya', PhD thesis, University of Cambridge, 1994.

Apter, David E. *The political kingdom in Uganda: a study in bureaucratic nationalism*. 2nd edn, Princeton, 1967.

Armstrong, Jill. *Uganda's AIDS crisis: its implications for development*, World Bank discussion paper no. 298. Washington, 1995.

Arnold, David (ed.) *Imperial medicine and indigenous societies*. Delhi, 1989.

Aruwa, W.A.K. 'A case of relapsing fever in a child of nine days old', *EAMJ*, 27 (1950), 176–7.

Ashby, Eric. *Universities: British, Indian, African: a study in the ecology of higher education*. London, 1966.

Atiman, Adrien. 'The dispensary at Karema', *The White Fathers in Africa* (November 1940), 114–15.

Atiman, Adrien. 'Adrien Atiman, by himself' (trans. L.B. Cane), *TNR*, 21 (June 1946), 46–76.

Avirgan, Tony, and Martha Honey. *War in Uganda: the legacy of Idi Amin*. Westport, 1982.

Babumba, Eria M. 'An African patient', *EAMJ*, 31 (1954), 373–6.

Bagshawe, A.F., G. Maina, and E.N. Mngola (eds.) *The use and abuse of drugs and chemicals in tropical Africa*. Nairobi, 1974.

Baker, Delbert W. *From exile to Prime Minister*. Washington, 1988.

Baraza, Richard. 'News and statistics', *Makerere Medical Journal*, 16 (September 1971), 46–9.

Barbour, Rosaline S. 'The impact of working with people with HIV/AIDS: a review of the literature', *SSM*, 39 (1994), 221–32.

Barkan, Joel D. *An African dilemma: university students, development and politics in Ghana, Tanzania and Uganda*. Nairobi, 1975.

Beck, Ann. *Medicine and society in Tanganyika 1890–1930*, Transactions of the American Philosophical Society, vol. 67, part 3. Philadelphia, 1977.

Beck, Ann. *Medicine, tradition, and development in Kenya and Tanzania, 1920–1970*. Waltham, 1981.

Bell, Heather. 'Medical research and medical practice in the Anglo-Egyptian Sudan, 1899–1940', DPhil thesis, University of Oxford, 1996.

Bennett, F.J., A.M. Nhonoli, and H. Nsanzumuhire (eds.) *Degenerative disorders in the African environment: epidemiology and consequences*. Nairobi, 1976.

Boesen, Jannik, Kjell J. Havnevik, Juhani Koponen, and Rie Odgaard (eds.) *Tanzania: crisis and struggle for survival*. Uppsala, 1986.

Bonner, Thomas Neville. *Becoming a physician: medical education in Britain, France, Germany and the United States, 1750–1945*. New York, 1995.

Bösch, Fridolin. *Les Banyamwezi*. Münster, 1930.

Bwengye, Francis A.W. *The agony of Uganda: from Idi Amin to Obote*. London, 1985.

Bwibo, N.O. 'Medical and paediatric clerkship', *Medicom*, 3 (1981), 47–8.

Bwibo, N.O. 'Medical education in a developing country', *EAMJ*, 64 (1987), 697–709.

Byaruhanga, D.B. 'Treatment and control of leprosy in Uganda with special reference to the Kingdom of Toro', DPH thesis, St Andrews (Dundee) University, 1962–3.

Bynum, W.F. *Science and the practice of medicine in the nineteenth century*. Cambridge, 1994.

Carr-Saunders, A.M., and P.A. Wilson. *The professions*. Oxford, 1933.

Carswell, J. Wilson, Roy Mugerwa, Nelson Sewankambo, Fred Kigozi, and Rick Goodgame. 'AIDS in Uganda: a special report by the Clinical Committee on AIDS', *Health Information Quarterly*, 2, 1 (February 1986), 11–20.

Chege, Michael. 'A tale of two slums: electoral politics in Mathare and Dagoretti', *Review of African Political Economy*, 20 (January 1981), 74–88.

Christie, James. *Cholera epidemics in East Africa*. London, 1876.

Clarke, Ian. *The man with the key has gone!* Chichester, 1993.

Clyde, David F. *History of the medical services of Tanganyika*. Dar es Salaam, 1962.

Clyde, David F. *Malaria in Tanzania*. London, 1967.

Cocks,Geoffrey, and Konrad H. Jarausch (eds.) *German professions, 1800–1950*. New York, 1990.

Colebatch, H.K. 'Government services at the district level in Kenya: roads, schools and health services', University of Nairobi Institute of Development Studies discussion paper no. 38, 1974.

Collins, D., J.D. Quick, S.N. Murau, D. Kraushaar, and I.M. Hussein. 'The fall and rise of cost sharing in Kenya: the impact of phased implementation', *Health Policy and Planning*, 11 (1996), 52–63.

Cook, Albert R. 'Notes on the diseases met with in Uganda', *Journal of Tropical Medicine*, 4 (1901), 175–8.

Cook, Albert R. *Uganda memories (1897–1940)*. Kampala, 1945.

Correa, P., and others. *Biomedical lectures: 1970–1973 series*, Afro Technical Papers No. 11. Brazzaville, 1975.

Davies, J.N.P. 'Endocardial fibrosis in Africans', *EAMJ*, 25 (1948), 10–14.

Davies, J.N.P. 'Pathology of central African natives: cardio-vascular diseases', *EAMJ*, 25 (1948), 454–67.

Davies, J.N.P. 'The history of the Uganda branch of the British Medical Association, 1913 to 1932', *EAMJ*, 31 (1954), 93–9.

Davies, J.N.P. 'The history of syphilis in Uganda', *Bulletin of the WHO*, 15 (1956), 1041–55.

Davies, J.N.P. 'The development of "scientific" medicine in the African kingdom of Bunyoro-Kitara', *Medical History*, 3 (1959), 47–57.

Davies, J.N.P., Sally Elmes, M.S.R. Hutt, L.A.M. Mtimavalye, R. Owor, and Lorna Shaper. 'Cancer in an African community, 1897–1956: an analysis of the records of Mengo Hospital, Kampala, Uganda', *British Medical Journal*, 1964/1, pp. 259–64, 336–41.

Davies, J.N.P., I.S. Kadama, and T. D'Souza. 'Pemphigoid eruption following burns', *EAMJ*, 23 (1946), 115–17.

Davies, J.N.P., J. Knowelden, and Barbara A. Wilson. 'Incidence rates of cancer in Kyadondo County, Uganda, 1954–1960', *Journal of the National Cancer Institute*, 35 (1965), 789–821.

Dawson, Marc H. 'Smallpox in Kenya, 1880–1920', *SSM*, 13B (1979), 245–50.

Dawson, Marc Harry. 'Socio-economic and epidemiological change in Kenya: 1880–1925', PhD thesis, University of Wisconsin-Madison, 1983.

de Bunsen, Bernard. *Adventures in education*. Kendal, 1995.

de Craemer, Willy, and Renée C. Fox. *The emerging physician: a sociological approach to the development of a Congolese medical profession*. Stanford, 1968.

de Zulueta, J., G.W. Kafuko, A.W.R. McCrae, J.R. Cullen, C.K. Pedersen, and D.F.B. Wasswa. 'A malaria eradication experiment in the highlands of Kigezi (Uganda)', *EAMJ*, 41 (1964), 102–20.

Dodge, Cole P. 'Uganda – rehabilitation, or redefinition of health services?' *SSM*, 22 (1986), 755–61.

Dodge, Cole P., and Paul D. Wiebe (eds.) *Crisis in Uganda: the breakdown of health services*. Oxford, 1985.

East African Institute of Social Research. 'One-day symposium on attitudes to health and disease among some East African tribes', duplicated, 1959.

Eraj, Yusuf Ali. 'The organization of doctors and the crisis in medicine', paper to the Commonwealth Medical Association Annual Conference, Nairobi, 1980.

Faya, S.S. 'HIV/AIDS – the real emergency of our times', *Medicus*, 12, 11 (November 1993), 338–41.

Feierman, Steven. 'Therapy as a system-in-action in northeastern Tanzania', *SSM*, 15B (1981), 353–60.

Feierman, Steven. *Peasant intellectuals: anthropology and history in Tanzania.* Madison, 1990.

Felkin, Robert W. 'Notes on labour in central Africa', *Edinburgh Medical Journal*, 29 (1884), 922–30.

Fendall, N.R.E. 'Planning health services in developing countries', *Public Health Reports*, 78 (1963), 977–88.

Ford, John. *The role of the trypanosomiases in African ecology*. Oxford, 1971.

Fortin, Alfred J. 'The politics of AIDS in Kenya', *Third World Quarterly*, 9 (1987), 906–19.

Foster, W.D. *The early history of scientific medicine in Uganda*. Nairobi, 1970.

Foster, W.D. *The Church Missionary Society and modern medicine in Uganda: the life of Sir Albert Cook*. N.p., 1978.

Fouquer, [Roger] *Le docteur Adrien Atiman, médecin-catéchiste au Tanganyika.* Condé-sur-Escaut, 1964.

Freers, J., and others. 'Echocardiographic diagnosis of heart disease in Uganda', *Tropical Doctor*, 26 (1996), 125–8.

Freidson, Eliot. *Profession of medicine: a study of the sociology of applied knowledge*. New York, 1972.

Freidson, Eliot. *Professional powers: a study of the institutionalization of formal knowledge*. Chicago, 1986.

Gatheru, R. Mugo. *Child of two worlds*. London, 1964.

Geison, Gerald L. (ed.) *Professions and the French state, 1700–1900*. Philadelphia, 1984.

Giddens, Anthony. *The consequences of modernity*. Cambridge, 1990.

Gilson, Lucy. 'Management and health care reform in sub-Saharan Africa', *SSM*, 40 (1995), 695–710.

Gilson, Lucy, Martin Alilio, and Kris Heggenhougen. 'Community satisfaction with primary health care services: an evaluation undertaken in the Morogoro Region of Tanzania', *SSM*, 39 (1994), 767–80.

Giraldo, G., E. Beth-Giraldo, N. Clumeck, M.R. Gharbi, S.K. Kyalwazi, and G. de Thé (eds.) *AIDS and associated cancers in Africa*. Basel, 1988.

Gish, Oscar. *Planning the health sector: the Tanzanian experience*. London, 1975.

Glatzel, Dr. '3 Monate im Sewa Hadji Hospital zu Dar es Salaam', *Archiv für Schiffs- und Tropen-Hygiene*, 10 (1906), 263–87.

Goldthorpe, J.E. *An African elite: Makerere College students, 1922–1960*. Nairobi, 1965.

Good, Charles M. *Ethnomedical systems in Africa: patterns of traditional medicine in rural and urban Kenya*. New York, 1987.

Great Britain. *Higher education in East Africa*, Colonial No. 142. London, 1937.

Great Britain: Colonial Office. *Report of the Commission on Higher Education in the Colonies*, Cmd 6647 of 1945. London, 1945.

Grmek, Mirko D. *History of AIDS*. Trans. R.C. Maulitz and J. Duffin, Princeton, 1990.

Grosskurth, Heiner, and others. 'Impact of improved treatment of sexually transmitted diseases on HIV infection in rural Tanzania: randomised controlled trial', *The Lancet*, 346 (1995), 530–6.

Gumodoka, B., I. Favot, Z.A. Berege, and W.M.V. Dolmans, 'Occupational exposure to the risk of HIV infection among health care workers in Mwanza Region, United Republic of Tanzania', *Bulletin of the WHO*, 75 (1997), 133–40.

Gutkind, Peter C.W. *The royal capital of Buganda*. The Hague, 1963.

Hackett, C.J. 'On the origin of the human treponematoses', *Bulletin of the WHO*, 29 (1963), 7–41.

Halmos, Paul (ed.) *Professionalisation and social change*. Keele, 1973.

Hampton, Janie. *Living positively with AIDS: The AIDS Support Organization (TASO), Uganda*. London, 1990.

Hansen, Holger Bernt, and Michael Twaddle (eds.) *Changing Uganda*. London, 1991.

Hauer, August. *Kumbuke: Erlebnisse eines Arztes in Deutsch-Ostafrika*. Berlin, 1922.

Heggenhougen, Kris, Patrick Vaughan, Eustace P.Y. Muhondwa, and J. Rutabanzibwa-Ngaiza. *Community health workers: the Tanzanian experience*. Oxford, 1987.

Henn, Albert E. *Tanzania: health sector strategy*. Dar es Salaam, 1980.

Herbert,Eugenia W. 'Smallpox inoculation in Africa', *JAH*, 16 (1975), 539–59.

Hicks, Andrew. 'Forty years of the British Medical Association (Kenya Branch)', *EAMJ*, 38 (1961), 43–53.

Holden, Pat. *Doctors and other medical personnel in the public health services in Africa 1930–1965*, Oxford Development Records Project Report 17. Oxford, 1984.

Holden, Pat, and Jenny Littelwood (eds.) *Anthropology and nursing*. London, 1991.

Hooper, Ed. *Slim: a reporter's own story of AIDS in East Africa*. London, 1990.

Hutt, M.S.R., D.P. Burkitt, J.J. Shepherd, B. Wright, J.K.G. Mati, and S. Auma. 'Malignant tumours of the gastrointestinal tract in Ugandans', *National Cancer Institute Monograph*, 25 (1967), 41–7.

Ibingira, Grace Stuart. *African upheavals since independence*. Boulder, 1980.

Iliffe, John. *A modern history of Tanganyika*. Cambridge, 1979.

Iliffe, John. *Africans: the history of a continent*. Cambridge, 1995.

Ingham, Kenneth. *Obote: a political biography*. London, 1994.

Ingman, Stanley R., and Anthony E. Thomas (eds.) *Topias and utopias in health: policy studies*. The Hague, 1975.

Jagwe, Jack G.M. 'Drug use in Uganda: a growing concern for the professional', *Medical Review (Uganda Edition)*, 2, 2 (April 1996), 16–20.

Jagwe, J.M. 'A retrospective study of causes of death among Ugandan African doctors', *Health Information Quarterly*, 3, 3 (September 1987), 12–13.

Janovsky, Gerlinde Katerina. 'Planning as organizational transaction and bargaining: the case of health in Kenya', EdD thesis, Harvard University, 1979.

Jeffery, R. 'Allopathic medicine in India: a case of deprofessionalization?' *SSM*, 11 (1977), 561–73.

Johnson, Terence J., and Marjorie Caygill. 'The British Medical Association and its overseas branches: a short history', *Journal of Imperial and Commonwealth History*, 1 (1972–3), 303–29.

Johnson, Urban. 'Ideological framework and health development in Tanzania 1961–2000', *SSM*, 22 (1986), 745–53.

Joinet, Bernard, and Theodore Mugolola. *Survivre face au sida en Afrique*. Paris, 1994.

Kaheru, Z.K.R. 'Statement in the National Resistance Council on the 1989/90 budget', duplicated, 1989 (UMOH library).

Kaheru, Z.K.R. 'Statement in the National Resistance Council on the 1990/91 budget', duplicated, 1990 (UMOH library).

Kajubi, S.K. 'Clinical and functional aspects of chronic pancreatic disease in Uganda', MD thesis, Makerere University, 1971.

Kaleeba, N., and others. 'Participatory evaluation of counselling, medical and social services of The AIDS Support Organization (TASO) in Uganda', *AIDS Care*, 9 (1997), 13–26.

Kalibala, S., and N. Kaleeba. 'AIDS and community-based care in Uganda: the AIDS support organization, TASO', *AIDS Care*, 1 (1989), 173–5.

Karasek, A. 'Beiträge zur Kenntnis der Waschambaa', *Baessler-Archiv*, 1 (1911), 155–222; 3 (1913), 69–131; 7 (1918–22), 56–98; 8 (1923–4), 1–53.

Kashagire, Harriet. 'The problems associated with health facilities in Ibanda County Mbarara District since 1900', BA thesis, Makerere University, 1993.

Kasili, Edward George. 'Leukaemia in Kenya', MD thesis, University of Nairobi, 1979.

Kasili, Edward G. 'Coping with cancer in sub-Saharan Africa', *World Health Forum*, 4 (1983), 149–52.

Kasili, Edward George. 'Childhood leukaemia: is it a problem in tropical Africa?' *Leukemia and Lymphoma*, 1 (1989–90), 187–93.

Kasili, Edward G. 'Palliative care of the terminally ill cancer patient in the Kenyan context', *Nairobi Journal of Medicine*, 16, 1 (February 1990), 5–8.

Kasili, E.G. *A synopsis of the management of some cancers in Kenya*. Nairobi, 1991.

Katabira, E.T. 'Looking after AIDS patients', *Health Information Quarterly*, 4, 4 (December 1988), 23–6.

Katabira, Elly, and Richard Goodgame. *AIDS care: diagnostic and treatment strategies for health workers*. Entebbe, 1989.

Keane, G.J., and D.G. Tomblings. *The African Native Medical Corps in the East African campaign*. London [?1920].

Kenya. *The economic development of Kenya: report of an economic survey mission, December 1962*. Nairobi, 1963.

Kenya. *A report by the Director of Medical Services on status of health in Kenya 1979*. Nairobi, 1982.

Kenya. *National development plan for the period 1989 to 1993*. Nairobi, n.d.

Kenya: Ministry of Health. *Medical Practitioners and Dentists Board: annual report 1978*. Nairobi, 1979.

Kenya: Ministry of Health. *National guidelines on counselling for HIV infection, December 1988*. Nairobi, 1988.

Kenya: Ministry of Health. 'Report of the proceedings of the first AIDS awareness seminar for traditional healers and herbalists', duplicated, 1989 (UNMS library).

Kibaya, A.K. 'Possible case of Crohn's Disease in a Ruanda native', *EAMJ*, 23 (1946), 317–20.

Kibukamusoke, J.W. 'Kidney disease in the tropics', *EAMJ*, 45 (1968), 632–7.

Kibukamusoke, John W. *Nephrotic syndrome of quartan malaria*. London, 1973.

Kibukamusoke, J.W. 'The nephrotic syndrome of quartan malaria', *Medical Journal of Australia*, 1978/1, pp. 187–91.

Kibukamusoke, John W. (ed.) *Tropical nephrology*. Canberra, 1984.

Kibukamusoke, J.W., M.S.R. Hutt, and N.E. Wilks, 'The nephrotic syndrome in Uganda and its association with quartan malaria', *Quarterly Journal of Medicine*, NS, 36 (1967), 393–408.

Kilama, W.L. *The war against mosquitoes and mosquito-borne diseases in Tanzania: some lost battles*. Dar es Salaam, 1994.

Killewo, Japhet, and others. 'Prevalence of HIV-1 infection in the Kagera Region of Tanzania: a population-based study', *AIDS*, 4 (1990), 1081–5.

Kimati, V.P. *The world's best medicine and a new health prescription*. Dar es Salaam, 1983.

King, Kenneth James. *Pan-Africanism and education*. Oxford, 1971.

King, Maurice (ed.) *Medical care in developing countries*. Nairobi, 1966.

Kinoti, S.N., P.G. Waiyaki, and J.B.O. Were (eds.) *Recent advances in medical research with a symposium on appropriate technology in disease control*. Nairobi, 1988.

Kipkorir, B.E. 'The Alliance High School and the origins of the Kenya elite 1926–1962', PhD thesis, University of Cambridge, 1969.

Kipkorir, B.E. 'The inheritors and successors: the traditional background to the modern Kenyan African elite: Kenya c.1890–1930', *Kenya Historical Review*, 2 (1974), 143–61.

Kirkaldy-Willis, W.H., and A.S. Mbuthia. 'Treatment of tuberculosis of bone and joint', *EAMJ*, 23 (1946), 326–44.

Kleine, Friedrich Karl. *Ein deutscher Tropenarzt*. Hannover, 1949.

Koech, Davy K. 'Challenges to health scientists in Africa', *African Journal of Health Sciences*, 1 (1994), 3–5.

Kohi, Thecla Wankuru. 'The knowledge, attitudes, and perceived support of Tanzanian nurses when caring for patients with AIDS', MNursing thesis, Dalhousie University, 1992.

Kohi, Thecla W., and Mona June Horrocks. 'The knowledge, attitudes and perceived support of Tanzanian nurses when caring for patients with AIDS', *International Journal of Nursing Studies*, 31 (1994), 77–86.

Koinange, K. 'Some reflections on development of health services in Kenya', *EAMJ*, 60 (1983), 599–602.

Kokwaro, J.O. *Medicinal plants of East Africa*. Nairobi, 1976.

Konde-Lule, Joseph K. 'The effects of urbanization on the spread of AIDS in Africa', *African Urban Quarterly*, 6 (1991), 13–18.

Konde-Lule, Joseph K., Seth F. Berkley, and Robert Downing. 'Knowledge, attitudes and practices concerning AIDS in Ugandans', *AIDS*, 3 (1989), 513–18.

Konde-Lule, Joseph K., M. Musagara, and S. Musgrave. 'Focus group interviews about AIDS in Rakai District of Uganda', *SSM*, 37 (1993), 679–84.

Konde-Lule, J.K., and A.I.N. Sebina. 'The impact of AIDS in a rural Ugandan community', *EAMJ*, 70 (1993), 725–9.

Konde-Lule, Joseph K., and others. 'Adolescents, sexual behaviour and HIV-1 in rural Rakai District, Uganda', *AIDS*, 11 (1997), 791–9.

Konde-Lule, Y.K. 'Syphilis in pregnant mothers at Mulago Hospital', DPH thesis, Makerere University, 1977.

Koponen, Juhani. *Development for exploitation: German colonial policies in mainland Tanzania, 1884–1914*. Helsinki, 1994.

Kroeber, Friedrich. *Der Doktor am Viktoriasee: 10 Jahre als Missionsarzt in Ostafrika*. Stuttgart, 1950.

Kyalwazi, S.K. 'Carcinoma of the penis: a review of 153 patients admitted to Mulago Hospital, Kampala, Uganda', *EAMJ*, 43 (1966), 415–25.

Kyalwazi, S.K. 'Treatment of Kaposi's sarcoma', *EAMJ*, 46 (1969), 450–8.

Kyalwazi, S.K. 'Kaposi's sarcoma', *Tropical Doctor*, 2 (1972), 68–72.

Kyalwazi, S.K. 'Problems of cancer treatment in Africa', *Uganda Medical Journal*, 3 (1974), 9–14.

Kyemba, Henry. *A state of blood: the inside story of Idi Amin*. New York, 1977.

Langseth, P., J. Katorobo, E. Brett, and J. Munene (eds.) *Uganda: landmarks in rebuilding a nation*. Kampala, 1995.

Last, Murray, and G.L. Chavunduka (eds.) *The professionalisation of African medicine*. Manchester, 1986.

Leakey, L.S.B. *The southern Kikuyu before 1903: volume II*. New York, 1977.

Lenoir, G.M., G.T. O'Conor, and C.L.M. Olweny (eds.) *Burkitt's lymphoma: a human cancer model*. Lyon, 1985.

Leslie, Charles (ed.) *Asian medical systems: a comparative study*. Berkeley, 1976.

Leslie, Charles, and Allan Young (eds.) *Paths to Asian medical knowledge*. Berkeley, 1992.

Leys, Colin. *Politicians and policies: an essay on politics in Acholi, Uganda, 1962–65*. Nairobi, 1967.

Lie, G.T., and P.M. Biswalo. 'HIV-positive patients' choice of a significant other to be informed about the HIV-test result: findings from an HIV/AIDS counselling programme in the regional hospitals of Arusha and Kilimanjaro, Tanzania', *AIDS Care*, 8 (1996), 285–96.

Lindblom, Gerhard. *The Akamba in British East Africa: an ethnological monograph*. Uppsala, 1920.

Lore, William. 'Some ethical issues in the medical profession in Kenya', *Medicus*, 12, 11 (November 1993), 321–3.

Lwamgira, F.X. 'The history of Kiziba and its kings', duplicated translation by E.R. Kamuhangire, 1969.

Lwihula, G., L. Dahlgren, J. Killewo, and A. Sandström. 'AIDS epidemic in Kagera Region, Tanzania – the experiences of local people', *AIDS Care*, 5 (1993), 347–57.

Macpherson, Margaret. *They built for the future: a chronicle of Makerere University College 1922–1962*. Cambridge, 1964.

Maina-Githinji, Elizabeth. 'The outpatient and the staff satisfaction with the treatment provided in a district hospital – Kiambu', MA thesis, University of Dar es Salaam, 1977.

Makene, W.J. 'Presiding Chairman's address to the opening of the Annual Scientific Conference of the Association of the Physicians of East Africa', *EAMJ*, 51 (1974), 822–3.

Makerere College. *Makerere College register 1922–53*. Kampala, 1955.

Makerere College. 'Makerere College register, vol. I, 1922–58 (confidential version)', manuscript (MUL UF.3).

Mamdani, Mahmood, and Joe Oloka-Onyango (eds.) *Uganda: studies in living conditions, popular movements, and constitutionalism*. Vienna, 1994.

Martin, David. *General Amin*. London, 1974.
Masara, S.K. (ed.) *Nairobi medical directory 93/94*. Nairobi, n.d.
Masawe, Aaron E. John. 'Syphilis in Uganda (the history, clinical features and cellular immunity)', MMed thesis, Makerere University, 1971.
Mati, J.K.G., and S. Auma. 'Cancer of the stomach', *Makerere Medical Journal*, 8 (May 1965), 38–40.
Maxwell, I.C.M. *Universities in partnership: the Inter-University Council and the growth of higher education in developing countries 1946–70*. Edinburgh, 1980.
Mbuthia, A.S., and W.H. Kirkaldy-Willis. 'Recent advances in orthopaedics', *EAMJ*, 31 (1954), 235–7.
McClelland, Charles E. *The German experience of professionalization*. Cambridge, 1991.
McGrath, J.W., and others. 'AIDS and the urban family: its impact in Kampala, Uganda', *AIDS Care*, 5 (1993), 55–70.
McIntosh, Brian G. 'The Scottish mission in Kenya, 1891–1923', PhD thesis, University of Edinburgh, 1969.
Menzel, Gustav. *Die Bethel-Mission: aus 100 Jahren Missionsgeschichte*. Neukirchen-Vluyu, 1986.
Merker, Moritz. *Die Masai*. Berlin, 1904.
Mfuko, Daudi. 'My job: VI – An African dispenser in the Zaramo', *Central Africa*, 57 (1939), 171–2.
Mhalu, F.S. 'AIDS and infections with the human immunodeficiency virus in Tanzania', *Tanzania Medical Journal*, 4, 1 (June 1989), 1–6.
Mhalu, F.S. 'Inter-relationships between HIV infection and other sexually transmitted diseases', *EAMJ*, 67 (1990), 512–17.
Mhalu, Fred, and others. 'Prevalence of HIV infection in healthy subjects and groups of patients in Tanzania', *AIDS*, 1 (1987), 217–21.
Motani, Nizaralli Abdulalli. 'The growth of an African civil service in Uganda, 1912–1940', PhD thesis, University of London, 1972.
Mshigeni, Keto E., and others (eds.) *Proceedings of an international conference of experts from developing countries on traditional medicinal plants*. Dar es Salaam, 1991.
Mtango, F.D.E., and M.T. Leshabari. 'Medical students performance: pre- and post-Musoma Resolution', *TNR*, 92 (1985), 89–94.
Mtawali, C.V. 'A health campaign in Tanganyika Territory', *Community Development Bulletin*, 2 (1951), 54–6.
Mugerwa, R.D., L.H. Marum, and D. Serwadda. 'Human Immunodeficiency Virus and AIDS in Uganda', *EAMJ*, 73 (1996), 20–6.
Muhangi, J. *Psychiatry in Kenya: new horizons in medical care*. Nairobi, 1980.
Mukoyogo, M. Christian, and Glen Williams. *AIDS orphans: a community perspective from Tanzania*. London, 1991.
Mulder, Daan, and others. 'Decreasing HIV-1 seroprevalence in young adults in a rural Uganda cohort', *British Medical Journal*, 311 (1995), 833–6.
Museveni, Yoweri Kaguta. *What is Africa's problem?* Kampala, 1992.
Musoke, Latimer K. 'An analysis of admissions to the paediatric division, Mulago Hospital in 1959', *Archives of Disease in Childhood*, 36 (1961), 305–15.
Muwazi, E.M.K. 'Penicillin in treatment of relapsing fever', *EAMJ*, 23 (1946), 55–64.

Muwazi, E.M.K., and H.C. Trowell. 'Neurological disease among African natives of Uganda: a review of 269 cases', *EAMJ*, 21 (1944), 2–19.

Muwazi, E.M.K., H.C. Trowell, and J.N.P. Davies, 'Congenital syphilis in Uganda', *EAMJ*, 24 (1947), 152–70.

Muwazi, E.M.K., H.C. Trowell, and R.S.F. Hennessey. 'Liver disease and jaundice in natives of Uganda', *EAMJ*, 19 (1942), 40–66.

Mwabu, Germano. 'Health care reform in Kenya: a review of the process', *Health Policy*, 32 (1995), 245–55.

Mwabu, German, James Mwanzia, and Wilson Liambila. 'User charges in government health facilities in Kenya: effect on attendance and revenue', *Health Policy and Planning*, 10 (1995), 164–70.

Mwaluko, G.M.P., W.L. Kilama, P.M. Mandara, M. Murru, and C.N.L. Macpherson (eds.) *Health and disease in Tanzania*. London, 1991.

Mwankemwa, Swedi A. 'Transcript of interview by John Iliffe, Dar es Salaam, 25 July 1995' (tape and typescript in University of Dar es Salaam Library, typescript in RH).

Mwesigwa, Robert J. 'Rural private clinics and health, a case study of Rwampara County Mbarara District', BA thesis, Makerere University, 1995.

Ndetei, P.M. 'Psychiatry in Kenya: yesterday, today and tomorrow: an overview', *Acta Psychiatrica Scandinavia*, 62 (1980), 201–11.

Ndirangu, Simon. *A history of nursing in Kenya*. Nairobi, 1982.

Nelson, G.S., and Y.B. Semambo. 'The treatment of tropical ulcers in the West Nile District of Uganda with special reference to an easily organised itinerant skin-grafting team', *EAMJ*, 33 (1956), 189–202.

Network of AIDS Researchers of Eastern and Southern Africa. *Focusing interventions among vulnerable groups for HIV infection: experiences from eastern and southern Africa*. Nairobi, 1994.

Newell, Kenneth W. (ed.) *Health by the people*. Geneva, 1975.

Nhonoli, A.M.M. 'An enquiry into the infant mortality rate in rural areas of Unyamwezi', *EAMJ*, 31 (1954), 1–12.

Nhonoli, Aloysius Mwessa. 'Hookworm disease and its cardio-vascular manifestations', MD thesis, University of East Africa, 1969.

Nhonoli, A.M. 'An analysis of the capacity of a university to act as an agent of socio-economic change', *Dar es Salaam Medical Journal*, 3, 2 (March 1971), 98–101.

Njenga, F.G. 'Doctors must stand up for human rights', *Nairobi Law Monthly*, 32 (April 1991), 34–5.

Nkinda, S.J. 'Fate of a "dream career"', *Makerere Medical Journal*, 8 (May 1965), 16–17.

Nkinda, Siegfried J. 'Traditional herbs for bronchial asthma in Tanga Region: an evaluation of their efficacy and bronchodilator activity', MMed thesis, University of Dar es Salaam, 1976.

Nordberg, E.M. 'The true disease pattern in East Africa: part 2', *EAMJ*, 60 (1983), 530–5.

Nsanze, Herbert. 'Sexually transmitted diseases', *Afya*, 18 (1984), 109–13.

Nsekela, Amon J., and Aloysius M. Nhonoli. *The development of health services and society in mainland Tanzania*. Nairobi, 1976.

Nyamwaya, David. 'Societal response to illness – the Pokot of Kenya', University of Nairobi Institute of African Studies paper no. 127, 1979.

Nyamwaya, David C. 'The management of illness in an East African society: a study of choice and constraint in health care among the Pokot', PhD thesis, University of Cambridge, 1982.

Nyamwaya, David. 'A case study of the interaction between indigenous and Western medicine among the Pokot of Kenya', *SSM*, 25 (1987), 1277–87.

Nyarango, P.M. 'Medical education for doctors in Kenya: an overview of its organisation and conduct', duplicated, London, 1987 (UNMS library).

Nyikal, James Wambura. 'Socio-economic background of children admitted to Kenyatta National Hospital with kwashiorkor', MMed thesis, University of Nairobi, 1984.

Nzioka, Charles B.K. 'The social construction and management of HIV and AIDS among low-income patients in Nairobi', PhD thesis, University of London, 1994.

Nzioka, C. 'Lay perceptions of risk of HIV infection and the social construction of safer sex: some experiences from Kenya,' *AIDS Care*, 8 (1996), 565–79.

Obbo, Christine. 'Healing: cultural fundamentalism and syncretism in Buganda', *Africa*, 66 (1996), 183–201.

Odenyo, Amos O. 'Professionalisation and change: the emergent Kenyan lawyer', duplicated, City University of New York, n.d. (KNA library).

Odhiambo, P.A. 'The first ten years of heart surgery in Kenya – aspirations, dilemmas and possibilities', *EAMJ*, 69 (1992), 520–4.

Odonga, A.M. 'Makerere Medical graduates' "Good old days"', *Makerere Medical Journal*, 7 (November 1964), 7–10.

Odonga, Alexander Mwa. *The first fifty years of Makerere University Medical School and the foundation of scientific medical education in East Africa*. Kisubi [?1990].

Odonga, Alexander M. *Practical medical ethics*. Kisubi, n.d.

Ogot, B.A., and W.R. Ochieng' (eds.) *Decolonization and independence in Kenya 1940–93*. London, 1995.

O'Hara, M. Louis, OSF. 'An unfinished canticle: the story of the Franciscan Missionary Sisters for Africa', typescript, 1980 (St Joseph's College Archives, Mill Hill).

Ojiambo, Hillary P. 'Postgraduate medical training in Kenya', *The Lancet*, 30 December 1967, pp. 1414–16.

Ojiambo, Hilary. *You and your health*. Nairobi, 1986.

Ojiambo, Hillary P. 'Medical education and research – an agenda for change and action', *Medicus*, 12, 11 (November 1993), 315–20.

Ojok, Omwony, and John Rwomushana. 'Uganda's response to the challenge of HIV/AIDS', *Uganda Journal*, 42 (December 1995), 1–15.

Okello, David A. 'The resource use patterns and the factors affecting the cost of care of patients with the Acquired Immunodeficiency Syndrome (AIDS) in Mulago Hospital, Kampala', MMedSci thesis, University of Newcastle (NSW), 1993.

Okuonzi, Sam Agatre, and Joanna Macrae. 'Whose policy is it anyway? International and national influences on health policy development in Uganda', *Health Policy and Planning*, 10 (1995), 122–32.

Olweny, Charles L.M. 'Hepatocellular carcinoma in Uganda', MD thesis, Makerere University, 1976.

Olweny, Charles L.M., Edward Katongole-Mbidde, David Otim, Stephen K. Lwanga, Ian T. Magrath, and John L. Ziegler. 'Long-term experience with

Burkitt's lymphoma in Uganda', *International Journal of Cancer*, 26 (1980), 261–6.
Olweny, Charles L.M., John L. Ziegler, Costan W. Berard, and A.C. Templeton. 'Adult Hodgkin's Disease in Uganda', *Cancer*, 27 (1971), 1295–301.
Orinda, Vincent Akoko, 'The mother of a sick child in a paediatric ward – her role in ward management', MMed thesis, University of Nairobi, 1982.
Ouko, W. 'Discussions on approaches to the African mind in effecting health education and hygiene matters (health education and the African)', *EAMJ*, 37 (1960), 167–70.
Owen, Hugh Brindley. 'Medical education in Uganda', *Tropical Diseases Bulletin*, 30 (1933), 659–68.
Owor, Raphael. 'The pathology of chronic pancreatic disease in Uganda', MD thesis, University of East Africa, 1970.
Owor, R., V.L. Ongom, and B.G. Kirya (eds.) *The child in the African environment: growth, development and survival*. Nairobi, 1975.
Parry, E.H.O. (ed.) *Principles of medicine in Africa*. 2nd edn, Oxford, 1984.
Peiper, [Otto]. 'Der Suaheli-Arzt', *Archiv für Schiffs- und Tropen-Hygiene*, 14 (1910), 561–73.
Perham, Margery. *East African journey: Kenya and Tanganyika 1929–30*. London. 1976.
Pickering, H., M. Okongo, B. Nnalusiba, K. Bwanika, and J. Whitworth, 'Sexual networks in Uganda', *AIDS Care*, 9 (1997), 199–207.
Pobee, J.O.M. 'Cardiovascular research: a luxury in tropical Africa?' *EAMJ*, 64 (1987), 396–410.
Power, d'Arcy, and J. Keogh Murphy (eds.) *A system of syphilis: volume II*. Oxford, 1908.
Pratt, Cranford. *The critical phase in Tanzania 1945–1968: Nyerere and the emergence of a socialist ideology*. Cambridge, 1976.
'Proceedings of the East African burden of disease, cost effectiveness of health care interventions and health policy regional workshop', duplicated, Nairobi, 1994 (UMOH library).
Raikes, Alanagh. 'Medical education in a developing country: a survey of Tanzanian medical students', MA thesis, University of Dar es Salaam, 1978.
Ranger, Terence O. 'Godly medicine: the ambiguities of medical mission in south-east Tanzania, 1900–1945', *SSM*, 15B (1981), 261–77.
Ranger, Terence, and Paul Slack (eds.) *Epidemics and ideas*. Cambridge, 1992.
Rankin, A.M. 'Dar es Salaam School of Medicine – the first five years', *Dar es Salaam Medical Journal*, 1, 1 (September 1968), 3–4.
Reiser, Stanley Joel. *Medicine and the reign of technology*. Cambridge, 1978.
Renault, François. *Lavigerie, l'esclavage africain, et l'Europe, 1868–92*. 2 vols., Paris, 1971.
Roles, N.C. 'Tribal surgery in East Africa during the XIXth century', *EAMJ*, 43 (1966), 579–94, and 44 (1967), 17–30.
Roscoe, John. *The soul of central Africa*. London, 1922.
Roscoe, John. *The Bakitara or Banyoro*. Cambridge, 1923.
Roscoe, John. *The Banyankole*. Cambridge, 1923.
Roscoe, John. *The Baganda*. 2nd edn, London, 1965.
Rosenthal, Marilynn M. *Health care in the People's Republic of China: moving towards modernization*. Boulder, 1987.

Routledge, W. Scoresby, and Katherine Routledge. *With a prehistoric people: the Akikuyu of British East Africa*. Reprinted, London, 1968.

Sabben-Clare, E.E., D.J. Bradley, and K. Kirkwood (eds.) *Health in Africa during the colonial period*. Oxford, 1980.

Seeley, J., E. Kajura, C. Bachengema, M. Okongo, U. Wagner, and D. Mulder. 'The extended family and support for people with AIDS in a rural population in south west Uganda: a safety net with holes?' *AIDS Care*, 5 (1993), 117–22.

Semali, Innocent Antony John. 'The opinions of allopathic health workers on traditional medicine/healers and degree of contact between the two in Tanzania', DPH thesis, University of Dar es Salaam, 1982.

Sembeguya, F.G. 'Presidential address 1962: the growth of an indigenous medical profession', *EAMJ*, 41 (1964), 39–45.

Senkubuge, Simon. 'The work of an African Assistant Medical Officer', *Uganda Teacher's Journal*, 1 (1939), 99–101.

Serwadda, David, Maria J. Wawer, Stanley D. Musgrave, Nelson K. Sewankambo, Jonathan E. Kaplan, and Ronald H. Gray. 'HIV risk factors in three geographic strata of rural Rakai District Uganda', *AIDS*, 6 (1992), 983–9.

Serwadda, D., and others. 'Slim disease: a new disease in Uganda and its association with HTLV-III infection', *The Lancet*, 1985/2, pp. 849–52.

Sewankambo, Nelson K. 'Care of HIV-infected people in the developing world: practical aspects', *AIDS*, 3 (1989), supplement, S195–S199.

Sewankambo, Nelson, and others. 'Enteropathic AIDS in Uganda: an endoscopic, histological and microbiological study', *AIDS*, 1 (1987), 9–13.

Sewankambo, Nelson K., and others. 'HIV infection through normal heterosexual contact in Uganda', *AIDS*, 1 (1987), 113–16.

Sezi, C.L. 'Theory: the cause of endomyocardial fibrosis', *Uganda Medical Journal*, 8, 3 (September 1991), 10–16.

Shaper, A.G., J.W. Kibukamusoke, and M.S.R. Hutt (eds.) *Medicine in a tropical environment*. London, 1972.

Shija, Joseph K. *Paediatric surgical care in developing countries: a handbook for doctors, nurses and students*. Nairobi, 1989.

Shija, J.K. *Surgery in Tanzania*. Reprinted, Dar es Salaam, 1990.

Sijaona, L. Nangwanda. 'Medical practice in the context of the socialist pattern of society', *Dar es Salaam Medical Journal*, 2, 1 (March 1970), 11–14.

Silcock, T.H. (ed.) *Professional structure in South-East Asia* (Canberra, 1977).

Sitel, Philip Wittman. 'Bo'n town life: youth, AIDS, and the changing character of adulthood in Kilimanjaro, Tanzania', PhD thesis, Boston University, 1995.

Soff, Harvey G. 'Sleeping sickness in the Lake Victoria region of British East Africa, 1900–1915', *African Historical Studies*, 2 (1969), 255–68.

Sonbol, Amira elAzhary. *The creation of a medical profession in Egypt, 1800–1922*. Syracuse, 1991.

Southall, R.J. *Parties and politics in Bunyoro*. Kampala, 1972.

Southall, Roger. *Federalism and higher education in East Africa*. Nairobi, 1974.

Ssali, C.L. 'A county practitioner's difficulties', *Medmak*, 1 (1958), 35–7.

Starr, Paul. *The social transformation of American medicine*. New York, 1982.

Stirling, Leader. *Tanzanian doctor*. London, 1977.

Swaka, Felix Lado. 'Practice of drug peddlers and health workers in relation to sexually transmitted diseases in Kenya', MPH thesis, University of Nairobi, 1992.

Tallack, R.J.K. 'Aspects of the public health of the Zanzibar Protectorate', DPH thesis, University of London, 1954 (Tallack papers, RH).

Tanzania. *Evaluation of the health sector 1979*. Dar es Salaam, 1980.

Tanzania. *Health profile 1991*. Dar es Salaam, 1991.

Tanzania: Bureau of Statistics. *Tanzania demographic and health survey 1991/92: summary report*. Dar es Salaam, 1993.

Tarimo, E. 'Primary health care in Tanzania, "Simultaneous Action on All Fronts"', *Tanzania Medical Journal*, special issue (September 1985), pp. 8–24.

Temu, A.J. *British Protestant missions*. London, 1972.

Thairu, Kihumbu. *The African civilization*. Kampala, 1975.

Thomas, Anthony E. 'Adaptation to modern medicine in lowland Machakos, Kenya: a controlled comparison of two Kamba communities', PhD thesis, Stanford University, 1970.

Thompson, B.G. 'Uganda and the Second World War: the limits of power in a colonial state', PhD thesis, University of London, 1990.

Thompson, Gardner. 'Colonialism in crisis: the Uganda disturbances of 1945', *African Affairs*, 91 (1992), 605–24.

Titmuss, Richard M., and others. *The health services of Tanganyika*. London, 1964.

Trowell, H.C. 'The medical training of Africans', *EAMJ*, 11 (1934–5), 338–53.

Trowell, H.C., and E.M.K. Muwazi. 'Severe and prolonged underfeeding in African children (the kwashiorkor syndrome of maligant malnutrition)', *Archives of Disease in Childhood*, 20 (1945), 110–16.

Turshen, Meredeth. *The political ecology of disease in Tanzania*. New Brunswick, 1984.

Turya, E. Baihireyo. 'Which way medical assistants of Uganda? A study of the evolution and management of medical assistants in Uganda', MSc thesis, University of London, 1980.

Uganda. *Report of the Commission of Inquiry into the Disturbances which occurred in Uganda during January, 1945*. Entebbe, 1945.

Uganda. *Report of the Commission of Inquiry into the Disturbances in Uganda during April 1949*. Entebbe, 1950.

Uganda. *Medical and health services in Uganda*. Entebbe, 1956.

Uganda. 'Report and recommendations of the Health Policy Review Commission under the chairmanship of Professor Raphael Owor', duplicated, Entebbe, 1987 (UMOH library).

Uganda: Ministry of Health. 'Report on the first meeting of District Medical Officers', duplicated, 1986 (UMOH library).

Uganda: Ministry of Health. 'AIDS Control Programme: proposals for a five year action plan (1987–1991)', duplicated, 1987 (UMOH library).

Uganda: Ministry of Health. *National health personnel study*. Entebbe, 1991.

Uganda: Ministry of Health. *The three year health plan frame 1993/94–1995/96*. Entebbe, 1993.

Uganda: Ministry of Health. *Approach and guidelines for health planning 1996/97 and 1997/98*. Entebbe, 1995.

Uganda: Ministry of Local Government. 'Report of the annual conference of DMOs, M/Ss and NGOs', duplicated, 1988 (UMOH library).

Uganda Medical Association. 'Private clinics owned by government employed doctors: memorandum submitted to H.E. the President of Uganda', duplicated, 1989 (UMOH library).

Valiathan, M.S., Krishna Somers, and C. Chandrasekharan Kartha (eds.) *Endomyocardial fibrosis*. Delhi, 1993.

Van der Geest, Sjaak, and Susan Reynolds Whyte (eds.) *The context of medicines in developing countries: studies in pharmaceutical anthropology*. Dordrecht, 1988.

Vaughan, Megan. *Curing their ills: colonial power and African illness*. Cambridge, 1991.

Vogel, Charles L., and Sebastian K. Kyalwazi. 'Recent advances in hepatocellular carcinoma research', *Makerere Medical Journal*, 16 (September 1971), 13–14.

Vogel, L.C., A.S., Muller, R.S. Odingo, Z. Onyango, and A. de Geus (eds.) *Health and disease in Kenya*. Nairobi, 1974.

Wallman, Sandra (ed.) *Kampala women getting by: wellbeing in the time of AIDS*. London, 1996.

Wandai, Karuga. *Thika leaders*. Thika, 1989.

Wawer, Maria J., and others. 'Trends in HIV-1 prevalence may not reflect trends in incidence in mature epidemics: data from the Rakai population-based cohort, Uganda', *AIDS*, 11 (1997), 1023–30.

Were, J.B.O., M.W. Mutugi, and J.I. Githure (eds.) *Recent advances in medical research with a symposium on the rational use of drugs*. Nairobi, 1992.

White, Luise. '"They could make their victims dull": genders and genres, fantasies and cures in colonial southern Uganda', *American Historical Review*, 100 (1995), 1379–1402.

Who's who in East Africa 1967–68. Nairobi, 1968.

Whyte, Susan Reynolds. 'Social implications of the interpretation of misfortune in Bunyole', PhD thesis, University of Washington, 1973.

Williams, A.D. 'The provision of hospitals for, and the medical training of Africans in Kenya', *Kenya Medical Journal*, 3 (1926–7), 46–51.

Wolff, Dr. 'Bilharzia in Deutsch-Ostafrika', *Archiv für Schiffs- und Tropen-Hygiene*, 15 (1911), 224–30.

World Bank. *Uganda population, health and nutrition sector review*. [Washington] 1985.

World Bank. *Tanzania: AIDS assessment and planning study*. Washington, 1992.

Zeller, Diane Leinwand. 'The establishment of Western medicine in Buganda', PhD thesis, Columbia University, 1971.

Zysk, Kenneth G. *Asceticism and healing in ancient India: medicine in the Buddhist monastery*. New York, 1991.

Index

OTHER BOOKS IN THE SERIES

64 *Bankole-Bright and Politics in Colonial Sierra Leone: The Passing of the 'Krio Era', 1919–1958* Akintola Wyse
65 *Contemporary West African States* Donal Cruise O'Brien, John Dunn and Richard Rathbone
66 *The Oromo of Ethiopia: A History, 1570–1860* Mohammed Hassen
67 *Slavery and African Life: Occidental, Oriental and African Slave Trades* Patrick Manning
68 *Abraham Esau's War: A Black South African War in the Cape, 1899–1902* Bill Nasson
69 *The Politics of Harmony: Land Dispute Strategies in Swaziland* Laurel Rose
70 *Zimbabwe's Guerrilla War: Peasant Voices* Norma Kriger
71 *Ethiopia: Power and Protest: Peasant Revolts in the Twentieth Century* Gebru Tareke
72 *White Supremacy and Black Resistance in Pre-Industrial South Africa: The Making of the Colonial Order in the Eastern Cape, 1770–1865* Clifton C. Crais
73 *The Elusive Granary: Herder, Farmer, and State in Northern Kenya* Peter D. Little
74 *The Kanyok of Zaire: An Institutional and Ideological History to 1895* John C. Yoder
75 *Pragmatism in the Age of Jihad: The Precolonial State of Bundu* Michael A. Gomez
76 *Slow Death for Slavery: The Course of Abolition in Northern Nigeria, 1897–1936* Paul E. Lovejoy and Jan S. Hogendorn
77 *West African Slavery and Atlantic Commerce: The Senegal River Valley, 1700–1860* James Searing
78 *A South African Kingdom: The Pursuit of Security in Nineteenth-Century Lesotho* Elizabeth A. Eldredge
79 *State and Society in Pre-Colonial Asante* T.C. McCaskie
80 *Islamic Society and State Power in Senegal: Disciples and Citizens in Fatick* Leonardo A. Villalon
81 *Ethnic Pride and Racial Prejudice in Victorian Cape Town: Group Identity and Social Practise* Vivian Bickford-Smith
82 *The Eritrean Struggle for Independence: Domination, Resistance and Nationalism, 1941–1993* Ruth Iyob
83 *Corruption and State Politics in Sierra Leone* William Reno
84 *The Culture of Politics in Modern Kenya* Angelique Haugerud
85 *Africans: The History of a Continent* John Iliffe
86 *From Slave Trade to 'Legitimate' Commerce* Robin Law

87 *Leisure and Society in Colonial Brazzaville* Phyllis M. Martin
88 *Kingship and State: the Buganda Dynasty* Christopher Wrigley
89 *Decolonization and African Life: The Labour Question in French and British Africa* Frederick Cooper
90 *Misreading the African Landscape: Society and Ecology in an African Forest–Savannah Mosaic* James Fairhead and Melissa Leach
91 *Peasant Revolution in Ethiopia: The Tigray Peoples Liberation Front, 1975–1991* John Young
92 *Senegambia and the Atlantic Slave Trade* Boubacar Barry
93 *Commerce and Economic Change in West Africa: The Oil Trade in the Nineteenth Century* Martin Lynn
94 *Slavery and French Colonial Rule in West Africa: Senegal, Guinea and Mali* Martin Klein